P9-DFF-217

ANNALS OF
THE NEW YORK ACADEMY
OF SCIENCES

Volume 601

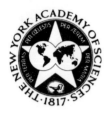

EDITORIAL STAFF
Executive Editor
BILL M. BOLAND
Managing Editor
JUSTINE CULLINAN
Associate Editor
SHEILA K. TREITLER

The New York Academy of Sciences
2 East 63rd Street
New York, New York 10021

THE NEW YORK ACADEMY OF SCIENCES
(Founded in 1817)

BOARD OF GOVERNORS, 1990

LEWIS THOMAS, *Chairman of the Board*
CHARLES A. SANDERS, *President*
DENNIS D. KELLY, *President-Elect*

Honorary Life Governors

H. CHRISTINE REILLY · IRVING J. SELIKOFF

Vice-Presidents

DAVID A. HAMBURG · CYRIL M. HARRIS
PETER D. LAX · CHARLES G. NICHOLSON

HENRY A. LICHSTEIN, *Secretary-Treasurer*

Elected Governors-at-Large

JOSEPH L. BIRMAN · FLORENCE L. DENMARK · LAWRENCE R. KLEIN
GERALD D. LAUBACH · LLOYD N. MORRISETT · GERARD PIEL

WILLIAM T. GOLDEN, *Past Chairman* · HELENE L. KAPLAN, *General Counsel*

OAKES AMES, *Executive Director*

ELECTROCARDIOGRAPHY
Past and Future

ANNALS OF THE NEW YORK ACADEMY OF SCIENCES
Volume 601

ELECTROCARDIOGRAPHY
Past and Future

Edited by Philippe Coumel and Oscar B. Garfein

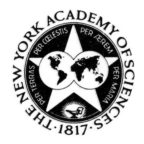

The New York Academy of Sciences
New York, New York
1990

Copyright © 1990 by the New York Academy of Sciences. All rights reserved. Under the provisions of the United States Copyright Act of 1976, individual readers of the Annals are permitted to make fair use of the material in them for teaching or research. Permission is granted to quote from the Annals provided that the customary acknowledgment is made of the source. Material in the Annals may be republished only by permission of the Academy. Address inquiries to the Executive Editor at the New York Academy of Sciences.

Copying fees: For each copy of an article made beyond the free copying permitted under Section 107 or 108 of the 1976 Copyright Act, a fee should be paid through the Copyright Clearance Center, 21 Congress St., Salem, MA 01970. For articles of more than 3 pages, the copying fee is $1.75.

ⓒ The paper used in this publication meets the minimum requirements of American National Standard for Information Sciences–Permanence of Paper for Printed Library Materials, ANSI Z39.48-1984.

Library of Congress Cataloging-in Publication Data

Electrocardiography : past and future / edited by Philippe Coumel and Oscar B. Garfein.
  p. cm. — (Annals of the New York Academy of Sciences ; ISSN 0077-8923 ; v. 601)
  Based on a conference held Sept. 7–9, 1989 in Nice, France, cosponsored by the New York Academy of Sciences and the European Society of Cardiology.
  Includes bibliographical references.
  Includes indexes.
  ISBN 0-89766-615-1 (cloth : alk. paper). — ISBN 0-89766-616-X (pbk. : alk. paper)
  1. Electrocardiography—Congresses. I. Coumel, Philippe.
II. Garfein, Oscar B. III. New York Academy of Sciences.
IV. European Society of Cardiology. V. Series.
  [DNLM: 1. Electrocardiography—trends—congresses. W1 AN626YL v.
601 / WG 140 E3747 1989]
Q11.N5 vol. 601
[RC683.5.E5]
500 s—dc20
[616.1'207547]
DNLM/DLC
for Library of Congress   90-6545
                                                              CIP

SP
Printed in the United States of America
ISBN 0-89766-615-1 (cloth)
ISBN 0-89766-616-X (paper)
ISSN 0077-8923

ANNALS OF THE NEW YORK ACADEMY OF SCIENCES

Volume 601
September 14, 1990

ELECTROCARDIOGRAPHY[a]
Past and Future

Editors and Conference Organizers
PHILIPPE COUMEL and OSCAR B. GARFEIN

CONTENTS

[a]This volume is the result of a conference entitled Electrocardiography: Past and Future held from September 7 to September 9, 1989 in Nice, France, cosponsored by The New York Academy of Sciences and the European Society of Cardiology.

Late Paper

Major European funding for this conference was provided by:
• KNOLL AG

Major United States funding for this conference was provided by:
• MEDTRONIC, INC.

Financial assistance was received from:
• HEWLETT PACKARD
• MARQUETTE ELECTRONICS, INC.
• SPACELABS

The New York Academy of Sciences believes it has a responsibility to provide an open forum for discussion of scientific questions. The positions taken by the participants in the reported conferences are their own and not necessarily those of the Academy. The Academy has no intent to influence legislation by providing such forums.

Preface

PHILIPPE COUMEL[a] AND OSCAR B. GARFEIN[b]

a Lariboisière Hospital
2, rue Ambroise-Paré
75010 Paris, France

b Division of Cardiology
St. Luke's-Roosevelt Hospital Center
Columbia University
College of Physicians & Surgeons
428 West 59th Street
New York, New York 10019

The birth of electrocardiography in the earliest days of this century marked a turning point in medicine. With this technique, precise measurements could be made of a biological and electrical event in humans and a whole area of clinical investigation was begun. Over the ensuing eight decades a great deal has been learned about cardiac physiology and pathology through electrocardiography using very little of the enormous potential of this technique. The basically crude measurements that were initially used to analyze the electrocardiographic waveform—utilizing an analog signal, and measuring by hand and eye the duration, polarity, and amplitude of the various electrical waves—have persisted to the present time. All this despite the revolution in recording and processing technologies, and the development of new types of investigation that permit highly sophisticated and sensitive invasive and noninvasive evaluation of cardiac function.

With the cosponsoring of the New York Academy of Sciences and the European Society of Cardiology, the conference Electrocardiography: Past and Future explored the various ways in which clinical electrocardiography will evolve in the second century of its existence. In six sessions over three days this conference reviewed different aspects of current technology that will enhance the diagnostic capabilities of electrocardiography in the future. The result of this conference, it is hoped, will be to encourage the widespread application of new and existing electrocardiographic techniques, computer and telecommunication technologies, and ancillary cardiology diagnostic techniques to improve the diagnosis of cardiac condition.

Experts first gave state of the art lectures about the three major components of the P-Q-R-S-T complex, namely P. Puech for the P wave, D. Krikler for the R wave, and A. J. Moss for the T wave. Other important aspects of the repolarization phase were addressed by M. B. Rosenbaum and A. Maseri, the former dealing with the still rather mysterious phenomenon of cardiac memory and its relationships with cardiac activation, the latter dealing with the pattern and significance of ischemic changes.

Then a variety of diagnostic techniques that assist in validating, modifying and understanding information derived from the electrocardiogram were discussed. Echocardiography, coronary angiography (E. M. Dwyer), positon emission tomography (M. Grover-McKay), nuclear magnetic resonance imaging (J. L. Weiss), thallium scintigraphy (B. Zaret) now supplant original correlations of electrocardiograms with postmortem specimens, with *in vivo* studies. The capability now exists to study myocardial hypertrophy and infarction, pump function, metabolism, perfusion, and structure of the human heart in living subjects, and to systematically cross-correlate these various diagnostic modalities with the electrocardiogram (ECG). Individually or in combination, they add a new measure of sophistication, specificity and sensitivity to electrocardiographic interpretation in the diagnosis of multiple physiologic, pathologic and anatomical entities. For the time being, such correlations are restricted to classical surface ECG recordings, but they will almost certainly be even more rewarding with further developments of the technique of electrocardiography itself.

Body surface mapping (N. C. Flowers) measures the electrical potential changes on the thorax that result from the generation of the cardiac electrical signal. While it has achieved almost no clinical status (in large meeasure due to the complexity of the technique) great amounts of unique information can be provided by the technique because it can demonstrate many of the individual vectoral components that vanish in the summated signal. Power spectrum analysis has been applied to the QRS complex (E. J. Berbari) and it can also unearth more complete information on the ventricular activation in normal and diseased myocardium. With signal-averaged electrocardiography (G. Breithardt), signals too small to be seen on the routine electrocardiogram can be visualized through the use of amplification, filtering, and averaging of the signal. With this technique His bundle recording is no longer reserved to endocavitary studies, and late systolic activity in the QRS complex which may herald the presence of potential arrhythmogenic substrates can be discerned. The latter, however, still have to be localized as the point of origin of arrhythmias by endocardial recordings in combination with epicardial mapping (M. E. Josephson). Endocavitary electrocardiography includes the recording of endocardial monophasic action potentials (S. B. Olsson) that make the bridge with intracellular electrophysiology but is restricted to experimental laboratories and *in vitro* techniques.

The autonomic nervous system has been largely ignored by clinicians for many reasons. The complexity of its physiology still makes this field difficult (M. N. Levy), but obstacles to obtaining information on the system through nonpharmacological, noninvasive techniques have been partially overcome. The circadian variations of the electrical properties of the heart (J. Cinca) are partially responsible for the behavior of arrhythmias, particularly the most severe ones that are responsible for sudden death of cardiac patients (P. J. Schwartz). This has important therapeutic implications, since arrhythmias and the autonomic nervous system are indeed interactive (M. B. Waxman). Analysis of sinus rate variability, an approach that was for a long time reserved to physiologists, has recently burst onto the clinical field (A. Malliani) with the advent of powerful minicomputers that give the ability to analyze the large amount of data provided by dynamic electrocardiography. The autonomic nervous system is, by definition, designed to sense all the physiological functions, and to react to any disturbance in order to activate the compensatory mechanisms. Monitoring these reactions is logically a good way to obtain valuable information on the cardiovascular system, with the corresponding prognostic implications.

The description of the cellular mechanisms of arrythmias 20 years ago concurrent with the origin of clinical electrophysiology led to the impressive and fruitful developments in the invasive exploration of cardiac arrhythmias. Clinicians have an ongoing need to refresh their knowledge of the cellular basis of arrhythmias (M. Arnsdorf) in order to best utilize the possibilities of endocavitary studies (H. J. J. Wellens). The autonomic nervous system is not the only factor that modulates the activity of the arrhythmogenic substrates. The prevailing rate as such is also operative at the cellular level (M. J. Janse), and extrapolating the observed phenomena into a computerized model of arrhythmias greatly helps in their understanding (J. Jalife). Conversely, studying the arrhythmia behavior as a function of the ambient heart rate is a very fruitful approach for the comprehension of mechanisms by noninvasive techniques (P. Coumel).

The electrocardiographic signal is well suited to the computer era, and it can be exploited in various ways. Surface recordings can be automatically processed in diagnostic terms, and quantitative electrocardiography is now a well-standardized discipline (J. Willems) the possibilities of which will certainly be extended in the future. Computer people (I. Rowlandson) and physicians (P. Kligfield) still have to cooperate closely to develop signal analysis in a dynamic way. Ideally, the global information concerning the electrical activity of the heart should be permanently monitored and the information stored for periods much longer than the 24-h recordings we are currently restricted to. Such an aim is most probably not as utopian as it might seem if one considers the fantastic acceleration that has been given to our knowledge in the last one or two decades by computer technology.

Progress can occur if, among other conditions, the coincidence exists between the technical possibilities and the demand from the scientists. Cardiologists are responsible for the latter condition, and the conference was held to study the various facets of the problem. We hope that these proceedings will suggest new ways of using electrocardiography in the coming decades.

PART I. PHYSIOLOGICAL, PATHOLOGICAL, AND PHARMACOLOGIC
CORRELATES OF ELECTROCARDIOGRAPHIC CHANGES

P Wave Morphology

P. PUECH

Cardiology Service B
Montpellier Hospital Center and University
34059 Montpellier Cedex, France

The P wave is the expression of the atrial depolarization and its morphology is influenced by many factors: the site of origin of atrial depolarization, the spread of activation through both atria, the thickness of the walls and the volume of the cavities, the position of the heart in the thorax, the propagation of the electrical field to the surface leads, and some transient factors, such as respiration changes, neurovegetative tone modulation, ischemic effect, or metabolic disorders.

FACTORS INFLUENCING P WAVE MORPHOLOGY

Site of Origin of Atrial Activation

The normal P wave depends on an impulse originating from the sinus node, located at the superior vena cava–upper right atrial junction. Direct recordings of the sinus node activity in man[1,2] have demonstrated the presence of a slow, prepotential activity, undetected by surface leads. The beginning of the P wave in surface leads corresponds to the primodepolarization of the common atrial tissue, in the area surrounding the sinus node, near the crista terminalis (FIGURE 1).

Ectopic atrial rhythms modify P wave configuration in a way that allows us to suggest the site of origin of the abnormal impulses. In most cases the whole activation process is reflected on surface leads, but in some cases of high-rate ectopic atrial rhythms, a part of the depolarization is concealed in surface leads and can only be detected using intracardiac or epicardial recordings.

Spread of Atrial Depolarization

In sinus rhythm, propagation of activation depends on the geometry of the atria. It is now established that the spread of excitation is not exactly uniform and radial but is influenced by disposition of the atrial fibers, facilitating conduction along three preferential (and not specific) pathways located in the right atrium, the so-called anterior, medial, and posterior internodal tracts. Bachmann's bundle, a branch of the anterior internodal tract, facilitates propagation of the excitation between the upper parts of both atria. Conduction through the atrial muscle is anisotropic, but, when homogeneous, anisotropic conduction seems not to influence the general process of activation and therefore the surface P wave.[4] The normal activation process evolves in three phases: isolated depolarization of the upper right atrium, followed by the simultaneous depolarization of the right and left atria, and finally isolated depolarization of the bottom part of the left atrium, in the vicinity of the distal coronary sinus. This activation sequence, demonstrated in man using intracardiac electrocardiography (ECG),[3] is illustrated in FIGURE 2.

The atria, having a very thin wall of negligible thickness in electrogenesis, are

1

assimilated to a bidimensional structure. Since the activation wave front arrives simultaneously at the endocardial and epicardial aspects, the intracavitary exploration of the endocardium is equivalent to the study of the epicardial surface of the atria.

Conduction disorders in the atrial wall modify P morphology in sinus rhythm. The best identified conduction disturbance is the conduction delay or block along Bachmann's bundle leading to asynchronal activation of the right and left atria. Intraatrial blocks secondary to anatomical lesions or nonhomogeneous anisotropic conduction (slow conduction in the transverse direction of the atrial fibers after block of the rapid conduction over the longitudinal axis in critical areas) play an important role in the genesis of atrial arrhythmias.

Atrial Overload

Hemodynamic conditions that impose an atrial systolic or diastolic overload lead to hypertrophy of the atrial wall and dilatation of the cavities. Both anatomic consequences are associated either with cases of obstacles to atrial ejection (valvular stenosis, impaired ventricular filling) or with cases of atrioventricular regurgitation and intra- or extracardiac shunts. Atrial hypertrophy is often difficult to assess on anatomical specimens, but is always present, as judged by the increase in atrial weight and the modification of the right over left atrial weight ratio.[3] Atrial dilatation is always predominant, due to the capacity of distension of the atria, depending upon wall elasticity, which is higher on the right side.

Since atrial thickness cannot be measured accurately *in vivo*, correlations between P wave morphology and anatomical changes have only taken into consideration atrial size. For this purpose echocardiography has been used for more than a decade, electroechocardiographic comparison being limited to the dimension of the left atrium for technical reasons.

Apart from Chirife *et al.*, who found a good electroechocardiographic correlation between left atrial size and P wave duration (all the patients with P wave duration

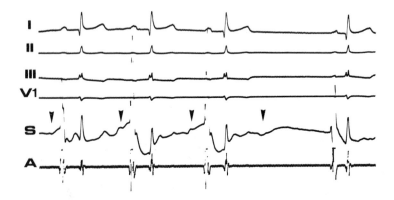

FIGURE 1. Direct recording of sinus node activity. A slow deflection (arrow) precedes the rapid atrial electrogram of the endocardial lead (A) and the onset of the P wave in surface leads. The fourth slow sinus potential is not followed by atrial activity (sinoatrial block). The last atrial beat is not preceded by a sinus prepotential, indicating a shift in the origin of the pacemaker after the atrial pause.

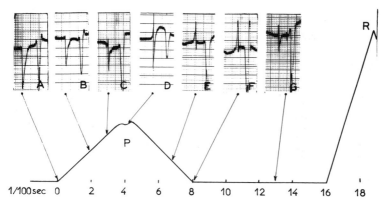

FIGURE 2. Unipolar recordings of atrial activity in the right and left atria through an interatrial septal defect. Negative electrograms in the upper and middle right atrium (A, B, and C), diphasic electrograms near the atrial septum (D), positive electrograms in the lower left atrium (E and F). The last panel (G) shows the His bundle potential recording obtained for the first time in 1957. The arrows indicate the timing of the intrinsecoid atrial and His bundle deflections with respect to the surface ECG.

superior to 105 mseconds had atrial enlargement more than 3.8 cm),[5] most authors have not observed a satisfactory correlation between P wave indexes suggesting left atrial enlargement and echocardiographic findings in various clinical conditions.[6-9] Josephson et al. noticed that only 52% of cases presenting abnormal P waves exhibited echocardiographic data of left atrial enlargement and 65% of patients with increased atrial size on echocardiogram had modified P wave.[10] Waggoner et al. concluded that the predictive index of ECG for left atrial enlargement was 63%, the sensitivity of the ECG criteria of left atrial enlargement increasing as left dilatation progresses (abnormal P waves in all instances of left atrial dimension greater than 5.0).[11] In a pediatric population, Maok and Krongrad estimated the overall sensitivity and predictive value of the ECG to detect atrial enlargement as 40% and 85% respectively, the ECG and echocardiogram failing to agree in 62% of the patients.[12] However, in pediatric[12] and adult[10] cohorts, P wave alterations are more sensitive as predicting left atrial dilatation in rheumatic valvular disease (especially mitral insufficiency) than in other cardiac diseases (congenital or acquired).

Atrial hypertrophy and dilatation lead to an increase in voltage and duration of the P wave and favor the occurrence of intraatrial conduction disturbances, the latter explaining the discrepancy between Elband echocardiographic findings.

FIGURE 3 is a schematic representation of the well-known consequences of the right and left atrial overloading on the surface P wave. Right atrial hypertrophy/dilatation increases the area of activation resulting from the depolarization of this cavity, which affects the first and the second components of the P wave, increasing the P voltage beyond physiologic values without prolonging the P duration. Left atrial hypertrophy/dilatation does not modify the initial portion of the P wave but affects the second and terminal portions of the P wave, leading to an increase in the P voltage and mainly to a lengthening of the P duration. Interatrial conduction delay is responsible for the notching of the P wave, with a peak to peak interval equal or superior to 0.04 second. The predominant pathologic atrial vectors are oriented downward and anteriorly in right atrial overload and upward to the left and posteriorly in left atrial overload.

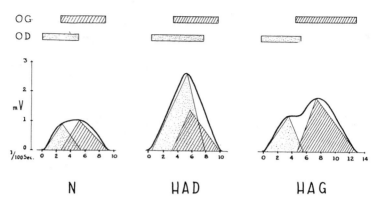

FIGURE 3. Schematic representation of the respective contribution of the right atrium (stippled area) and left atrium (hatched area) to the shape of the surface P wave. N = normal. HAD = right atrial hypertrophy. HAG = left atrial hypertrophy. (After Puech.)[3]

Examples of changes in P wave morphology as a consequence of right and left atrial hypertrophy/dilatation are reported in FIGURES 4 and 5.

Intracardiac recordings in atrial hypertrophy/dilatation have been useful in defining the respective contribution of each atrium in the configuration of the surface P wave.

In left atrial overload the prolongation of left atrial depolarization is well documented by coronary sinus recordings which show the last inscriptions of the atrial intrinsic deflections occurring at 110 mseconds or more (FIGURE 6). The conduction time from the upper right atrium to the area of the His bundle recording has a normal time interval (less than 50 mseconds) and the endpoint of the P wave is more or less synchronous with the His bundle spike. Esophageal leads show the increase in amplitude of unipolar atriograms and the delayed inscription of the deflections (FIGURE 7).

In right atrial overload the prolongation of right atrial depolarization, as demonstrated by intracavitary leads, is usually not sufficient to lengthen the total duration of atrial depolarization. Thus, the end of right atrial activation may be recorded near that of the left atrium.

In combined atrial overload, intracavitary recordings show delayed right and left atrial activation.

Position of the Heart in the Thorax

The projection of the main atrial vector on the frontal plane is influenced by the position of the heart. Vertical position associated with dextrorotation leads to preferential orientation of the atrial vector in inferior leads, and conversely, horizontal position and levorotation tends to direct the atrial vector to the left side. The relationship between the anatomical situation of the right atrium and the right precordial leads contributes to the variations of P wave morphology in V1, observed for instance in cases of right atrial overloads (FIGURE 4).

Propagation of the Current to Surface Electrodes

Resistance to propagation of the electrical field in the body (pulmonary emphysema, pericarditis) reduces the amplitude of the P wave, without affecting its morphology. Close proximity of the atrial cavity to the chest wall, as a consequence of dilatation of the atria, is responsible, in association with increased intrinsic voltage of atriograms, for the high amplitude of P waves in precordial leads.

Transient Factors Influencing P Wave Morphology

Respiratory Influences

Deep inspiration and the Valsalva maneuver significantly increase the amplitude of the P wave in inferior leads in normal subjects and patients with atrial overload. According to recent experimental data, the major mechanism of this increased voltage is related to a transient increase in right atrial volume, independent of variations in right atrial phasic or mean pressures.[13] The voltage change is dependent on autonomic control, as demonstrated by the persistent increase in amplitude of the P wave after

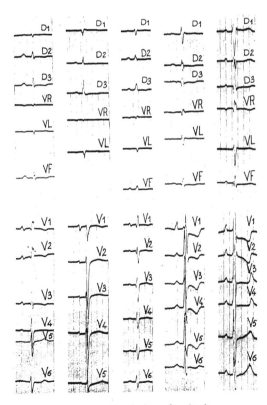

FIGURE 4. Examples of right atrial hypertrophy in surface leads.

pharmacologic autonomic nervous system denervation, achieved by administration of atropine and beta blocker.

Variation of Neurovegetative Tone

Variations in autonomic nervous system tone may influence P wave morphology indirectly through changes in atrial rate and directly in modifying the amplitude of atrial action potentials. Activation of orthosympathetic nervous system discharge increases P wave amplitude, while increase in vagal tone tends to reduce P wave voltage.

Atrial Infarction

Acute myocardial infarction impinges on P wave morphology in two ways: ischemic alterations of atrial activation when the necrotic process is extended to the atrium, and hemodynamic consequences of ventricular dysfunction. Most atrial infarctions involve the right side: 81% to 98% of right atrial, 2% to 19% of left atrial, and 19% to 24% of biatrial involvement.[14]

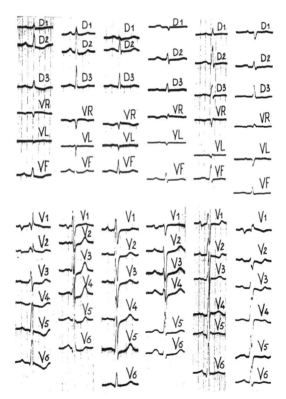

FIGURE 5. Examples of left atrial hypertrophy in surface leads.

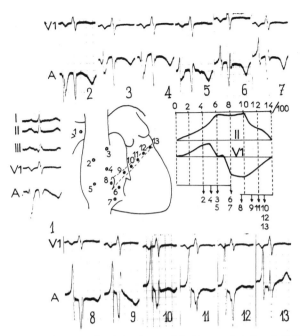

FIGURE 6. Left atrial hypertrophy (mitral stenosis). P wave duration is 0.14 second. The coronary sinus leads from the ostium (8) to the left border of the heart (14) record the delayed left atrial activation.

The major diagnostic criteria of atrial infarction are represented by changes in the PTa segment, while abnormal P waves (W- or W-shaped, notched) are included in minor criteria.[15] Evolutionary changes in P wave contour and in the J (A) point and PR segment in serial tracings and concurrent appearance of atrial arrhythmias are additional useful criteria of atrial involvement in acute myocardial infarction.[16] PTa shift is not a specific sign of ischemic atrial injury; primary changes in atrial repolarization have been reported in pericarditis, atrial trauma, orthohypersympathicotony, and after tricyclic antidepressant intoxication.[17]

Acute hemodynamic overload chiefly involves the left atrium, the increase in the atrial pressure being responsible for abnormal terminal P-terminal force in V1, without concomitant left atrial enlargement, as judged by echocardiography. The P wave often reverts to normal when the left atrial pressure returns to normal.[18]

Metabolic Disorders

Hyperkaliemia reduces the P wave amplitude until the atrial activity disappears in surface leads, when plasmatic K concentration reaches 10 mEq/l or more. Persistent activity of the sinus node, more resistant to hyperkaliemia than the common atrial muscle, is concealed in conventional ECG.

The opposite effect of hypokaliemia (increase of amplitude of the P wave) is less obvious, but has been documented by careful analysis of clinical tracings.[19]

P Wave Alternans

Alternation of the P wave in sinus rhythm is usually associated to alternans of other ECG components (QRS, T) in the setting of cardiac tamponade. Isolated P wave alternans is extremely rare, and the few published cases have been submitted to critical analysis.[20] Electrical alternans limited to the P wave could be explained by differences in refractory periods (and recuperation of excitability) between a small atrial region and the rest of the atria, the former having a longer refractoriness than the latter.

INTRA- AND INTERATRIAL CONDUCTION DEFECTS

The prolongation of atrial conduction in sinus rhythm can be observed independently of any hemodynamic atrial overload. These isolated intra- or interatrial conduction disturbances may be due to ischemic, degenerative, or infiltrative disorders, such as amyloidis or lipomatous hypertrophy of the interatrial septum, a finding associated with obesity and advancing age.[21] Minor intraauricular conduction disturbances could be better identified using high magnification, high-frequency vectocardiography of the P loop,[22] but this method is not commonly used and lacks validation as far as the location of the conduction disorders is concerned.

Right intraatrial conduction delay cannot be identified by surface ECG. The demonstration of the intraatrial disturbance is brought about by endocardial recordings, which show the prolongation of the interval between the beginning of the surface P wave (or the primodepolarization in the upper right atrium) and the atrial deflection recorded in the vicinity of the His bundle, marking the arrival of the atrial excitation process at the lower and anterior part of the interatrial septum. The PA interval, or

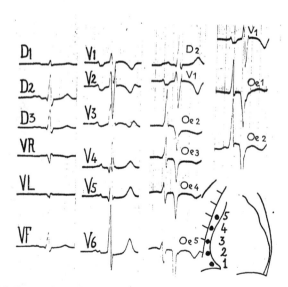

FIGURE 7. Unipolar esophageal recordings in a case of left atrial hypertrophy. The normal atrial activation process is preserved: negative atrial electrograms in the upper part, positive in the lower part of the left atrium. The amplitude of the electrograms is increased, and the time of inscription of the intrinsic deflections delayed.

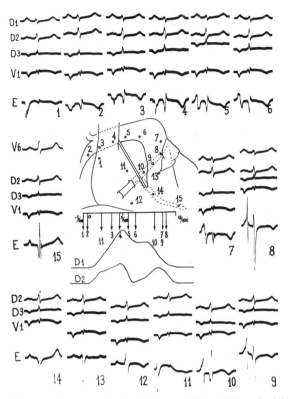

FIGURE 8. Partial interatrial conduction block in a case of left atrial overload (mitral stenosis). Recordings from the right pulmonary artery above Bachmann's bundle (5, 6) show the activation delay of the upper part of the left atrium. The depolarization of Bachmann's bundle precedes that of the lower left atrium (coronary sinus leads).

internodal conduction time, is considered as abnormal when superior to 55 mseconds. This prolongation of the PA interval can be responsible for a pseudo-first-degree AV block on surface leads (prolongation of PR interval).

Partial interatrial block refers to conduction delay over Bachmann's bundle, impairing the propagation of the impulse between both cephalic portions of the atria. The duration of the P wave is prolonged beyond 0.12 second, and the P wave is notched with two components separated by an interval of more than 0.04 second. The delay in activation of the roof of the left atrium is well demonstrated by esophageal leads recorded in an upper position (FIGURE 7) and atrial recordings obtained from the pulmonary artery (FIGURE 8). The activation delay of the left atrial cephalic portion is followed by a uniform descending activation wave front of the rest of the left atrium. Indeed esophageal recordings show the progressive delay of inscription of unipolar atriograms from the top to the bottom of the paraseptal left atrium (FIGURE 7). Intracavitary recordings show that activation of the lower part of the left atrium (coronary sinus leads) follows that of upper regions (FIGURE 8).

Advanced interatrial block is characterized by the inversion of the activation process over the left atrium, following depolarization of the right atrium. The P wave is considerably enlarged (130 to 170 mseconds) and is divided into two parts: the first one corresponds to the cephalic-to-caudal right atrial depolarization, and the second one to the oppositely directed left atrial activation. The right atrial vector (first portion of the P wave) is directed downward (between 45° and 90°) and forward (initial positivity in V1). The left atrial vector (second portion of the P wave) is directed upward and to the left (between −30° and −90° in the frontal place) and slightly backward (terminal negativity of P in V1). Esophageal leads and intracavitary recordings[3,23,24] demonstrate the caudocranial activation of the left atrium (FIGURE 9). Patients with advanced interatrial block and retrograde activation of the left atrium are prone to develop atrial tachyarrhythmias and, according to Bayes de Luna *et al.*,[25] atypical atrial flutter.

ECTOPIC ATRIAL RHYTHMS

Atrial Pace Mapping

The best correlative approach to the electrical propagation in the atria and the corresponding morphology of P waves in surface leads can be obtained by pacing

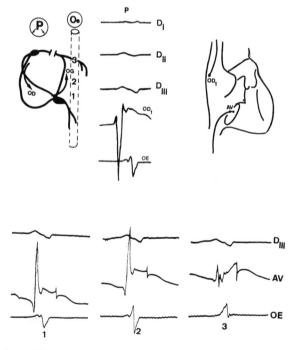

FIGURE 9. Advanced interatrial conduction block. The esophageal leads (Oe) show the inversion of the activation process in the left atrium: first inscription of the atrial electrogram in the lower esophageal lead and progressive delay of the atrial deflections from the bottom to the top of the left atrium (1 to 3). The electrogram recorded in the His bundle lead (AV) precedes the atrial activation of the left side and coincides with the polarity change of the surface P wave in lead III.

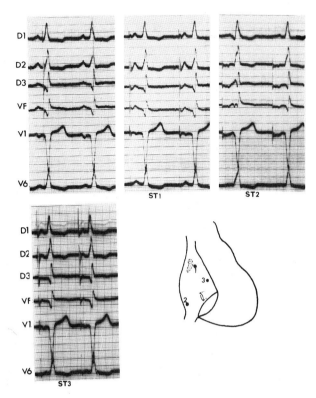

FIGURE 10. Right atrial pacing. Upper left panel: S-A node rhythm. Pacing (ST) in the vicinity of the S-A node (1) gives P waves resembling those of the control tracing. P waves resulting from pacing of the lower part of the free wall (2) are negative in leads II, III, and V1, flat in V6. Pacing of the middle anterior part of the atrial septum (3) results in P waves whose polarity is the same as in S-A node rhythm, in frontal and precordial leads, but the amplitude of the P waves that originate from atrial septum pacing is reduced, in comparison to the normal P waves.

multiple points of the endocardial or epicardial aspects of the atria and the coronary sinus, the value of this atrial pace mapping being obviously submitted to the precise location of the stimulated areas. Under radiologic supervision, the topography of intracavitary electrodes is easy to identify in the frontal plane but is more difficult for the sagittal projection. The atrial pace mapping provides the opportunity to evaluate the criteria employed in the diagnosis of atrial extrasystoles and monomorphic atrial tachycardias.

Illustrations of atrial pace mapping are given in FIGURES 10, 11, 12, and 13.

Right Atrial Pacing

P waves induced by endocardial or epicardial pacing of the upper and middle part of the right atrial wall, in the vicinity of the crista terminalis, present with minor changes in polarity and morphology from the spontaneous rhythm in the standard and

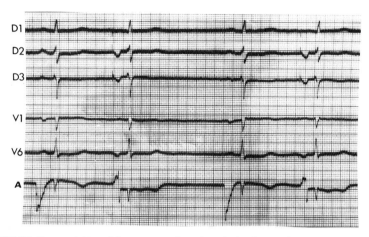

FIGURE 11. Lower right atrial septum pacing. A, unipolar intraatrial lead recorded in the vicinity of the S-A node. Pacing of the posteroinferior part of the atrial septum near the coronary sinus ostium (second and fourth beats) results in P waves that are negative in leads II, III, and V6, and flat in V1. During the induced inferior atrial rhythm, the intrinsic deflection at the superior vena cava–right atrium junction is recorded 80 mseconds after the spike.

precordial leads.[26-28] Pacing the caudal part of the right atrium, in front of the inferior vena cava, results in P waves with mean vector oriented upward and to the left; the P waves are of low voltage, always negative in leads II, III, and aVF, and negative in most or all precordial leads.[26-30]

Interatrial Septum Pacing

The P waves produced by pacing the upper and middle part of the interatrial septum are positive in leads I, II, and III, the mean vector of the atrial depolarization being oriented more inferiorly and to the right than that of the sinus rhythm. Pacing of the posteroinferior portion of the septum, close to the coronary sinus ostium, results in P waves that are usually negative and sometimes biphasic (− + with predominant negative fraction) in leads II, III, and aVF,[27,31] the P wave atrial vector usually having a slight forward orientation.

Pacing in the region of the His bundle recording (low anterior interatrial septum) most often produces negative P waves in leads II, III, and aVF; on rare occasions, atrial activity is biphasic with a terminal positive deflection of low amplitude. P waves, in our experience, are never positive in this situation.

Left Atrial Pacing

Epicardial pacing of the middle part of Bachmann's bundle results in positive P waves in leads II, III, and aVF, flat or positive in lead I, negative in the right precordial leads.[28,31]

Stimulation of the left atrial appendage gives rise to P waves whose mean vector is oriented from left to right, inferiorly (negative P waves in leads I and aVL) and anteriorly (positive in V1).

P waves produced by pacing the posterior wall of the left atrium have different shapes, depending on the high or low position of the stimulating electrodes and the proximity of the atrial septum.[29,30] Negative P waves in lead I (and aVL) result from excitation beginning in the vicinity of the left pulmonary veins.[28]

Pacing the posteroinferior aspect of the left atrium through the coronary venous system gives rise to P waves with mean vector oriented upward, between $-80°$ and $-120°$.[32,33] The P waves, always negative in leads II, III, and aVF, are flat in lead I when pacing is performed in the proximal portion of the coronary sinus and become negative in lead I when pacing at a more distal position, near the lateral wall of the left

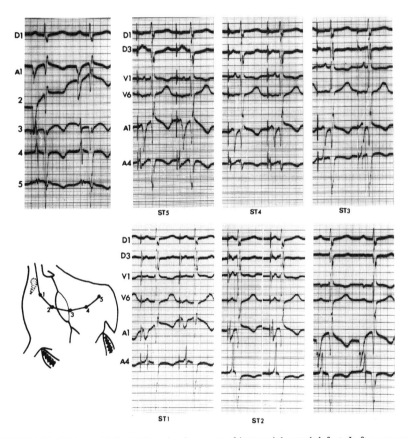

FIGURE 12. Right and left atrial pacing in a case of interatrial septal defect. Left upper and right lower panels: sinus rhythm. The P waves resulting from the pacing of point 1 (vicinity of S-A node) are positive in surface leads. Pacing of the middle part of the right atrium (2) produces negative P waves in lead III and positive in V1 and V6. Pacing in the vicinity of the left lower atrial septum results in flat P waves in leads I a,d V6, negative P waves in lead III, and "dome and dart" shaped P waves in V1. Pacing in the middle left atrium (4) gives an atrial vector directed downward, anteriorly, and to the right. Pacing at the root of the left atrial appendage (5) induces negative P waves in leads I and V6, positive P waves in leads III and V1.

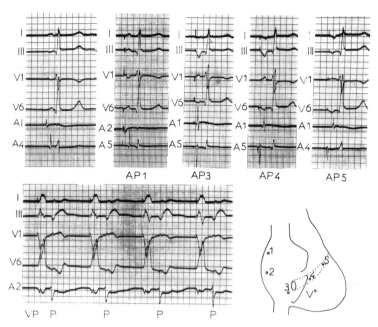

FIGURE 13. Atrial and ventricular pacing. Upper left panel: S-A node rhythm. Bipolar atrial electrograms recorded in the region of the S-A node (A1) and in the coronary sinus (A4). Other upper panels: atrial pacing (AP) by close bipolar electrodes at the points indicated by the diagram, with corresponding surface, right (A1 or A2), and left (coronary sinus, A4 or A5) leads. The atrial vector in the frontal plane resulting from the pacing of the lower portions of both atria is directed upward, from −85° (site 3) to −130° (site 5). The precordial P waves in the posteroinferior right and left ectopic rhythms are positive in V1 and negative in V6. Lower panel: right ventricular pacing (VP) followed by retrograde atrial activation. The R-P interval measured from the spike to the earliest atrial activity is 0.16 second. The retrograde P waves are negative in leads III and V6, and late positive in leads I and V1.

atrium (FIGURE 13). In the horizontal plane, the mean atrial vector is oriented forward and to the right, resulting in P waves negative in left precordial leads and positive, often biphasic, in V1 (V2). Sometimes the P waves in right precordial leads have the "dome and dart" shape described by Mirowski[34] as suggestive of ectopic rhythms originating from the posteroinferior left atrial wall. The duration of the P wave resulting from direct or indirect pacing (through the coronary sinus) of the lower left atrium is about 20 mseconds longer than that observed in spontaneous rhythm.

In conclusion, P waves produced by pacing different atrial sites have a vectorial orientation that corresponds to the position of the pacing electrodes with respect to the origin of the atrial activation.

Negative P waves in lead I (aVL) in the absence of atrial situs inversus and malposition of the limb electrodes are the best criteria of an ectopic left atrial rhythm.

Positive P waves in lead I with mean atrial vector oriented downward, anteriorly, and to the right can be produced by ectopic activities originating from the upper or middle right atrium and atrial septum and from the upper left atrium.

Negative P waves in the right precordial leads result from right ectopic atrial activities but can also occur in rhythms originating from Bachmann's bundle.[28]

Negative P waves in the left precordial leads are observed in left ectopic atrial rhythms but also when the abnormal impulse originates from the low right atrium, in the vicinity of the inferior vena cava orifice. However negative P waves in V6 are associated with negative P waves in all precordial leads when the ectopic rhythm begins in the right atrium, and with positive P waves in V1 (V2) in left ectopic atrial activities.

Retrograde Atrial Activation

The retrograde activation of the atria is the consequence of an atrial depolarization originating either from the normal conducting tissue (AV node, His bundle) or its vicinity (septal accessory pathways), leading to a "symetrical" depolarization of the atria, or from an accessory pathway (free wall Kent's bundle) responsible for "asymetrical" activation of the atria.

The chief difficulty in analyzing P wave morphology in retrograde atrial depolarization is the frequent concealment of the atrial activity into the QRS complex or the ventricular repolarization.

Retrograde atrial depolarization from the AV node or its approaches results in inverted P waves or, less often, biphasic (− +) with dominant negativity in leads II, III, aVF, and V6 and biphasic (− +) or upright in V1 (FIGURES 13 and 14). In lead I, the P wave is flat or slightly positive. In cases of biphasic (− +) P waves in leads II, III, and aVF the initial negative portion may be concealed in the preceding QRS complex, mimicking an upright P wave in these leads.[31]

Retrograde atrial activation resulting from a primodepolarization located at a distance from the normal conducting tissue (parietal Kent's bundle) gives rise to abnormal P waves, whose morphology depends upon the site of insertion of the accessory pathway. The occurrence of an inverted P wave in lead I in the course of a reentrant supraventricular tachycardia or during ventricular pacing is a valuable criterion for the presence of a left lateral accessory pathway with overt (WPW

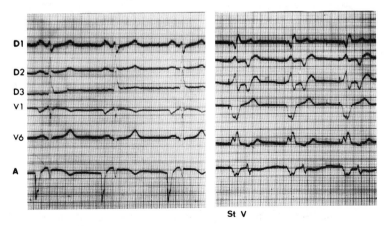

St V

FIGURE 14. Right ventricular pacing. Retrograde atrial conduction. A, unipolar auriculogram in the vicinity of the S-A node. D1, D2, D3 = leads I, II, III. Left panel: control tracing. Right panel: pacing of the right ventricle (St V) at a rate of 85/minute followed by 1 retrograde conduction to the atria (R-P interval 0.20 second). The retrograde P waves are deeply negative in leads II and III, negative in V6, flat in V1.

syndrome) or concealed preexcitation (normal QRS) in sinus rhythm.[35] This is illustrated in FIGURE 15.

Atrial Tachycardias

Monomorphic Atrial Tachycardias

In its paroxysmal (dependent on intraatrial reentry or triggered activity) or chronic (automatic focus) varieties, the P wave pattern is linked to the site of origin of the ectopic depolarization. Surface ECG suggests the location of the ectopy according to

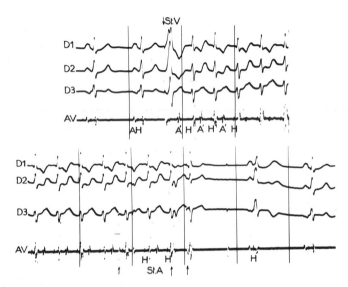

FIGURE 15. Reciprocating supraventricular tachycardia in a case of concealed left-sided Kent's bundle. Upper panel: initiation of supraventricular tachycardia after a single ventricular premature beat. Note the deeply inverted retrograde P wave in lead I in tachycardia. Lower panel: arrest of the supraventricular tachycardia by two atrial stimuli (arrows). In tachycardia the primodepolarization site of the atria was located near the distal coronary sinus lead (not reproduced).

the guidelines suggested above. Intraatrial recordings define the spread of activation in tachycardia, and stimulation techniques are of great help in approaching the mechanism of the atrial tachycardia. In the chronic (permanent or incessant) form, it is possible to record a prepotential activity, preceding the onset of the surface P wave and the initial component of the intraatrial electrogram (FIGURES 16 and 17). Thus the small area of activation in the vicinity of the atrial focus is concealed in the distant leads. This pathological zone is important to identify when an ablative method (fulguration or surgery) is considered in order to prevent an arrythmia-dependent cardiomyopathy.

FIGURE 18 is an example of chronic automatic atrial activity dependent on an atrial focus localized in the left atrium (vicinity of the left pulmonary veins), with negative P

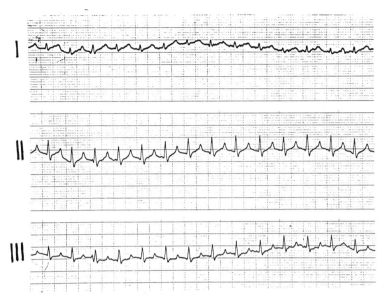

FIGURE 16. Automatic chronic atrial tachycardia. Atrial rate 150 per minute, positive P wave in surface leads, 1/1 AV conduction.

wave in lead I in tachycardia. The automatic focus was successfully removed by open-heart surgery.

Polymorphic Atrial Tachycardia

The incessant change in P wave morphology with the presence of at least three different P wave shapes reflects the change in the site of origin of the atrial pacemaker,

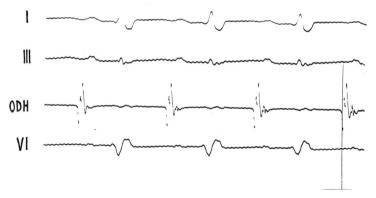

FIGURE 17. (same case as FIGURE 16). Right intraatrial recording showing a prepotential activity corresponding to the focus discharge in the upper atrium (ODH). Successful ablation of the atrial focus guided by the atrial mapping.

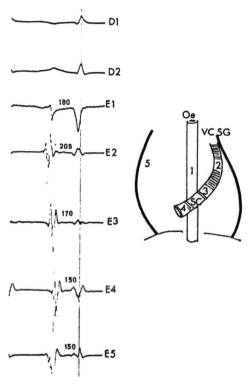

FIGURE 18. Automatic chronic atrial tachycardia. Negative P wave in lead I, positive in lead II. Atrial mapping from the esophagus (Oe), a persistent left vena cava (VCSG) opening onto the coronary sinus and the right atrium demonstrates the origin of the ectopic atrial activity in position 2. Successful removal of the left atrial focus by surgery.

usually associated with intraatrial conduction disturbances, as expressed by the differences in duration and notching of the atrial waves.

Atrial Flutter

Common Atrial Flutter (Type I)

The characteristic "sawtooth" appearance of the flutter (F) waves corresponds to a particular spread of the depolarization wave front, which has been depicted by selective esophageal and endocavitary atrial leads. The negative fraction of the F waves recorded in leads II, III, aVF, and V6 corresponds to depolarization of the atrial septum and the left atrium, proceeding in an ascendant way. The positive fraction of the F waves recorded in leads II, III, aVF, and V1 refers to the cephalic to caudal depolarization of the free wall of the right atrium.[36,37] FIGURE 19 is an example of right and left atrium mapping showing that the atrial depolarization process covers the whole cycle of the atrial flutter. The flat portion of the F wave in leads II, III, and aVF (pseudo isoelectric line) is due to the fact that the potentials generated from a small area of the low right atrium have an amplitude too low to be transmitted to distant leads. Macroreentry with an excitable gap in the right atrium is the mechanism currently accepted for the common atrial flutter. The area of the reentry is located in the posteroinferior right atrium,[38,39] and the rotation of the loop is counterclockwise (FIGURE 20). The presence of two "pivoting" zones on the reentrant circuit is suggested by the inscription of fragmented (double-spike) atrial electrograms recorded in the low right atrium (Koch's triangle) and in the middle intercaval region, as illustrated in FIGURE 21. The double-spike electrogram recorded in the low right atrium overrides the projection of the initial negativity of the F wave in leads II, III, and aVF, while the fragmented activity recorded in an upper zone corresponds to the change in polarity of the F wave, becoming positive in leads II, III, and aVF (FIGURE 21).

Detailed mapping in atrial flutter allows discovery of other fragmented activities, not incorporated in the reentrant circuit and which correspond to localized intraatrial conduction defects in zones more or less distant from the flutter loop. These fragmented activities are undetected by surface leads. Spontaneously or during rapid atrial pacing, these "bystander areas" of depressed conduction exhibit dissociation from the flutter mother wave.

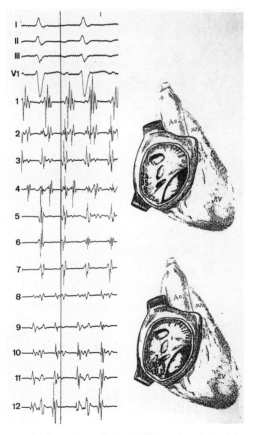

FIGURE 19. Common atrial flutter (type I). Detailed mapping of the right atrium showing that rapid atrial deflections are recorded during the whole cycle of the atrial flutter. The vertical line indicates the onset of the negative fraction of the flutter wave in leads II and III.

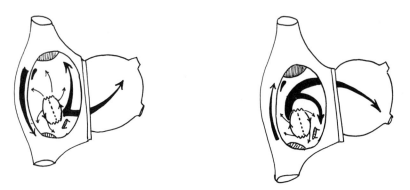

FIGURE 20. Schematic representation of the activation process in common (left) and uncommon (right) atrial flutter.

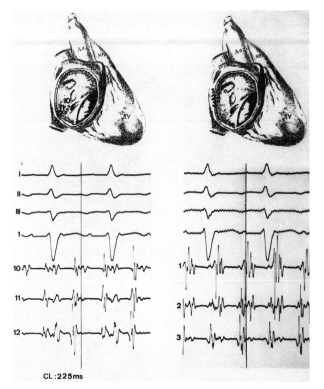

FIGURE 21. Recording of the "pivoting zones" of the reentrant circuit in a case of common atrial flutter. Left panel: double spike electrograms in the lower location recorded across the line indicating the onset of the negative fraction of the surface F wave in leads II and III. Right panel: fragmented electrograms in an upper part of the intercaval region, corresponding to the change in polarity of the F wave in surface leads.

Uncommon Atrial Flutter (Type II)

The atrial rate is in the same range as that of type I (over 250 per minute), but the morphology of the F waves is different, predominantly positive in the frontal plane and the precordial leads.

Selective atrial mapping of type II atrial flutter is in favor of a macroreentry in the right atrium with clockwise rotation of the flutter loop (FIGURE 20). As illustrated in

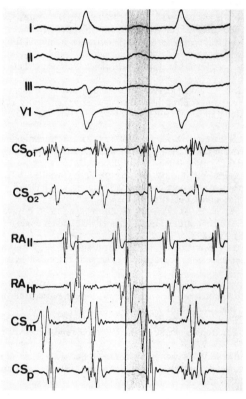

FIGURE 22. Uncommon atrial flutter. Mapping of the right atrium (RA) in low lateral (ll) and high lateral (hl) positions, the atrial septum (As) at middle (m) and lower (l) levels, the coronary sinus (Cs) near the ostium (o1 and o2) and inside its proximal (p) and middle part (m) . Atrial activity is recorded during all the atrial flutter cycle. The overt fraction of atrial depolarization in surface leads (between the vertical lines) corresponds to the descending activation of the atrial septum and the left atrium. Part of the right atrial depolarization is concealed in surface leads.

FIGURE 22 the activation process is descending along the interatrial septum and the left atrium. A fragmented, prolonged atrial electrogram is recorded in the vicinity of the coronary sinus (area of slow conduction incorporated in the circuit). In spite of the fact that the atrial depolarization recorded in intracavitary leads spans the whole cycle of the atrial flutter, a part of the right atrial depolarization is concealed in surface leads, the positive configuration of the F waves reflecting the septal and left atrial activation. In type II atrial flutter, the left atrium seems to be a bystander (macroreentry located in the right atrium), but its cephalic to caudal depolarization is the chief determinant of F wave morphology in surface leads.

REFERENCES

1. CASTILLO FENOY, A., J. F. THEBAUT, F. ACHARD & B. DELANGENHAGEN. 1979. Identification du potentiel sinusal chez l'homme. Critères d'identification, résultats préliminaires. Arch. Mal. Coeur 72(9): 948–956.
2. HARIMAN, R. F., E. KRONGRAD, R. A. BOXER, H. B. WEISS, C. N. STEEG & B. F. HOFFMAN. 1980. Method for recording electrical activity of the sino-atrial node and autonomic atrial foci during cardiac catheterization in human subjects. Am. J. Cardiol. 45(4): 775–781.
3. PUECH, P. 1956. L'Activité Électrique Auriculaire Normale et Pathologique. Masson Ed. Paris, France.
4. SPACH, M. S. & P. C. DOLBER. 1985. The relation between discontinuous propagation in anisotropic cardiac muscle and the "vulnerable period" of reentry. In Cardiac Electrophysiology and Arrhythmias. D. P. Zipes & J. Jalife, Eds.: 241–252. Grune and Stratton. Orlando, Fla.
5. CHIRIFE, R., G. S. FEITOSA & W. S. FRANKL. 1975. Electrocardiographic detection of left atrial enlargement. Correlation of P wave with left atrial dimension by echocardiography. Br. Heart J. 37(12): 1281–1285.
6. ORLANDO, J., M. DEL VICARIO, W. S. ARONOW & J. CASSIDY. 1977. Correlation of mean pulmonary artery wedge pressure, left atrial dimension, PTF-V1 in patients with acute myocardial infarction. Circulation 55(4): 750–752.
7. SHETTIGAR, U. R., W. H. BARRY & H. N. HULTGREN. 1977. P wave analysis in ischemic heart disease. An echocardiographic, haemodynamic and angiographic assessment. Br. Heart J. 39(8): 894–899.
8. DI BIANCO, R., J. S. GOTTDIENER, R. D. FLETCHER & H. V. PIPBERGER. 1979. Left atrial overload: a hemodynamic, echocardiographic and vectocardiographic study. Am. Heart J. 98(4): 478–489.
9. GONZALEZ PLIEGO, J. A., G. SANCHEZ TORRES & J. F. GUADALAJARA BOO. 1988. La onda P en la hipertension arterial sistemica. Correlation con el ecocardiograma y el apexcardiograma. Arch. Inst. Cardiol. Mex. 58: 115–119.
10. JOSEPHSON, M. E., J. A. KASTOR & J. MORGANROTH. 1977. Electrocardiographic left atrial enlargement. Electrophysiologic, echocardiographic and hemodynamic correlates. Am. J. Cardiol. 39(7): 967–971.
11. WAGGONER, A. D., A. V. ADYANTHAYA, M. A. QUINONES & K. F. ALEXANDER. 1976. Left atrial enlargement. Echocardiographic assessment of electrocardiographic criteria. Circulation 54(4): 553–557.
12. MAOK, J. & E. KRONGRAD. 1984. Assessment of electrocardiographic criteria in left atrial enlargement in childhood. Am. J. Cardiol. 53(1): 215–217.
13. SARDI-SCHOONEWOLF, E. G., P. L. FERRER, A. S. PICKOFF, A. CASTELLANOS JR., N. F. SARDI & H. GELBAND. 1989. Right atrial pressure and P wave voltages during normal breathing and deep inspiration. An experimental study. Rev. Lat. Cardiol. 10(2): 112–117.
14. GARDIN, J. M. & D. H. SINGER. 1981. Atrial infarction: importance, diagnosis and localization. Arch. Intern. Med. 141: 1345–1348.
15. LIU, C. K., G. GREENSPAN & R. T. PICCIRILLO. 1961. Atrial infarction of the heart. Circulation 23: 331–338.
16. MAYUGA, R. D. & D. H. SINGER. 1985. Atrial infarction: clinical significance and diagnostic criteria. Pract. Cardiol. 11: 142–160.
17. FRIART, A. 1989. Alterations of atrial repolarization after tricyclic antidepressant drug absorption. Acta Cardiol. 44(1): 15–18.
18. CHANDRARATNA, P. A. N. 1978. On the significance of an abnormal P-terminal force in lead V1. Am. Heart J. 95(2): 267–268.

19. SURAWICZ, B. & E. LEPESCHKIN. 1953. The electrocardiographic pattern of hypopotassemia with and without hypocalcemia. Circulation 8(6): 801–828.
20. DONATO, A., G. ORETO & L. SCHAMROTH. 1988. P wave alternans. Am. Heart J. 116(3): 875–877.
21. ISNER, J. M., C. S. SWAN, J. P. MIKUS & B. L. CARTER. 1982. Lipomatous hypertrophy of the interatrial septum: in vivo diagnosis. Circulation 66(2): 470–473.
22. ZONERAICH, O. & S. ZONERAICH. 1976. Intra-atrial conduction disturbances: vectocardiographic patterns. Am. J. Cardiol. 37(5): 736–742.
23. WARIN, J. F. & J. P. FAUCHIER. 1978. Les troubles de la conduction intra-auriculaire. In Les Troubles du Rythme Cardiaque. P. Puech & R. Slama, Eds.: 95–107. Corbière. Nanterre, France.
24. CASTILLO, A. & P. VERNANT. 1973. Troubles de conduction inter-auriculaire par bloc du faisceau de Bachmann. Etude de 3 cas par électrocardiographie endo-auriculaire et oesophagienne. Coeur 4(1): 31–39.
25. BAYES DE LUNA, A., M. CLADELLAS, R. OTER, P. TORNER, J. GUINDO, V. MARTI, I. RIVERA & P. ITURRALDE. Eur. Heart J. 9(10): 1112–1118.
26. LEON, D. F., J. F. LANCASTER, J. A. SHAVER, F. W. KROETZ & J. J. LEONARD. 1970. Right atrial ectopic rhythms. Experimental production in man. Am. J. Cardiol. 25: 6–10.
27. PUECH, P. 1974. The P wave: correlation of surface and intra-atrial electrograms. In Complex Electrocardiography 2. Cardiovascular Clinics. C. Fisch & N. Brest, Eds.: 43–46. F. A. Davis Company. Philadelphia, Pa.
28. MACLEAN, W. A., R. B. KARP, N. T. KOUCHOUKOS, T. N. JAMES & A. L. WALDO. 1975. P waves during ectopic atrial rhythms in man. Circulation 52(3): 426–434.
29. HARRIS, B. C., J. A. SHAVER, S. GRAY, F. W. KROETZ & J. J. LEONARD. 1968. Left atrial rhythms. Experimental production in man. Circulation 37: 1000.
30. MASSUMI, R. & A. A. TAWAKKOL. 1967. Direct study of left atrial P waves. Am. J. Cardiol. 20(3): 331–340.
31. WALDO, A. L., K. J. VITIKAINEN, G. A. KAISER, J. R. MALM & B. F. HOFFMAN. 1970. The P wave and PR interval: effects of the site of origin of atrial depolarization. Circulation 42(4): 653–671.
32. GIRAUD, G., H. LATOUR & P. PUECH. 1954. L'électrocardiographie du sinus coronaire II: etude électrocardiographique endocavitaire des dysrythmies du sinus coronaire chez l'homme. Arch. Mal. Coeur 47(12): 1008–1025.
33. LAU, S. H., S. I. COHEN, E. STEIN, J. J. HAFT, K. M. ROSEN & A. N. DAMATO. 1970. P waves and P loops in coronary sinus and left atrial rhythms. Am. Heart J. 79(2): 201–214.
34. MIROWSKI, M. 1966. Left atrial rhythm. Diagnostic criteria and differentiation from nodal arrhythmias. Am. J. Cardiol. 17(2): 203–210.
35. PUECH, P. & R. GROLLEAU. 1977. L'onde P rétrograde négative en D1, signe de faisceau de Kent postéro-latéral gauche. Arch. Mal. Coeur 70(1): 49–60.
36. PUECH, P., H. LATOUR & R. GROLLEAU. 1970. Le flutter et ses limites. Arch. Mal. Coeur 63(1): 116–144.
37. CHAUVIN, M., C. BRECHENMACHER & J. R. VOEGTLIN. 1983. Applications de la cartographie endocavitaire à l'étude du flutter auriculaire. Arch. Mal. Coeur 76(9): 1020–1030.
38. KLEIN, G. J., G. M. GUIRAUDON, A. D. SHARMA & S. MILSTEIN. 1986. Demonstration of macro-reentry and feasibility of operative therapy in the common type of atrial flutter. Am. J. Cardiol. 57(8): 587–591.
39. COSIO, F. G., F. ARRIBAS, J. M. BARBERO, C. KALLMEYER & A. GOICOLEA. 1988. Validation of double-spike electrograms as markers of conduction delay or block in atrial flutter. Am. J. Cardiol. 61(10): 775–780.

The QRS Complex

DENNIS M. KRIKLER

Cardiovascular Division
Royal Postgraduate Medical School
Du Cane Road
London W12 0NN, United Kingdom

The first recordings of cardiac activity from the surface of the intact human were made in 1857 by Marey[1] and of course reflected mechanical function; these attracted much interest so that by 1870 there were at least 10 such studies.[2] That simultaneous recordings of several pulses, using drums of smoked paper for the recordings, were valuable was shown by Mackenzie,[3] but he was already being overtaken by the nascent electrocardiograph with which Waller used Lippmann's capillary electrometer to produce electrical, as opposed to or as well as, mechanical tracings.[4] But these were crude recordings, though for their purpose they did indeed show ventricular activity. By 1900 Einthoven was able to define the QRS complex using the capillary electrometer[5] but he did much better with the string galvanometer[6] that he was developing,[7] and was now able more clearly to depict the various waveforms of the electrocardiogram. Various letters had been attached to the waves seen on the capillary electrometer tracings, e.g., A, B, C, D; Einthoven had already in 1900 decided to use letters from the latter part of the alphabet[5] and had not only named but also defined the P, QRS, and T waves (FIGURE 1), reflecting, respectively, atrial and ventricular activity.[5] The U wave, the precise origin of which remains open to debate,[8] came later.[9]

An early aspect of Einthoven's work was the derivation of the electrical axis of the heart; by means of the famous equilateral triangle he did in effect produce the first vectorial representation of the direction of ventricular depolarization.[10] From this one could deduce, using the standard limb leads, that the magnitude of the complex (in this case, the QRS) showed the relationship: lead I + lead III = lead II. But at that time knowledge of the electrical axis was not yet correlated with conduction disturbances; this was still to come. A little earlier, however, Samojloff had demonstrated changes in QRS shape with respiration, affecting lead III,[11] which provided evidence of extracardiac influences on the vector derived from the Einthoven equation.

NORMAL VENTRICULAR ACTIVATION

Empirical observations of the normal QRS appearances often suffice as the basis for diagnostic deductions, but the studies in dogs reported by Lewis indicated that the impulse reaching the ventricles from the atria commenced its further progress from the upper part of the interventricular septum, crossing it to the right while also moving distally.[12] This and many other animal studies were finally corroborated, and the basis for the configuration of the normal QRS complex validated, by the seminal experiments on ventricular excitation performed some 20 years ago by Durrer and his colleagues.[13] Reference will not be made to the many texts that describe the normal QRS complex, but whether written from an empirical basis or derived from observations on large groups, they must all depend on the knowledge acquired by observers from Lewis to Durrer. However, at an early stage, Kraus and Nicolai[14] had revived earlier mechanistic concepts that, though the ventricles contract synergistically, they produce individual QRS patterns, and that separate contraction of one ventricle could cause an appearance that they described, as had others in preelectrocardiographic days, as hemisystole. As it became appreciated that extrasystoles could be initiated from different parts of the ventricle and then invade and depolarize the rest of the chambers, this concept was discarded as an explanation for varying QRS patterns. Extrasystoles and their patterns, the appearances seen in escape complexes such as occur distal to complete atrioventricular block, and the QRS configuration in ventricu-

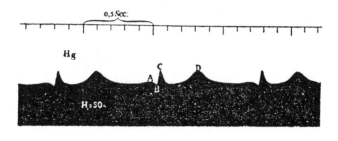

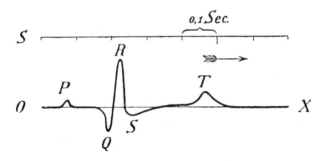

FIGURE 1. Capillary electrometer recording (above) and string galvanometer recording (below), from same patient; reproduced from Einthoven.[6] While the PQRST complexes are clearly evident in the string galvanometer recording, the corresponding A (=P) and B (=Q) waves in the capillary electrometer tracings are barely visible and C (=R) is small.

lar tachycardias and the less common tachycardias associated with preexcitation, constitute a separate topic from the present paper.

It is 65 years since Lewis summarized the then current state of knowledge "the ventricular complex is modified by three chief known factors:- (a) by the lie of the heart in the chest, (b) by the manner in which the excitation wave is distributed to the ventricle, and (c) by the relative weights of muscle in the right and left ventricle."[15] Already seen, but not recognized at the time, the effects of myocardial infarction on the QRS complex, and the Wolff-Parkinson-White syndrome, must be added to the above though in theory they could be subsumed within his headings.

BUNDLE BRANCH BLOCK

Electrocardiographic abnormalities of rhythm first received attention, but early experiments with dogs in whom silver nitrate was injected into the interventricular septum produced appearances labeled as block of the right and left bundle branches;[16,17] these propositions were accepted by Lewis in his own studies in dogs in which he cut the branches,[12] and were extensively extrapolated to man.[15] The whole story has been well analyzed by Hollman,[18] who shows that Lewis's initial errors were compounded by others, including Wilson,[19] though George Fahr—who had worked with Einthoven before returning to Minneapolis—used the Einthoven triangle to contradict Lewis.[20] The correct terminology, as now used, became recognized after Mann's depiction of derived vectorcardiographic loops[21] and, most importantly, Wilson's use of multiple precordial leads.[22]

A separate aspect, where Lewis's original assessment proved correct, was his use of the term aberration when a patient seen in 1912 had paroxysmal supraventricular tachycardia, sometimes with normal QRS complexes and sometimes with wide and altered appearances of the QRS. "Thus the wave spreads abnormally to the ventricles . . . consequently I term the resultant beats *aberrant*."[15] As we now well recognize, even in sinus rhythm as opposed to supraventricular tachycardia, the appearances of bundle branch block may be intermittent and often dependent upon relative differences in the heart rate—slow or fast—or the coupling interval between sinus complexes and subsequent supraventricular extrasystoles.

FASCICULAR BLOCKS AND AXIS DEVIATION

Lewis's comment on the "lie of the heart in the chest" came after a long discussion on the rotation of the electrical axis.[15] This, as originally defined by Einthoven, reflected changes in the frontal plane, such as could have been calculated from the limb leads, though he referred to clockwise and anticlockwise rotation and to the effects of respiration and posture. The relation between electrical axis and ventricular hypertrophy attracted interest early on and is alluded to in that section; on the other hand, Wilson and his colleagues expressed the view in 1941 that "the exact position of the mean electrical axis of the heart is of no clinical important."[23] Strangely enough, within a few years, new relevance for the electrical axis in terms of conduction disturbances was indeed found. Actually, the roots of this work could be seen, according to Rosenbaum,[24] in an earlier paper from Wilson and his colleagues[25] in which they had postulated that deep S waves in leads II and III, in three patients with right bundle branch block, could be due to a lesion of the anterior division of the left bundle branch. Grant was the first clearly to suggest that lesions affecting the anterior division of the left bundle branch block were responsible for some cases of left axis deviation, and of the posterior division, for some examples of right axis deviation.[26] He and others subsequently analyzed the specific changes in the initial vectors that enabled distinctions to be made between axis deviation due to such blocks and other causes, but the importance of this concept, and its dissemination, is largely dependent on Mauricio Rosenbaum and his colleagues, from Buenos Aires.[24] They applied the term hemiblocks to such appearances; a task force of the World Health Organization and the International Society and Federation of Cardiology considered that anterior and posterior fascicular blocks were more appropriate terms.[27] The useful concept does not however, in the clinical context, indicate the presence of a specific focal anatomical lesion. As with bundle branch blocks, such fascicular blocks may also be intermittent, and may also occur transiently, in response, for example, to rate changes, and constitute an expression of aberration.

VENTRICULAR HYPERTROPHY

Initially, the interpretation of the electrical axis of the heart was clouded by the misunderstandings mentioned above regarding bundle branch block. The first associations with right and left axis deviation can be linked with the early descriptions of the appearances of right and left ventricular hypertrophy by Einthoven,[9] to which Lewis added the rider of ventricular preponderance associated with hypertrophy.[28] Lewis's electrocardiographic observations were underpinned by measurement of the weight of the ventricles at necropsy;[15] Herrmann and Wilson confirmed the correlation between electrocardiographic signs of hypertrophy and the weight of the ventricles only for relatively heavy hearts.[29]

The problem of the correct diagnosis of ventricular hypertrophy on the electrocardiogram could not be taken further using limb leads only. As single precordial leads were introduced individual reports of better criteria for the electrocardiographic diagnosis of ventricular hypertrophy appeared, but a significant step forward was taken by Wood and Selzer, with multiple precordial leads that they devised.[30] It was however the advent of the multiple lead precordial electrocardiogram by Wilson that enabled systems for the recognition, and later the attempted quantification of the degree, of ventricular hypertrophy to come into clinical use on an accepted basis.[31] But an important rider must be added in that standard criteria for QRS amplitude for hypertrophy must be tempered by the knowledge that they may normally be greater than acceptable for white adults in juveniles as well as those of African or other ethnic origin,[32] whether seen in isolation or combined with ST segment changes.

MYOCARDIAL INFARCTION

Very soon after the clinical diagnosis of coronary thrombosis had been made in life[33,34] it was shown that ligation of branches of the left coronary artery in dogs[35] produced ST-T changes, and that similar electrocardiographic findings could be detected clinically.[36,37] In their systematic analysis of the electrocardiographic changes in cardiac infarction, Parkinson and Bedford drew no specific conclusions about "changes in the initial ventricular deflections (QRS)"[38] but mentioned the presence of Q waves in five patients who displayed T wave inversion in lead III. Several of their illustrations, however, that show T inversion in I, have small Q waves also. Only later, and with the advent of multiple precordial leads, did the significance of the development of Q waves in anterior infarction become appreciated, and the progressive study of patients with myocardial infarction using unipolar chest leads enabled Wilson and his colleagues to synthesize the data and classify infarcts according to their location as determined by the changes in specific leads.[31] For this they depended heavily on a series of studies on experimental infarction in dogs conducted over a decade and reprinted in his collected works;[39] it is only since Wilson's work on QRS changes in chest as well as limb leads that the electrocardiogram has attained its key diagnostic value in myocardial infarction.

PREEXCITATION

The bizarre QRS patterns seen in the Wolff-Parkinson-White syndrome were at first thought to reflect bundle branch block; not at all surprising then, in 1930,[40] when the true nature of left and right bundle branch block was only just becoming clearly recognized. The broad QRS complexes became narrow when the complicating atrioventricular tachycardia occurred as had already been observed in the earliest cases;[41,42] it was not long before these features were linked with the short PR interval and defined as preexcitation, in which an accessory atrioventricular pathway carries the earliest part of the signal from atrium to ventricle more quickly than does the atrioventricular node.[43] Anatomical corroboration of the presence of such pathways soon followed, and the normalization of the QRS in tachycardia was shown to reflect circus movement using the atrioventricular node in the anterograde direction. Clues to the location of the pathway arose out of the observation in right precordial leads that the QRS could be upright (group A) or inverted (group B), possibly linked to differences in the order of ventricular activation,[44] later shown generally to correspond to left or right sided pathways respectively.[45] This development has led in due course to surgical or endocavitary ablation of the responsible pathway, where warranted, success being attended by the restoration of a QRS pattern reflecting atrioventricular nodal conduction. As with other conduction disturbances mentioned earlier, preexcitation may be intermittent; one cannot here discuss concealed preexcitation as by definition it reflects the presence of the pathway, and of the tendency to arrhythmia, without overt abnormality of the QRS configuration; latent preexcitation is probably best defined as the occurrence of preexcited complexes only in the presence of an atrial arrhythmia.[46]

Bundle branch block was, as indicated, an original, though erroneous, part of the definition of the Wolff-Parkinson-White syndrome;[40] on the electrocardiogram one may be able to detect the coexistence of preexcitation and bundle branch block on the basis of the QRS configuration and verify this electrophysiologically[47] as well as by pathological study.[48]

REFERENCES

1. MAREY, E-J. 1863. Physiologie Médicale de la Circulation du Sang Basée sur l'Étude Graphique des Mouvements du Coeur et du Pouls Artériel, avec Applications aux Maladies de l'Appareil Circulatoire. Adrien Delahaye. Paris, France.
2. LORAIN, P. 1870. Le Pouls. Ses Variations et Ses Formes Diverses dans les Maladies. J-B Baillière et fils. Paris, France.
3. MACKENZIE, J. 1894. The venous and liver pulses, and the arythmic contraction of the cardiac cavities. J. Pathol. Bacteriol. 2: 84–154, 273–345.
4. WALLER, A. D. 1887. A demonstration on man of electromotive changes accompanying the heart's beat. J. Physiol. 8: 229–234.
5. EINTHOVEN, W. & K. DE LINT. 1900. Über das normale menschliche Elektrokardiogramm und über die capillar-elektrometrische Untersuchung einiger Herzkranken. Pflügers Arch. ges. Physiol. 80: 139–160.
6. EINTHOVEN, W. 1903–4. The string galvanometer and the human electrocardiogram. K. Akad. Wet. Amst. Proc. Sect. Sci. 6: 107–115.
7. EINTHOVEN, W. 1901. Un nouveau galvanomètre. Archives Néerlandaises des Sciences Exactes et Naturelles. Sér. 2 6: 625–633.
8. LEPESCHKIN, E. 1972. Physiologic basis of the U wave. In Advances in Electrocardiography. R. C. Schlant & J. W. Hurst, Eds.: 431–447. Grune & Stratton. New York, N.Y.
9. EINTHOVEN, W. 1906. Le télécardiogramme. Arch. Int. Physiol. 4: 132–164.
10. EINTHOVEN, W., G. FAHR & A. DE WAART. 1913. Über die Richtung und die manifest Grösse der Potentialschwankungen im menschlichen Herzen und über den Einfluss der

Herzlage auf die Form des Elektrokardiogramms. Pflügers Arch. ges. Physiol. 150: 275–315.

11. SAMOJLOFF, A. 1908. Elektrokardiogrammstudien. Beitrage zur Physiologie und Pathologie. O. Weiss, Ed.: 171. Enke. Stuttgart, Germany.

12. LEWIS, T. 1916. The spread of the excitatory process in the vertebrate heart. Phil. Trans. R Soc. Lond. Ser. B 207: 221–310.

13. DURRER, D., R. TH. VAN DAM, G. E. FREUD, M. J. JANSE, F. L. MEIJLER & R. C. ARZBAECHER. 1970. Total excitation of the isolated human heart. Circulation 41: 899–912.

14. KRAUS, F. & G. F. NICOLAI. 1910. Das Elektrokardiogramm des gesunden und kranke Menschen. Veit & Comp. Leipzig, Germany.

15. LEWIS, T. 1925. The Mechanism and Graphic Registration of the Heart Beat. 3rd edit. Shaw and Sons. London, England.

16. EPPINGER, H. & C. J. ROTHBERGER. 1909. Zur Analyse des Elektrokardiogramms. Wien. klin. Wschr. 22: 1091–1098.

17. ROTHBERGER, C. J. & H. WINTERBERG. 1913. Zur Diagnose der einseitigen Blockierung der Reitzleitung in den Tawaraschen Schenkeln. Zbl. Herz Gefasskrankh. 5: 206–208.

18. HOLLMAN, A. 1985. The history of bundle branch block. Med. Hist. Suppl. 5: 82–102.

19. WILSON, F. N. & G. R. HERRMANN. 1920. Bundle branch block and arborization block. Arch. Intern. Med. 26: 153–191.

20. FAHR, G. 1920. An analysis of the spread of the excitation wave in the human ventricle. Arch. Intern. Med. 25: 146–173.

21. MANN, H. 1931. Interpretation of bundle branch block by means of the monocardiogram. Am. Heart J. 6: 447–457.

22. WILSON, F. N., A. G. MACLEOD & P. S. BARKER. 1932. The order of ventricular excitation in human bundle branch block. Am. Heart J. 7: 305–330.

23. WILSON, F. N., F. D. JOHNSTON, N. COTRIM & F. F. ROSENBAUM. 1941. Relations between the potential variations of the ventricular surfaces and the form of the electrocardiogram in leads from the precordium and the extremities. Trans. Assoc. Am. Phys. 56: 258–271.

24. ROSENBAUM, M., M. V. ELIZARI & J. O. LAZZARI. 1970. The Hemiblocks. Tampa Tracings. Oldsmar, Fla.

25. WILSON, F. N., F. D. JOHNSTON & P. S. BARKER. 1934. Electrocardiograms of an unusual type in right bundle branch block. Am. Heart J. 9: 472–479.

26. GRANT, R. P. & E. H. ESTES, JR. 1952. Spatial Vector Electrocardiography. Clinical Electrocardiographic Interpretation. Blakiston Co. New York, N.Y.

27. WILLEMS, J. L., E. O. ROBLES DE MEDINA, R. BERNARD, P. COUMEL, C. FISCH, D. KRIKLER, N. A. MAZUR, F. L. MEIJLER, L. MOGENSEN, P. MORET, Z. PISA, P. M. RAUTAHARJU, B. SURAWICZ, Y. WATANABE & H. J. J. WELLENS. 1985. Criteria for intraventricular conduction disturbances and pre-excitation. J. Am. Coll. Cardiol. 5: 1261–1275.

28. LEWIS, T. 1913–14. Observations upon ventricular hypertrophy, with especial reference to preponderance of one or other chamber. Heart 5: 367–402.

29. HERRMANN, G. R. & F. N. WILSON. 1921–22. Ventricular hypertrophy. A comparison of electrocardiographic and post mortem observations. Heart 9: 91–147.

30. WOOD, P. & A. SELZER. 1939. Chest leads in clinical electrocardiography. Br. Heart J. 1: 49–80.

31. WILSON, F. N., F. D. JOHNSTON, F. F. ROSENBAUM, H. ERLANGER, C. E. KOSSMAN, H. H. HECHT, N. COTRIM, R. MENEZES DE OLIVEIRA, R. SCARSI & P. S. BARKER. 1944. The precordial electrocardiogram. Am. Heart J. 27: 19–85.

32. KRIKLER, D. M. 1974. The electrocardiogram. In Cardiovascular Diseases in the Tropics. A. G. Shaper, M. S. R. Hutt & Z. Fejfar, Eds.: 160–169. British Medical Association. London, England.

33. OBRASTZOW, W. B. & N. D. STRASCHENKO. 1910. Zur Kenntnis der Thrombose der Koronararterien des Herzens. Z. klin. Med. 71: 116–132.

34. HERRICK, J. B. 1912. Clinical features of sudden obstruction of the coronary arteries. J. Am. Med. Assoc. 59: 2015–2020.

35. SMITH, F. M. 1918. The ligation of coronary arteries with electrocardiographic study. Arch. Intern. Med. **22:** 8–27.
36. HERRICK, J. B. 1919. Thrombosis of the coronary arteries. J. Am. Med. Assoc. **72:** 387–390.
37. PARDEE, H. E. B. 1920. An electrocardiographic sign of coronary artery obstruction. Arch. Intern. Med. **26:** 244–257.
38. PARKINSON, J. & D. E. BEDFORD. 1927–28. Successive changes in the electrocardiogram after cardiac infarction (coronary thrombosis). Heart **14:** 195–212.
39. JOHNSTON, F. D. & E. LEPESCHKIN, Eds. 1954. Selected papers of Dr. Frank N. Wilson. J. W. Edwards. Ann Arbor, Mich.
40. WOLFF, L., J. PARKINSON & P. D. WHITE. 1930. Bundle branch block with short P-R interval in healthy young people prone to paroxysmal tachycardia. Am. Heart J. **5:** 685–699.
41. COHN, A. E. & F. R. FRASER. 1913–14. Paroxysmal tachycardia and the effect of stimulation of the vagus nerves by pressure. Heart **5:** 93–105.
42. WILSON, F. N. 1915. A case in which the vagus influenced the form of the ventricular complex of the electrocardiogram. Arch. Intern. Med. **16:** 1008–1027.
43. ÖHNELL, R. F. 1944. Pre-excitation, a cardiac abnormality. Acta Med. Scand. Suppl 152.
44. ROSENBAUM, F. F., H. H. HECHT, F. N. WILSON & F. D. JOHNSTON. 1945. The potential variations of the thorax and the esophagus in anomalous atrioventricular excitation (Wolff-Parkinson-White syndrome). Am. Heart J. **29:** 281–326.
45. GIRAUD, G., H. LATOUR, P. PUECH & J. ROUJON. 1956. Les troubles de rythme du syndrome de Wolff-Parkinson-White. Analyse électrocardiographique endocavitaire. Arch. Mal. Coeur **49:** 101–133.
46. ROBINSON, K., E. ROWLAND & D. M. KRIKLER. 1988. Latent pre-excitation: exposure of anterograde accessory pathway conduction during atrial fibrillation. Br. Heart J. **59:** 53–55.
47. KRIKLER, D., P. COUMEL, P. CURRY & C. OAKLEY. 1977. Wolff-Parkinson-White syndrome type A obscured by left bundle branch block. Eur. J. Cardiol. **5:** 49–62.
48. ROBINSON, K., M. J. DAVIES & D. M. KRIKLER. 1988. Type A Wolff-Parkinson-White syndrome obscured by left bundle branch block associated with a vascular malformation of the coronary sinus. Br. Heart J. **60:** 352–354.

Multidimensional Quantitation of Ventricular Repolarization[a]

Static and Dynamic Characteristics

ARTHUR J. MOSS, MARIO MERRI, JESAIA BENHORIN,
MICHELA ALBERTI, AND EMANUELA LOCATI

Heart Research Follow-up Program
Department of Preventive and Community Medicine
University of Rochester School of Medicine and Dentistry
Rochester, New York 14642

INTRODUCTION

The electrocardiographic recording of ventricular repolarization includes the time interval from the end of the QRS complex to the completion of the T-U wave. Ventricular repolarization duration is traditionally quantified by measuring the QT interval with correction for the heart rate by the Bazett algorithm[1] or equivalent formulae.[2,3] The axis of the repolarization T wave and the magnitude of the T wave can be quantitated by vectorial analysis,[4] and a variety of primary and secondary factors may affect the T wave configuration. Ventricular repolarization is a complex electrical phenomenon. Precordial mapping of the repolarization forces can be performed,[5] but the complexity of the procedure has precluded its use in clinical medicine. With the advent of digital electrocardiographic recordings, accurate quantitation of various repolarization characteristics can now be accomplished. This report details our recent experience in the multidimensional quantitation of ventricular repolarization involving digitized 12-lead electrocardiographic recordings and 24-hour ambulatory Holter recordings.

METHOD

Population

The study population consisted of 423 normal individuals (200 females and 223 males) aged 10–81 years who had digitized 12-lead electrocardiographic recordings obtained on a MAC-12 recorder (Marquette Electronics, Inc.), and a separate population of 11 normal subjects who had 24-hour ambulatory electrocardiographic recordings obtained on a Marquette 8500 series recorder.

Data Acquisition and Processing

Data acquisition and processing for the 12-lead electrocardiogram have been previously reported.[6,7] In brief, digitized 12-lead electrocardiograms were recorded on

[a]Supported in part by research grant HL-33843 from the National Institutes of Health and by funds from Marquette Electronics, Inc. (Milwaukee, Wis.) and the Daisy-Marquis-Jones Foundation.

a MAC-12 system at a sampling frequency of 250 Hz. Lead specific median beats were processed and analyzed by a validated wave-detection computer algorithm which determines T-wave maximum, T-wave offset, and U-wave offset. The algorithm relates the time of occurrence of these repolarization waves to the earliest P-wave onset, earliest Q-wave onset, and latest S-wave offset in the 12-lead recording. For the 24-hour ambulatory electrocardiographic recording, a sampling frequency of 128 Hz per channel was utilized, and a validated wave-detection algorithm identified the peak of the R-wave and the maximum amplitude of the T-wave.

Repolarization Characteristics and Variables

For the 12-lead electrocardiogram, the repolarization characteristics and the corresponding variables included (1) early duration (SoTm, SoTmc) the S-wave offset (So) to T-wave maximum amplitude (Tm) interval (SoTm), and the Bazett heart rate corrected[1] early duration (SoTmc); (2) late duration (TmTo)—Tm to T-wave offset (To) interval; (3) area (Atot)—total absolute repolarization area from So to the end of the repolarization signal or to the next P-wave onset (whichever occurs first); and (4) late phenomena (% A@To)—% Atot accumulated at To. All variables were measured in lead V5. The QT interval (QT) and the Bazett heart rate corrected QT interval (QTc) were utilized as conventional reference variables.

For the 24-hour ambulatory electrocardiographic recording, the variables were (1) early repolarization (RTm)—the interval from the peak of the R-wave to the maximum amplitude of the T-wave; (2) heart rate cycle length (RR)—the interval between two consecutive R-waves in the beat preceding RTm. The regression of RTm on RR was obtained for all recorded heart beats on each of the normal subjects; only subjects with a correlation relationship $(r) \geq 0.69$ were included in the analysis. This criterion was utilized to eliminate patients with a large amount of nonphysiologic data that were verified as being artifacts. Ten of the 11 normal subjects met this criterion. The slope, RTm/RR, that provided the best fit to the RTm versus RR relationship was computed for each normal subject.

Statistical Analysis

Values of the selected variables in the two populations were summarized by standard descriptive statistics. Differences between mean values in gender subsets were tested for statistical significance by the T-test, allowing for multiple comparisons when assessing statistical significance.

RESULTS

12-Lead Electrocardiogram

TABLE 1 summarizes the distributions of the principle electrocardiographic variables among the total population and by gender. Females had faster heart rates, longer repolarization duration (SoTm) and smaller total repolarization area (Atot) than males did.

24-Hour Ambulatory Electrocardiogram

The pertinent findings relating to the relationship between ventricular repolarization duration and heart rate during the 24-hour ambulatory electrocardiographic recording are presented in TABLE 2. More than 77,000 beats were recorded and analyzed in each of the patients. Of note, a log transformation of the RR cycle length did not improve the fit of the regression between RTm and RR.

DISCUSSION

Multidimensional quantitation of ventricular repolarization is now easily obtained on digitized electrocardiographic recordings. The findings from the 12-lead electrocar-

TABLE 1. Static Ventricular Repolarization Characteristics from 12-Lead Digitized Electrocardiogram[a]

	Total Population ($n = 423$)	Male ($n = 223$)	Female ($n = 200$)	p Value[b]
Heart cycle				
RR mseconds	912 ± 142	948 ± 146	873 ± 126	<0.0001
Total duration				
QT mseconds	394 ± 29	397 ± 30	392 ± 27	NS
QTc mseconds$^{1/2}$	415 ± 17	409 ± 14	421 ± 18	<0.0001
Early duration				
SoTm mseconds	213 ± 27	205 ± 25	222 ± 26	<0.0001
SoTmc mseconds$^{1/2}$	224 ± 23	212 ± 18	238 ± 21	<0.0001
Late duration				
TmTo mseconds	113 ± 19	114 ± 16	112 ± 21	NS
Area				
A$_{tot}$ mv · mseconds	47 ± 22	54 ± 24	38 ± 15	<0.0001
Late phenomena				
% A@To percent	89 ± 6	89 ± 6	89 ± 7	NS

[a]Values are mean ± standard deviation (SD). See text for abbreviations. This table is derived from Tables 5 and 6 in the article by Merri *et al.*[7]
[b]p value comparing males with females.

diogram indicate that the interval from the R-wave to the maximum amplitude of the T-wave (RTm) contains the heart rate dependency of the ventricular repolarization duration. We were able to apply this information to the 24-hour Holter recording. It has always been difficult to identify the termination of the T-wave on the Holter recording accurately, and until now this has precluded the use of the Holter recording in evaluating ventricular repolarization duration. However, the R-wave and the maximum amplitude of the T-wave are easily identified by computer algorithm on digitized Holter recordings, and this information should be useful in the evaluation of patients with cardiac arrhythmias.

This approach to the quantitation of ventricular repolarization must be considered empiric. Ventricular electrical repolarization is a complex ionic process that is represented on the surface electrocardiogram as the ST-T-U complex. The relationship of

TABLE 2. Dynamic Ventricular Repolarization-Cycle Length Relationship from 24-Hour Digitized Ambulatory Electrocardiogram[a]

Subject	Number of Heartbeats	Correlation Coefficient RTm vs. RR	Slope RTm/RR
MA	85,322	0.75	0.11
PB	96,031	0.70	0.14
AD	100,678	0.89	0.18
AE	115,035	0.88	0.14
ZK	99,592	0.75	0.14
SAM	109,481	0.69	0.13
SVM	77,859	0.80	0.13
MO	95,355	0.76	0.12
AP	116,036	0.82	0.17
LS	77,313	0.82	0.17
Mean	97,270	0.79	0.14
±SD	13,972	0.07	0.02

[a]See text for abbreviations.

the surface electrocardiographic parameters to the complex repolarization process is inadequately understood, and we are reluctant to attach any specific electrophysiologic interpretations to the repolarization parameters that we have quantitated. Nevertheless, the findings presented in this study provide a descriptive normal data base that will be useful for evaluating disordered repolarization in a variety of known or suspected disorders. For example, preliminary data suggest a significant difference in several of the presented repolarization characteristics between normal subjects and patients with the Long QT Syndrome. Furthermore, the slope relationship between ventricular repolarization duration and heart rate on the 24-hour Holter recording (RTm/RR) appears to be significantly increased in patients with the Long QT Syndrome when compared to normal subjects,[8] a finding that indicates an exaggerated delay in repolarization at long RR cycle lengths in this disorder.

In conclusion, we believe that the multidimensional quantitation of static and dynamic ventricular repolarization characteristics conveys more morphologic information than the conventionally measured QT interval. These new quantified electrocardiographic characteristics should prove useful in the evaluation of patients with known abnormal repolarization.

REFERENCES

1. BAZETT, H. C. 1920. An analysis of time relations of electrocardiograms. Heart 7: 353–370.
2. ASHMAN, R. 1942. The normal duration of the QT interval. Am. Heart J. 23: 522–531.
3. AHNVE, S. 1985. Correction of the QT interval for heart rate. Am. Heart J. 109: 568–574.
4. HOFFMAN, B. F. & P. F. CRANEFIELD. 1960. Electrophysiology of the Heart. McGraw-Hill. New York, N.Y.
5. AMBROGGI, L., T. BERTONI, E. LOCATI, M. STRAMBA-BODIALE & P. SCHWARTZ. 1986. Mapping of the body surface potentials in patients with idophatic long QT syndrome. Circulation 74: 1334–1345.
6. MERRI, M., M. MERRI, J. BENHORIN, J. W. HALL, E. LOCATI & A. J. MOSS. 1988. Multidimensional quantitation of ventricular repolarization. In Proceedings of the Annual

International Conference of IEEE Engineering in Medicine and Biology Society, New Orleans, La., November 4–7. IEEE/EMBS Press.

7. MERRI, M., J. BENHORIN, M. ALBERTI, E. LOCATI & A. J. MOSS. 1989. Electrocardiographic quantitation of ventricular repolarization. Circulation **80**: 1301–1308.

8. MOSS, A. J., M. MERRI, M. MERRI, J. BENHORIN, E. CARLEEN, J. ROBINSON, E. LOCATI & P. J. SCHWARTZ. 1989. Relationship between ventricular repolarization duration and heart rate during 24-hour Holter ECG recordings: findings in normal and LQTS patients. Circulation **80**(2): 37.

Electrocardiographic Characteristics and Main Causes of Pseudoprimary T Wave Changes[a]

Significance of Concordant and Discordant T Waves in the Human and Other Animal Species

MAURICIO B. ROSENBAUM, HORACIO H. BLANCO,[b]
AND MARCELO V. ELIZARI[b]

Medical School
University of Buenos Aires
Buenos Aires, Argentina
[b]Division of Cardiology
Ramos Mejía Hospital
Buenos Aires, Argentina

For many years it has been dogmatically accepted that T wave changes are either primary or secondary in nature,[1,2] and that this simple classification covers all T wave abnormalities occurring in the human electrocardiogram (ECG).[3] However, we have recently reported the existence of abnormal T waves that do not fit into either of these two categories.[4-6] These abnormal T waves look like primary changes, but in contrast to the latter, do not imply any clinical abnormality per se. Because of this they were termed *pseudoprimary T wave changes*.[4] These changes are caused by a shift in ventricular activation and tend to persist long after the provoking cause has subsided. This has obvious diagnostic connotations, and serious mistakes may often result from inappropriate knowledge of the electrocardiographic characteristics and circumstances in which pseudoprimary T wave changes are likely to occur. Furthermore, the mechanism underlying such changes is of great biological interest, and can be considered as a new opening to a more comprehensive understanding of the T wave in general. These two aspects will be discussed separately.

THE ELECTROCARDIOGRAPHIC CHARACTERISTICS AND MAIN CAUSES OF PSEUDOPRIMARY T WAVE CHANGES

The "Postponed" Effects of Left Bundle Branch Block

The ECG in FIGURE 1 was recorded from a 50-year-old man during a checkup. The negative T waves in leads II, III, and V1 to V6 suggested a possible non–Q wave myocardial infarction and the patient was hospitalized. Various studies, including cardiac catheterization and coronary angiography, failed to show any abnormality, but a simple acceleration of the heart rate revealed that the abnormal T waves were related

[a]Supported in part by "Fundación de Investigaciones Cardiológicas Einthoven."

to a rate-dependent left bundle branch block (LBBB).[4,5] Why should LBBB result in the subsequent occurrence of grossly abnormal T waves? A first clue is apparent in FIGURE 2, which in each panel shows side by side a normally conducted beat and an LBBB beat. It is indeed remarkable that in each one of the 12 leads, the abnormal T waves (during normal conduction) show the same direction as that of the QRS complex during LBBB. In classical terms, the T waves are *concordant,* not with their own QRS but with the one determined by the LBBB.

This is even more striking in the vectorcardiograms (VCGs) shown in FIGURE 3. It is extremely unlikely that perfect concordance of the T waves such as the one illustrated

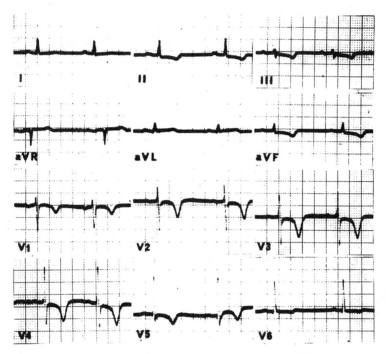

FIGURE 1. Pseudoprimary T wave changes (see text and FIGURES 2 and 3).

in FIGURES 2 and 3 should be fortuitous. In fact, a similar response was documented in over 85 cases of intermittent LBBB.[4] From these very simple electrocardiographic observations, it was clearly apparent that (a) a change in the sequence of ventricular activation such as the one induced by LBBB caused the *subsequent* occurrence of pseudoprimary T wave changes, the direction of which was concordant with the QRS forces of the LBBB; (b) the T wave changes persisted long after the LBBB had ceased to occur; and (c) these effects were masked *during* the LBBB because of predominance of the well-known secondary effects causing discordant T waves, and could only become manifest when normal conduction was restored. The latter may explain why for so many years these pseudoprimary T wave changes failed to be understood.

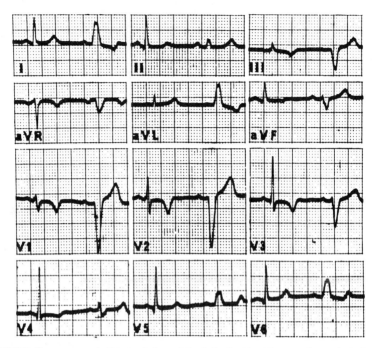

FIGURE 2. Same case as in FIGURE 1. In each lead, the first beat is normally conducted and the second shows LBBB. The T waves of the normally conducted beats are concordant with the QRS of the LBBB beats. (Reproduced from Reference 4, with permission.)

Effects of Right Ventricular Pacing

From our clinical studies it was also apparent that the magnitude of the T wave changes was proportional to the time during which the LBBB had been persistently present.[4,5] To obtain further insight into this relationship, it was necessary to define more accurately for how long the LBBB had been present, but this proved to be nearly impossible even with the help of repeated Holter recordings. To overcome this difficulty we decided to study the effects of right ventricular pacing (RVP), because (a) this procedure is accessible and easy to perform; (b) the induced activation sequence is similar to the one caused by LBBB; (c) the duration as well as the rate of pacing can be monitored; and (d) previous studies had shown that RVP does indeed provoke marked T wave changes.[7] The effects of RVP were shown to be similar in eight subjects with a normal heart and a normal ECG[4] and a representative example is illustrated in FIGURES 4 and 5. The upper panel in FIGURE 4 shows a normal ECG recorded before pacing; the lower panel shows the ECG obtained while pacing from the outflow tract of the right ventricle, resulting in an "LBBB pattern" with right axis deviation; and the middle panel shows the effects of 48 hours of continuous RVP. Deeply inverted T waves occurred in leads V1 to V4, and the overall direction of the T waves was concordant with that of the QRS of the paced beats. This response was not much different from the one previously observed in spontaneously occurring LBBB.

In the same study, the RVP was periodically interrupted (for about one minute) in order to record a nonpaced ECG. Thus, progression of the T wave changes could be

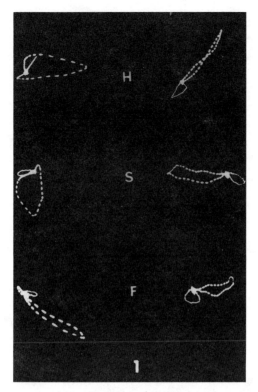

FIGURE 3. Vectocardiogram from the same patient. In each of the three planes, the T loop during normal conduction (left) and the QRS loop during LBBB (right) exhibit a similar direction. F, frontal plane; S, sagittal plane; H, horizontal plane. (Reproduced from reference 4, with permission.)

charted as a function of the pacing time, as illustrated in FIGURE 5. In the eight similar studies, the T wave changes were shown to progress gradually and uniformly during the first 30 to 60 hours of pacing, whereas regression took a much longer time, as also illustrated in FIGURE 5. In general, the greater the magnitude of the induced T wave changes, the longer was the time required for full dissipation of the effect. Faster rates of RVP induced T wave changes in relatively shorter times. In several studies, the first discernible changes were observed after 10 to 15 minutes of RVP, depending on the pacing rate.

Accumulation and Memory

We have shown that during continuous RVP (or LBBB) marked T wave changes develop in a gradually cumulative fashion. The fact that the response to a repeated but constant sequence of abnormal activation showed this gradual increment suggested to us the idea that the heart was in some way "learning" to react with greater intensity to the same perturbation.[4] To test this hypothesis, in two cases we performed *discontinu-*

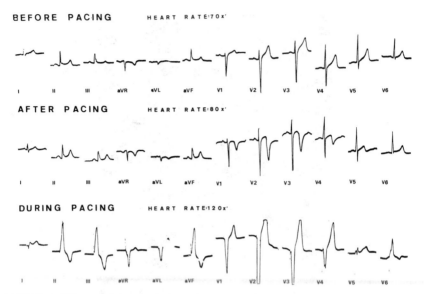

FIGURE 4. Effects of right ventricular pacing. Pacing from the outflow tract (bottom panel) induced a "left bundle branch block" pattern with right axis deviation. Postpacing T waves (middle panel) show a similar direction to that of the QRS complex of paced beats. (Reproduced from Reference 4, with permission.)

ous trains of pacing lasting 15 minutes each, separated by nonpacing intervals lasting as long as needed for the pacing-induced changes to revert to the control condition. In one of these studies in which 10 trains of RVP were administered (FIGURE 6), each successive train induced a greater change than the preceding trains, and the 10th train

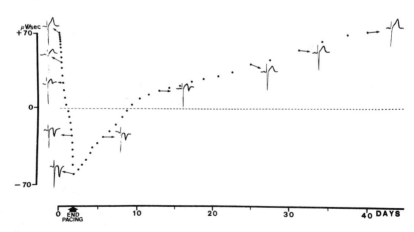

FIGURE 5. Same case as in FIGURE 4. Progression and regression of the T wave changes (lead V2) induced by right ventricular pacing. (Reproduced from Reference 4, with permission.)

caused in 15 minutes as much change as that seen in other cases after several hours of continuous RVP. Similar results were obtained in the second study. These results suggest that, after the provoking stimulus is discontinued and its effects are no longer apparent, the myocardial cells involved in this process seem to keep a memory of the previous effect, or to behave as though they had been conditioned by previous exposure to the same stimulus.

Clinical Implications

We have seen that the change in cardiac activation induced by LBBB or RVP causes pseudoprimary T wave changes which are concordant in direction with that of the abnormal QRS, and show accumulation and memory. It can equally be demon-

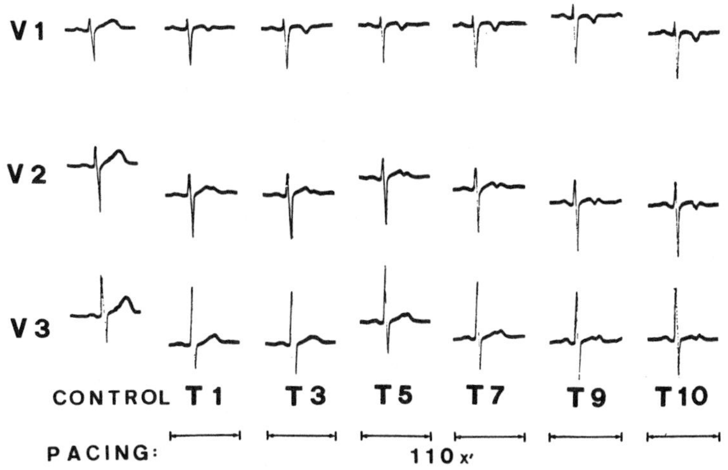

FIGURE 6. T wave changes induced by 10 discontinuous trains (T) of right ventricular pacing (see text). Only the effects of trains 1, 3, 5, 7, 9 and 10 are shown. Each pacing train induces a greater degree of change than the preceding trains. (Reproduced from Reference 4, with permission.)

strated that *any* shift in the spread of excitation will cause similar effects.[4] This has been shown to be the case for the abnormal T waves that occur in some cases of complete AV block with a wide QRS complex,[8] in single or combined forms of fascicular block,[4,5] in cases of ventricular preexcitation,[4,5] the so-called posttachycardia syndrome,[9-11] Gallavardin's tachycardia,[12,13] and some postextrasystolic T wave changes.[14-16] The following two examples are particularly instructive.

A 32-year-old man was referred to us with a history of recurrent paroxysmal tachycardia which was shown to be supraventricular in origin, with aberrant ventricular conduction. In all the episodes the aberrancy showed a pattern of right bundle branch block (RBBB) with left anterior hemiblock (LAH). The ECG recorded during one of these episodes is reproduced in panel A of FIGURE 7. The cardiac rate was 155 beats per minute, and the episode lasted 16 hours. Panel B shows the ECG recorded the next day. Inverted T waves can be seen in leads II, III, aVF, and V3 to V6, concordant in direction with that of the QRS complex during the tachycardia. ECGs recorded at daily intervals showed that the T wave changes reverted back to normal slowly and gradually in about 15 days (panel C). This sequence is illustrated for a single lead in panel D. All the episodes recorded from the same patient resulted in similar T wave changes, but the magnitude and persistence of the changes was proportional to the duration of the tachycardia. In this case, a sequence of ventricular activation entirely different from that seen in LBBB or RVP also resulted in grossly abnormal and concordant T waves, supporting the concept that any shift in the spread of excitation may cause pseudoprimary T wave changes.

A 30-year-old man was found to have frequent ventricular extrasystoles (VEs) and abnormal T waves. Several studies, including cardiac catheterization and coronary angiography failed to discover any abnormality. A 24-hour Holter recording showed frequent unifocal VEs and ventricular bigeminy was present most of the time. As shown in FIGURE 8A, the VEs exhibited a pattern of RBBB with LAH, and the abnormal T waves were concordant in direction with that of the QRS complex of the ectopic beats. This strongly suggests that the abnormal T waves were simply a consequence of the nearly continuous presence of the ventricular ectopy and not a manifestation of cardiac disease per se. In fact, when the VEs practically disappeared after four weeks of treatment with amiodarone, the T waves showed a strong tendency to normalization (FIGURE 8B), whereas discontinuance of amiodarone resulted in reappearance of both the VEs and the abnormal T waves, which were again suppressed by the prolonged administration of the same drug. In this case, the shift in the activation sequence causing pseudoprimary T wave changes was not continuously present (as in the case in FIGURE 7), but only in every other beat. This is consistent with the cumulative character of such changes.

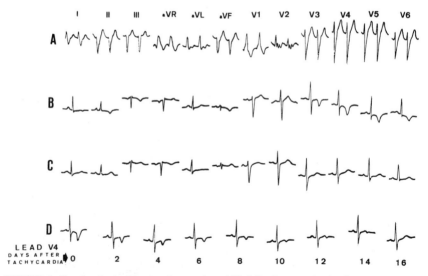

FIGURE 7. Pseudoprimary T wave changes (panel B) following an episode of supraventricular tachycardia with aberrant ventricular conduction showing a pattern of right bundle branch block with left anterior hemiblock (panel A). The abnormal T waves are concordant in direction with that of the QRS during the tachycardia. Regression of the T wave changes took about 15 days (panels C and D). See text for further details.

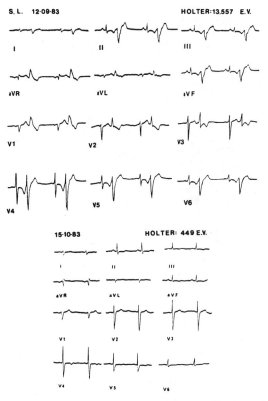

FIGURE 8. Pseudoprimary T wave changes caused by frequent unifocal ventricular extrasystoles showing a pattern of right bundle branch block with left anterior hemiblock (upper panel). The abnormal T waves are concordant in direction with that of the QRS of the ectopic beats. Treatment with amiodarone resulted in nearly complete disappearance of the extrasystoles and a strong tendency to normalization of the T waves (lower panel). See text for further details.

SIGNIFICANCE AND MECHANISM OF CONCORDANT VERSUS DISCORDANT T WAVES

Pseudoprimary T wave changes imply the existence of two new and apparently interrelated electrophysiologic manifestations: concordance with a previously abnormal QRS, and accumulation and memory. According to classical electrocardiographic theory,[2] T wave concordance means that ventricular repolarization proceeds in a general direction contrary to the spread of excitation, whereas T wave discordance indicates just the opposite. Keeping this concept in mind, it is worthwhile to ask ourselves which circumstances other than pseudoprimary changes also result in concordant (or discordant) T waves in the ECG of man and other animal species. For example, in the ECG recorded from a small armadillo (FIGURE 9), the T waves were perfectly concordant. In contrast, the T waves were discordant in the ECG of a large turtle (FIGURE 10). The ECG recorded from an iguana (also a cold-blooded animal)

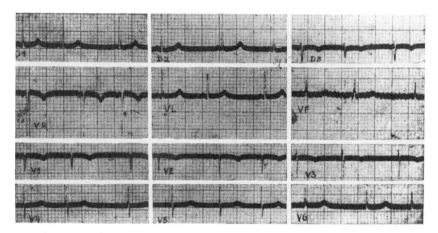

FIGURE 9. Twelve-lead ECG recorded from a small armadillo. Cardiac rate, 85–122/minute; P-R interval, 0.06 second; QRS interval, 0.03 second; Q-T interval, 0.26 second, ÂQRS, +20°; ÂT, +20°. T waves are perfectly concordant in direction (in each one of the 12 leads) with that of the QRS complex. (Reproduced from Reference 20, with permission.)

showed, however, concordant T waves (FIGURE 11), whereas the single bipolar lead recorded from a domestic fly revealed that the T wave was discordant (FIGURE 12). FIGURE 13 shows two VCGs recorded from a 40-year-old man without any evidence of cardiac disease but for the presence of unifocal VEs. The T waves were concordant during sinus beats (panel A) and discordant during the VEs (panel B). From this limited and selective sampling, it is clear that both concordant and discordant T waves may occur under "natural" conditions. Why and when one or the other?

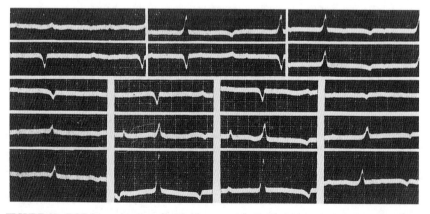

FIGURE 10. ECG from a large turtle. The first two rows: leads I, II, III, aVR, aVL, and aVF, at 1.5 cm/millivolt. Last three rows: various chest leads at different levels, at 1.0 cm/millivolt. Heart rate, 33/minute; P-R, 0.60 second; QRS, 0.14 second; Q-T, 1.00 second; ÂQRS, +90°; ÂT, −90°. The T waves are clearly discordant. (Reproduced from Reference 20, with permission.)

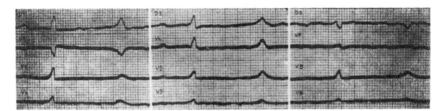

FIGURE 11. ECG from a medium-sized iguana. Limb leads, at 1.00 cm/millivolt; chest leads, at 0.50 cm/millivolt. Heart rate, 30/minute; P-R, 0.50 second; QRS, 0.12 second; Q-T, 1.20 seconds; ÂQRS, +15°; ÂT, +10°. The T waves are perfectly concordant. (From Reference 20, with permission.)

Discordant T Waves in the Human

It is well known that in the normal human ECG the T waves are essentially concordant, but can become discordant in a wide variety of circumstances. The extensive electrocardiographic experience of the last 50 years is probably the best collective source of information regarding the causes determining whether T waves will be concordant or discordant, or when one will change to the other as in the example in FIGURE 13. The following analysis is based on such experience, as reported in classical textbooks.[9,17-20]

Discordant T waves in the human are related to an increase of the ventricular mass being activated in the same direction and/or an increase in the conduction time. An increase of ventricular mass generally implies an increase in conduction time. On the other hand, processes that primarily prolong the conduction time, commonly imply an increase of the ventricular mass being activated in the same direction due to loss of cancellation effects.[19] Therefore, the effects of mass and conduction time cannot be entirely dissociated. In more specific terms, the main causes of discordant T waves are bundle branch block, ventricular preexcitation, VEs, ventricular tachycardia, idioventricular rhythms, supraventricular arrhythmias with aberrant ventricular conduction, and advanced right or left ventricular hypertrophy. In all these conditions, the QRS complex tends to grow both in duration and amplitude, and therefore in area. As a practical rule, it may be said that whenever the QRS interval measures 100 mseconds or more, and particularly if the amplitude is also increased, the T waves will be or tend to be discordant. In other words, if the mass of ventricular tissue and/or the conduction

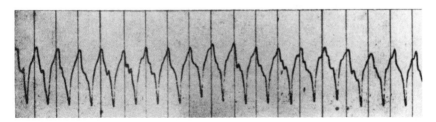

FIGURE 12. Bipolar (caudocraniale) lead recorded from a domestic fly, at 1.8 cm/millivolt. Rate: 480/minute. The T wave is discordant.

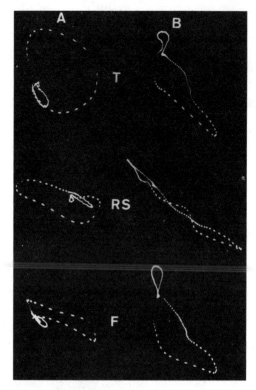

FIGURE 13. Vectocardiogram from a 40-year-old man. The T loop is essentially concordant with the QRS loop during a sinus beat (A), and grossly discordant during a ventricular extrasystole (B). T, transverse plane; RS, right sagittal plane; F, frontal plane.

time are increased beyond a given limit, the tendency for repolarization to proceed in the same direction as that of depolarization will predominate over any "local factor" that might otherwise dictate a different or even opposite direction.

Discordant T Waves in Other Animal Species

In most animal species the T waves are or tend to be discordant, from small insects with a tiny and simple cardiac tube, to the largest mammals with a huge and complex heart. It is beyond the scope of this paper to discuss the possible direction of the T wave in all animal species, and the following guidelines should only be considered as a preliminary approach to the problem. They are based on what we have learned from the causes of discordant T waves in the human, and from the records reported in the atlas published by Zuckerman in 1955,[20] in which the ECGs of some 80 different animal species were illustrated.

1. Whenever the QRS interval measures 100–120 mseconds or longer, the T waves are or tend to be discordant, as in the human. The difference is that in man this only occurs under abnormal conditions. A wide QRS complex may be observed

in (a) large mammals with big hearts. These big hearts are usually provided with a more widely distributed Purkinje network, which results in the QRS duration increasing less than would be expected from the large cardiac mass itself. But even so, the QRS interval commonly measures 100–120 mseconds or more; (b) cold-blooded animals, in which all ECG intervals are extremely long. The wide QRS results in part from a less developed or absent Purkinje network; (c) insects and arthropods, in which the QRS is wide due to the slow response type of tissue of which their hearts are composed. All these diversities of animals tend to show discordant T waves. There is no reason to think that the basic mechanism is different from the one causing discordant T waves in the human.

2. The T waves are or tend to be discordant whenever the Q-T interval is extremely short (150–200 mseconds or less). Under such conditions repolarization is so "fast" that it necessarily follows the same order of depolarization. A Q-T interval of 200 mseconds or less is observed in (a) Small mammals with high metabolic activity and very rapid heart rates (200–400 beats per minute); (b) birds, which in addition to having extremely rapid heart rates, exhibit a body temperature higher than all other species. It is interesting that at very rapid heart rates, the normally concordant T wave of the human ECG tends to become discordant.[9]

Concordant T Waves in the Human and Other Animal Species

In biological terms, concordant T waves are rather the exception than the rule, and appear to be restricted to a group of species, including man, in which the mass of ventricular tissue is not "exceedingly" large, the conduction time is below 100 mseconds, and the Q-T interval above 200 mseconds. The fact that the majority of animal species fail to show concordant T waves is not surprising. If T wave discordance means that repolarization proceeds in the same direction as that of the spread of excitation, this is the *natural* response to be expected. The apparently *unnatural* event is that repolarization should proceed in a diametrically opposite direction, resulting in T wave concordance. What causes the natural sequence of repolarization to be totally reversed? Many years ago this was taken as an indication that duration of the excited state was not uniform throughout the ventricular muscle,[2] and the most recent evidence seems to indicate that action potential duration is indeed shorter in subepicardial than in subendocardial layers of the ventricle.[21] The reason for this departure from uniformity in action potential duration is still under discussion, and is related in our view to what we call "directional differences in action potential duration."

Directional Differences in Action Potential Duration

The experiment illustrated in FIGURE 14 is representative of a series of unpublished studies from our laboratory. A subepicardial strip from the left ventricle of a cat was stimulated from one or the other end of the preparation, while a microelectrode impaled at one end recorded the transmembrane potential. Essentially the action potential duration was shown to shorten when stimulation was shifted from the proximal to the distal end of the strip (in relation to position of the microelectrode), and this process could be repeatedly reversed just by changing the direction of stimulation. These results strongly support the view that the mere spread of excitation in a given direction results in a prolongation of the action potential duration in fibers where the process begins, and in a shortening in fibers where the process terminates. Theoretically, it can be shown that this "deformation" of the action potential as it travels along a given pathway is the result of electrotonic interactions which occur during the process of repolarization, in such a way that a local circuit current set up during phases 2 and 3 flows as a depolarizing current "upstream" and as repolarizing current "downstream" with reference to the direction of conduction of the impulse. Evidence supporting the existence of this mechanism has previously been reported.[22,23]

It is interesting that several authors, independently, attributed various teleological advantages to the directional differences in action potential duration, long before they were directly demonstrated. According to Lepeschkin, a longer duration of the excited

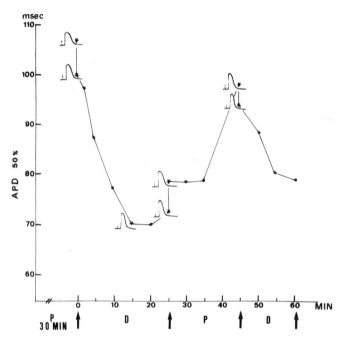

FIGURE 14. Action potential duration measured at 50% of maximal amplitude (APD), as related to the direction of stimulation from a proximal (P) or distal (D) stimulating site. The action potential duration is prolonged when activation moves away from the recording microelectrode, and is shortened when activation moves toward the recording site. Rate of stimulation was 120/minute. See text for further details.

state in subendocardial layers may serve the "purpose" of the papillary muscles remaining contracted longest of all other ventricular muscle in order to prevent the mitral and tricuspid valves from being inverted into the auricles.[9] According to Burgess *et al.,* the fact that areas activated early have the longest refractory periods while areas activated late have the shortest tends to make all portions of the ventricles complete recovery at about the same time and may play a protective role in the prevention of reentrant arrhythmias.[24] Similarly Cohen *et al.* suggest that "an important function of such a difference is that the longer action potential at early points in the conducting pathway may prevent reexcitation and reentry."[25] Whether or not these possible advantages are physiologically meaningful, the directional differences in action potential duration represent a general response of cardiac tissues, and probably of all excitable tissues in which repolarization lasts long enough for significant electrotonic interactions to occur during the process of impulse propagation.

The directional differences in action potential duration may serve to explain *both* the concordant T waves that normally occur in man and other animal species, and the concordant pseudoprimary T wave changes that occur after any shift in the activation sequence. It is remarkable that two such disparate events as the positive T waves of the normal human ECG and the grossly negative T waves that for example follow LBBB or RVP should share a common mechanism. This supports the idea that any sequence of ventricular activation, whether normal or abnormal, must necessarily result in a tendency to produce *its own* directional changes in action potential duration. In each case, direction of the waves will be different, but in all cases, the T waves will be concordant.

FUTURE DIRECTIONS

Many questions still remain unanswered, as shown by the following list: (1) Is the normally concordant T wave of the human ECG the result of a process showing accumulation and memory, as was shown to occur with the concordant pseudoprimary T wave changes? (2) What are the cellular bases of the directional changes in action potential duration? (3) What is the basic mechanism underlying the existence of a cardiac memory? (4) Is the effect of the electrotonic interactions causing a change in action potential duration a merely passive response of the cardiac tissue, or does it include an "active" and enduring change of membrane properties? (5) Which is the upper limit that a directional difference in action potential duration may attain, and how does it relate to the conduction time and to the "intrinsic" action potential duration? As in many other fields of science, small advances may multiply the number of problems that require further study.

REFERENCES

1. WILSON, F. N. & R. FINCH. 1923. The effect of drinking iced water upon the form of the T deflection of the electrocardiogram. Heart **10:** 275–278.
2. WILSON, F. N., A. G. MacLEOD & P. S. BARKER. 1931. The T deflection of the electrocardiogram. Trans. Assoc. Am. Physicians. **46:** 29–38.
3. SURAWICZ, B. 1972. The pathogenesis and clinical significance of primary T wave abnormalities. *In* Advances in Electrocardiography. R. C. Schlant & J. W. Hurst, Eds.: 377–421. Grune & Stratton. New York & London.
4. ROSENBAUM, M. B., H. H. BLANCO, M. V. ELIZARI, J. O. LAZZARI & J. M. DAVIDENKO. 1982. Electrotonic modulation of the T wave and cardiac memory. Am. J. Cardiol. **50:** 213–222.
5. ROSENBAUM, M. B., H. H. BLANCO, M. V. ELIZARI, J. O. LAZZARI & H. M. VETULLI. 1983. Electrotonic modulation of ventricular repolarization and cardiac memory. *In* Frontiers of Cardiac Electrophysiology. M. B. Rosenbaum & M. V. Elizari, Eds.: 67–99. Martinus Nijhoff Publishers. Boston & the Hague.
6. ROSENBAUM, M. B., S. J. SICOURI, J. M. DAVIDENKO & M. V. ELIZARI. 1985. Heart rate and electrotonic modulation of the T wave: a singular relationship. *In* Cardiac Electrophysiology and Arrhythmias. D. P. Zipes & J. Jalife, Eds.: 485–488. Grune & Stratton, Inc. Orlando, Fla.
7. CHATTERJEE, K., A. HARRIS, G. DAVIES & A. LEATHAM. 1969. Electrocardiographic changes subsequent to artificial ventricular depolarization. Br. Heart J. **31:** 770–779.

8. WARENBOURG, H., M. BAUCHANT, G. DUCLOUX, *et al.* 1969. Les troubles de repolarisation ventriculaire des blocks auriculo-ventriculaires complets. Les inversions "massives" de l'onde T. Arch. Mal. Coeur **62:** 1219–1240.

9. LEPESCHKIN, E. 1951. Modern Electrocardiography. Williams & Wilkins. Baltimore, Md.

10. COSSIO, P., R. VEDOYA & I. BERCONSKY. 1944. Modificaciones del electrocardiograma después de ciertas crisis de taquicardia paroxística. Rev. Arg. Cardiol **11:** 164–184.

11. KERNOHAN, R. J. 1944. Post-paroxysmal tachycardia syndrome. Br. Heart J. **31:** 1803–1806.

12. GALLAVARDIN, L. 1922. Extrasystolie ventriculaire a paroxysmes taquicardiques prolongés. Arch. Mal. Coeur **15:** 298–306.

13. PARKINSON, J. & C. PAPP. 1947. Repetitive paroxysmal tachycardia. Br. Heart J. **9:** 241–262.

14. LEVINE, H. D., B. LOWN & R. B. STREEPER. 1944. The clinical significance of post-extrasystolic T wave-changes. Circulation **6:** 538–548.

15. SCHERF, D. 1944. Alterations in the form of the T wave with changes in heart rate. Am. Heart J. **28:** 332–347.

16. JANSE, M. F., A. B. M. VAN DER STEEN, R. T. VAN DAM & D. DURRER. 1969. Refractory period of the dog's ventricular myocardium following sudden changes in frequency. Circ. Res. **24:** 251–262.

17. BARKER, J. M. 1952. The Unipolar Electrocardiogram. A Clinical Interpretation. Appleton-Century-Crofts, Inc. New York, N.Y.

18. GARDBERG, M. 1957. Clinical Electrocardiography. Interpretation on a Physiologic Basis. A Hoeber-Harper Book. New York, N.Y.

19. SCHAEFER, H. & H. G. HAAS. 1962. Electrocardiography. *In* Handbook of Physiology. Section 2. Circulation: 323–415. American Physiological Society. Washington, D.C.

20. ZUCKERMAN, R. 1955. Atlas der Elektrokardiographie. VEG Georg Thieme. Leipzig, GDR.

21. LITOVSKY, S. H. & C. ANTZELEVITCH. 1988. Transient outward current present in canine ventricular epicardium but not endocardium. Circ. Res. **62:** 116–126.

22. MENDEZ, C. & G. K. MOE. 1966. Some characteristics of transmembrane potentials of AV nodal cells during propagation of premature beats. Circ. Res. **19:** 993–1006.

23. CRANEFIELD, P. F., H. O. KLEIN & B. F. HOFFMAN. 1971. Conduction of the cardiac impulse. I. Delay, block, and one-way block in depressed Purkinje fibers. Circ. Res. **28:** 199–219.

24. BURGESS, M. J., L. S. GREEN, K. MILLAR, R. WYATT & J. A. ABILDSKOV. 1972. The sequence of normal ventricular recovery. Am. Heart J. **84:** 660–669.

25. COHEN, I., W. GILES & D. NOBLE. 1976. Cellular basis for the T wave of the electrocardiogram. Nature **262:** 657–661.

Electrocardiographic Diagnosis of Transient Myocardial Ischemia

Sensitivity, Specificity, and Practical Significance

ATTILIO MASERI, JUAN CARLOS KASKI, FILIPPO CREA,
AND LUIS ARAUJO

Cardiovascular Research Unit
Royal Postgraduate Medical School
Hammersmith Hospital
Ducane Road
London W12 ONN, United Kingdom

The electrocardiogram is by far the most widely available method of documenting objectively the presence of transient myocardial ischemia, whether occurring spontaneously or induced by effort and other provocative tests. However, to determine the ischemic or nonischemic nature of transient changes of ventricular repolarization is not always straightforward, particularly in the general population, as the interpretation of electrocardiographic (ECG) changes is heavily dependent on the pretest probability of the individual having ischemic heart disease.[1] Thus in general, unless the shear magnitude of the transient changes is obviously diagnostic, when the changes are not accompanied by angina pectoris, they are much more likely to represent myocardial ischemia in patients with known ischemic heart disease than in apparently healthy individuals.

In this presentation we will consider (a) the sensitivity and specificity of ECG changes for the diagnosis of transient myocardial ischemia in patients with known ischemic heart disease; (b) the possibility of improving the specificity and sensitivity of the ECG diagnosis of ischemia by more accurate or additional measurements; and (c) the practical significance of the ECG diagnosis of ischemia.

ASSESSMENT OF THE SENSITIVITY AND SPECIFICITY OF THE ECG DIAGNOSIS OF MYOCARDIAL ISCHEMIA

The specificity and sensitivity of the electrocardiogram have traditionally been assessed by comparison of the results of exercise stress testing with those of coronary arteriography. The use of coronary arteriography as gold standard is clearly inappropriate, as coronary stenoses may not cause myocardial ischemia if the collateral circulation is well developed and, conversely, ischemia may develop in the absence of stenoses.[2] Comparisons of ischemic changes on the ECG with other objective and independent markers of ischemia are more appropriate. Anginal pain is an additional, valuable element for the interpretation of ischemic ECG changes, but it usually develops late compared to the ECG changes, and is frequently absent altogether.

The major determinants of the sensitivity of ECG changes are reported in TABLE 1.

The sensitivity and specificity of the ECG to detect transient myocardial ischemia can be evaluated by:

1. Assessing the presence or absence of ST segment changes and the temporal

51

evolution of the ECG changes during episodes in which ischemia is independently documented.

2. Assessing the relationship between the distribution of ECG changes and the distribution of regional myocardial ischemia assessed by positron emission tomography (PET).

TEMPORAL ECG CHANGES DURING TRANSIENT ISCHEMIC EPISODES

Continuous hemodynamic and ECG monitoring in patients with frequent spontaneous ischemic episodes provides the opportunity to assess the sequence of ECG changes during objectively documented myocardial ischemia. We have analyzed the ECG lead showing the greatest ischemic changes at the very onset and during the waning phase of transient ischemic episodes of different severity in patients with variant angina.[2–5] The examples taken from these studies, reported in FIGURES 1–4, show the temporal changes of the ECG observed during continuous monitoring of left ventricular pressure, left ventricular dp/dt, and coronary sinus blood oxygen saturation. Such recordings provide typical illustrations of how variable the changes can be, even in the most affected lead, during the various phases of an ischemic episode documented by simultaneous transient increase of diastolic pressures and volumes, fall of the dp/dt, and drop of coronary sinus blood oxygen saturation.

At the onset of these objectively documented ischemic episodes and also during episodes of mild ischemia, the ischemic changes in the ECG are so minimal that it would seem rather adventurous to consider them indicative of myocardial ischemia in the absence of independent evidence of ischemia such as that provided by hemodynamic or coronary sinus blood oxygen saturation monitoring. These typical examples clearly suggest that episodes of spontaneous, transient myocardial ischemia, with or without pain, but severe enough to affect left ventricular function and coronary sinus blood oxygen saturation, can occur in the absence of, or with only minimal, ECG changes. Thus, if ischemic episodes are of very short duration, or if they are prolonged but not severe, the ECG changes of even the most affected lead may not be sufficiently pronounced to diagnose myocardial ischemia according to accepted criteria.

Another intriguing example of the lack of sensitivity of the ECG in detecting myocardial ischemia is provided by some patients with syndrome x.[6] FIGURE 5 shows an example of a patient with syndrome x who during exercise testing consistently developed angina and diagnostic ST segment depression. However, during pacing he developed his typical anginal pain with large, diagnostic reduction of coronary sinus oxygen saturation, in the absence of ECG changes on the lead with ischemic changes during the effort test.

In patients with chronic stable angina, the ECG can also fail to show "diagnostic" changes during the progressive development of effort-induced ischemia. This possibility is illustrated by the results of the exercise stress test in a patient with angiographically documented coronary atherosclerosis and severe angina (FIGURE 6). The ST segment changes observed in this patient at peak exercise are clearly diagnostic of ischemia. However, considering that ischemia develops gradually, it is most likely that

TABLE 1. Myocardial Ischemia: Sensitivity of ECG Changes

1. The severity, extension location of ischemia.
2. The position of the exploring electrodes.
3. The signal to noise ratio.
4. The presence of intraventricular conduction abnormalities.

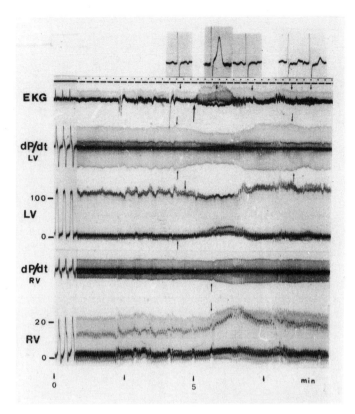

FIGURE 1. Continuous recording of the ECG, lead V5, left ventricular pressure (LV), right ventricular pressure (RV), and left and right ventricular dP/dt (dP/dt LV and dP/dt RV) in the coronary care unit (CCU). Two transient ischemic attacks occurred during the recording: one characterized by ST elevation, followed about two minutes later by one characterized by ST depression. Both are associated with obvious changes in diastolic LV pressure and dP/dt. The very different pattern of the ST and T wave changes on the ECG during the evolution of the two ischemic episodes compared to the resting morphology indicate the difficulties in establishing strict diagnostic criteria for a tracing taken at a single point in time, at the very beginning or end of the episodes. (Reproduced from Reference 3 with permission.)

the upsloping ST segment observed earlier was also ischemic in origin. Had the exercise test been terminated earlier, it would have failed to show "diagnostic ischemic changes" according to the standard criteria. On the other hand, if similar changes are to be considered diagnostic of ischemia, in order to increase the sensitivity of the test, its specificity would be greatly decreased, particularly in populations with low prevalence of myocardial ischemia.

ECG CHANGES DURING DIPYRIDAMOLE-INDUCED
MYOCARDIAL ISCHEMIA

In patients with obstructive coronary artery disease, dipyridamole is commonly believed to cause subendocardial ischemia in the myocardial territory distal to an

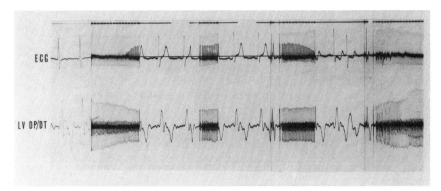

FIGURE 2. Continuous recording of the ECG lead V_4 and of left ventricular dP/dt in another patient during a spontaneous ischemic attack in CCU. Note the variability of the ischemic changes on the ECG during the episode, characterized by marked reduction of peak positive and negative LV dP/dt. (Reproduced from Reference 2 with permission.)

obstructed vessel due to coronary "steal." In 11 patients, each with a single coronary artery obstruction and no previous infarction, regional myocardial perfusion was assessed by whole heart PET in control condition and following the dipyridamole test. The 15 tomographic slices obtained and reconstructed tridimentionally provide a 3D

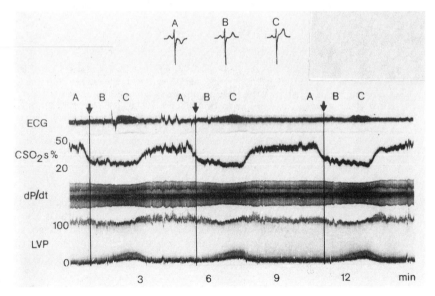

FIGURE 3. Three spontaneous ischemic episodes recorded in CCU. Top ECG, coronary sinus blood oxygen saturation (CSO_2), left ventricular pressure (LVP), and dP/dt. During each episode the ECG shows a gradual change from the resting pattern A to patterns B and C. It would be difficult to establish the ischemic nature of the ECG changes recorded only at the very beginning or end of each episode in the absence of independent evidence provided by the obvious, consistent changes in CSO_2 dP/dt, and LVP. (Reproduced from Reference 4 with permission.)

image of the heart cavities (labeled by an intravascular tracer—^{15}O carbon monoxide) and myocardial perfusion measured by ^{15}O water. In resting conditions myocardial blood flow was similar in both areas perfused by normal arteries and in those supplied by obstructed arteries, as all patients had normal ventricular function. Following dipyridamole, transmural flow in poststenotic areas increased only 30% of that in normal areas (coronary blood flow in normal areas increased 2.45 times the resting

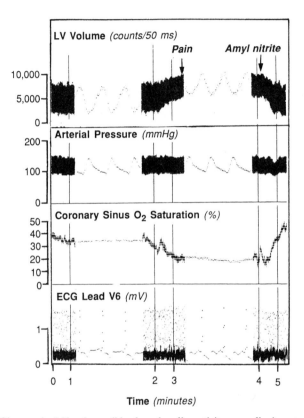

FIGURE 4. Changes in LV volume (blood pool radio activity recording), arterial pressure, coronary sinus O₂ saturation, and ECG during a spontaneous ischemic episode. The ST segment is already abnormal in the resting state and becomes only slightly more abnormal in spite of the severity of myocardial ischemia indicated by the doubling of end-systolic ventricular volume, halving of the ejection fraction and of coronary sinus oxygen saturation.

values whereas in poststenotic areas it increased only 1.38 times the resting values). On the basis of experimental studies it is likely that this small increase in flow in poststenotic areas is only an average value resulting from a large increase in subepicardial zones and a decrease of subendocardial zones,[7] which cannot be detected separately because of the limited spatial resolution of available PET technology. Following the dipyridamole test, 5 patients developed their typical anginal pain with diagnostic

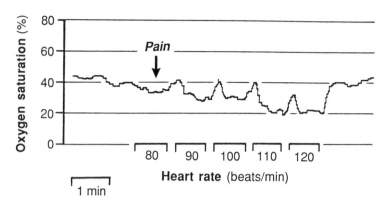

FIGURE 5. Monitoring of coronary sinus O_2 saturation during pacing in a patient with syndrome x. The marked progressive reduction of O_2 saturation with increasing heart rate is similar to that observed in patients with critical coronary stenosis and indicates severe myocardial ischemia. Yet the patient had no detectable ECG changes. (Reproduced from Reference 6 with permission.)

ST segment depression, 5 developed angina but no ECG changes, and 1 developed neither angina nor ECG changes. However, independently of the presence of ST segment changes, localized, intense uptake of ^{19}F deoxyglucose was observed in all patients in the area of myocardium distal to the obstructed coronary artery which exhibited only a small increase of average myocardial blood flow during the dipyridamole test. This enhanced regional myocardial uptake of glucose indicates that ischemia had actually developed during the test according to previous studies in patients with

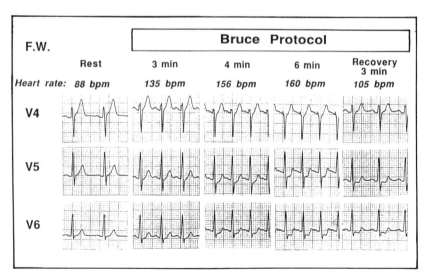

FIGURE 6. Result of ECG exercise stress testing in a patient with documented coronary atherosclerosis and severe angina. The test is clearly positive at end of exercise, but the ascending ST-segment depression in the middle period is also likely to represent ischemia.

chronic stable angina. Therefore, dipyridamole-induced ischemia, severe enough to cause anginal pain and postischemic myocardial glucose uptake, can occur in the absence of any detectable ECG changes.

SPECIFICITY OF ECG CHANGES

We have seen that the ECG can fail to show ischemic changes in the presence of objective evidence of myocardial ischemia caused by epicardial coronary spasm, small vessel disease, and obstructive coronary artery disease, even when ischemia is severe enough to cause major impairment of global left ventricular function, a large drop of coronary sinus blood oxygen saturation, and obvious changes in regional myocardial metabolism.

The specificity of ischemic ECG changes is more difficult to assess than their sensitivity because it requires the application of extremely sensitive independent techniques capable of objectively detecting ischemia in large numbers of individuals, under different conditions. The specificity of the ECG changes during exercise testing is usually reported to be about 80%. However, it is worth noting that this figure expresses the incidence of false positives, on the assumption that the true positives are patients with coronary atherosclerosis. It is not yet known how many of these false positives are "true" false positives or, rather, patients with myocardial ischemia and normal coronary arteries.

The specificity of transient ischemic changes during Holter monitoring was investigated in our institution in 100 asymptomatic subjects. By defining transient ischemic changes as transient episodes of at least 1 mm ST segment depression, lasting at least 1 minute, with gradual onset and termination, only 1 subject resulted to be positive. However, the observation that patients with syndrome x can have transient episodes of ST segment depression[8] indistinguishable from those in patients with coronary atherosclerosis[9] highlights the fact that the specificity of ECG changes has to be established not on the basis of the presence of coronary atherosclerosis, but on the basis of the objective documentation of myocardial ischemia, frequently difficult to achieve.

HOW TO IMPROVE THE SENSITIVITY AND SPECIFICITY OF THE ECG FOR THE DETECTION OF TRANSIENT MYOCARDIAL ISCHEMIA

Attempts have been made to improve the sensitivity of the ECG for the diagnosis of myocardial ischemia. It has been observed that an increase of the R and S wave voltages frequently precedes or accompanies the alterations of the ST segments.[10,11] However, these changes are unlikely to provide further diagnostic information compared to ST segment changes. It has also been suggested that the presence of an inverted U wave after exercise can be a clue to ischemia.[12] However, this is not a frequent finding and, furthermore, cardiac hypertrophy rather than myocardial ischemia appears to be a far more frequent cause of inverted U waves than angina.[13] The measurement of the QX/QT ratio has also been found to be a weak predictor of coronary artery disease.[14]

An increase in septal Q waves (when present) has been observed in normals during exercise. A lack of this response in subjects with ST segment depression has been proposed as a good indicator of transient anterior myocardial ischemia.[15]

More recently, Okin *et al.*[16] have quantified observations made by Bruce *et al.*[17] more than 20 years ago, and provided evidence that certain recovery phase patterns of

ST segment depression can markedly enhance the accuracy of the exercise electrocardiogram for the identification of coronary artery disease. Hollenberg *et al.* have
proposed a score based on the integral of the ST shifts (assessed in two leads) during
exercise test and 10 minute recovery and on exercise duration and peak heart rate.[18]
The difficulty of these studies lies in the selection of the gold standard of myocardial
ischemia. Indeed, the simple utilization of the coronary anatomy to this end can be, as
previously discussed, rather misleading.

While it is likely that more accurate, objective measurements of the ST-T wave,
their temporal relationship and correlation with QRS changes could provide diagnostic
criteria with greater sensitivity, this seems difficult to achieve without decreasing their
specificity. This is suggested by the fundamental observation that even major ischemic
changes in global ventricular function can be associated with only minor or no
detectable changes on the ECG.

THE PRACTICAL SIGNIFICANCE OF THE ECG IN THE
ASSESSMENT OF MYOCARDIAL ISCHEMIA

Short of absolute ECG criteria to detect transient myocardial ischemia, it is useful
first to consider when an accurate diagnosis of ischemia is essential for therapeutic
and/or prognostic reasons, second to establish whether or not currently used ECG
criteria are adequate for the diagnosis and for risk stratification of myocardial
ischemia.

Diagnostic "uncertainties" can be more easily tolerated when the diagnosis of
myocardial ischemia does not carry immediate vital therapeutic or prognostic implications. Conversely, diagnostic uncertainties are not acceptable when a prompt diagnosis
is important in order to make life-saving therapeutical decisions.

Ischemic episodes severe enough to cause acute left ventricular failure, necrosis, or
arrhythmias strongly influence short-term prognosis. Such episodes are very unlikely to
be unaccompanied by currently accepted diagnostic ECG changes. In these cases, the
ECG is a simple and efficient tool that allows us to both establish the diagnosis of
ischemia and monitor its treatment. However, even when ischemic episodes are not
severe enough to threaten by themselves the patient's life, they may have a prognostic
significance.

If long-term prognosis is the major concern, which is usually the case in patients
with ischemic heart disease, because of the possible unpredictable occurrence of
infarction and sudden death, then the prognostic significance of ischemic episodes
should be assessed. The significance of ischemic episodes for long-term prognosis is
extremely variable depending on (a) the cause of ischemia; (b) the severity of a
preexisting impairment of left ventricular function; and (c) the severity of coronary
atherosclerosis.

At one extreme of the spectrum, patients with syndrome x appear to have normal
life expectancy.[19] In this case acute myocardial ischemia requires treatment only
because it produces unpleasant symptoms. Their disappearance, either spontaneous, or
as a result of rational or even empirical treatment, would completely solve the patient's
problem.

At the other extreme of the spectrum, patients with unstable angina have the worst
prognosis.[20] In these patients ischemic episodes can not only be inherently dangerous
because of their extension and severity, but may also represent a marker of an acute
evolutive tendency of coronary lesions. The latter need not necessarily be represented
by severe stenoses. In between these two extremes, patients with stable ischemic
episodes (with or without angina), no previous infarction, normal ventricular function,
and good effort tolerance have a fairly good prognosis.

In totally asymptomatic individuals, the risk of infarction or death is largely determined by the presence of risk factors. The MRFIT study demonstrated that about 12% of the 12,500 individuals who are in the upper 10% of the risk stratification (out of a total of 361,000 individuals screened) had a positive exercise test according to standard criteria (but no angina).[21] In this study a positive test was associated with a threefold increase in cardiovascular mortality (54 deaths in seven years per 1000 individuals versus 15 in individuals with negative test). It is of great interest to note that no excess mortality was observed in the group with positive exercise test randomized to special risk reduction intervention but without specific antiischemic treatment. More specific criteria for detecting the severity of ischemia such as the degree of the ST segment depression and the duration of exercise testing might have increased the prognostic information of the test. Conversely, the adoption of more sensitive criteria for the detection of ischemia would have reduced its prognostic discriminatory power.

In asymptomatic individuals a normal or uncertain maximal effort test does not rule out the presence of coronary atherosclerotic disease or even obstruction. It only indicates that they are not severe enough to cause diagnostic ECG signs according to current criteria even at maximal workload. In these individuals ambulatory ECG monitoring is also most likely to be negative.

In individuals with known ischemic heart disease and stable angina, the prognosis is strongly dependent on information not derived from the ECG; however, some results of the CASS study seem to indicate that the response to exercise testing appears to carry important additional prognostic information.[22] In fact, this study showed that patients with a positive exercise test—with or without angina—had a worse prognosis than those with a negative test. The study also showed that an improved survival rate after surgical treatment was present in patients who, prior to surgery, could exercise for less than 6 minutes on the Standard Bruce Protocol, but not in patients who could exercise longer than 6 minutes, irrespective of the results of the test.

These findings indicate that coupling of commonly accepted ECG criteria with quantitative data, like exercise duration, heart rate, and heart rate–blood pressure product at the onset of ischemia, as indicators of residual coronary flow reserve, could provide additional valuable prognostic information.

CONCLUSIONS

Electrocardiographic changes, as currently assessed, are not always sensitive markers of ischemia. It might be possible to improve the sensitivity of ECG changes in order to detect ischemia, but it remains to be established whether this can be achieved without reducing diagnostic specificity. From the practical point of view, currently available criteria are sufficiently reliable to detect myocardial ischemia that represents an immediate risk for the patient because of its severity. For the long-term prognosis, it is essential to interpret the results of ECG stress testing together with the global, clinical information available, as myocardial infarction can often develop as a result of occlusion of coronary arteries without critical stenoses as documented by a series of recent studies.

REFERENCES

1. DIAMOND, G. A. & J. S. FORRESTER. 1979. Analysis of probability as an aid in the clinical diagnosis of coronary artery disease. N. Engl. J. Med. **300:** 1350–1358.
2. MASERI, A. & S. CHIERCHIA. 1982. Coronary artery spasm: demonstration, definition, diagnosis and consequences. Prog. Cardiovasc. Dis. **25:** 169–192.

3. MASERI, A., R. MIMMO, S. CHIERCHIA, C. MARCHESHI, A. PESOLA & A. L'ABBATE. 1975. Coronary spasm as a cause of acute myocardial ischemia in man. Chest **68:** 625–629.
4. CHIERCHIA, S., C. BRUNELLI, I. SIMONETTI, M. LAZZARI & A. MASERI. 1980. Sequence of events in angina at rest: primary reduction in coronary flow. Circulation **61:** 759–768.
5. DAVIES, G. J., W. BENCIVELLI, G. FRAGASSO, S. CHIERCHIA, F. CREA, J. CROW, P. CREAN, T. PRATT, M. MORGAN & A. MASERI. 1988. Sequence and magnitude of ventricular volume changes in painful and painless myocardial ischemia. Circulation **78:** 310–319.
6. CRAKE, T., R. CANEPA-ANSON, L. SHAPIRO & P. A. POOLE-WILSON. 1988. Continuous recording of coronary sinus oxygen saturation during atrial pacing in patients with coronary artery disease or with syndrome x. Br. Heart J. **59:** 31–38.
7. GOULD, K. L., R. K. WESTCOTT, P. C. ALBRO & G. W. HAMILTON. 1978. Noninvasive assessment of coronary stenosis by myocardial imaging during pharmacologic coronary vasodilation. II. Clinical methodology and feasibility. Am. J. Cardiol. **41:** 279–287.
8. KASKI, J. C., F. CREA, P. NIHOYANNOPOULOS, D. HACKETT & A. MASERI. 1986. Transient myocardial ischemia during daily life in patients with syndrome x. Am. J. Cardiol. **58:** 1242–1247.
9. DEANFIELD, J. E., A. P. SELWYN, S. CHIERCHIA, A. MASERI, P. RIBEIRO, S. KRIKLER & M. MORGAN. 1983. Myocardial ischaemia during daily life in patients with stable angina: its relation to symptoms and heart rate changes. Lancet **2:** 753–758.
10. DE CAPRIO, L., S. BUOMO & P. BELLOTTI. 1980. R wave amplitude changes during stress testing: comparison with ST segment depression and angiographic correlation. Am. Heart J. **99:** 413–418.
11. GALLINO, A., S. CHIERCHIA, G. SMITH, M. CROOM, M. MORGAN, C. MARCHESI & A. MASERI. 1984. Computer system for analysis of ST segment changes on 24 hour Holter monitor tapes: comparison with other available systems. J. Am. Coll. Cardiol. **4(2):** 245–252.
12. FARIS, S. V., P. L. MCHENRY & S. N. MORRIS. 1978. Concepts and applications of treadmill exercise testing and the exercise electrocardiogram. Am. Heart. J. **95:** 102–107.
13. KISHIDA, H., J. S. COLE & B. SURAWICZ. 1982. Negative U wave: a highly specific but poorly understood sign of heart disease. Am. J. Cardiol. **49:** 2030–2036.
14. ROMAN, L. & S. BELLET. 1965. Significance of the QX/QT ratio and the QT ratio (QTr) in the exercise electrocardiogram. Circulation **32:** 435–440.
15. FAMULARO, M. A., Y. PALIUAL & R. REDD. 1983. Identification septal ischemia during exercise by Q wave analysis: correlation with coronary angiography. Am. J. Cardiol. **51:** 440–443.
16. OKIN, P. M., O. AMEISEN & P. KLIGFIELD. 1989. Recovery-phase patterns of ST segment depression in the heart rate domain. Circulation **80:** 533–537.
17. BRUCE, R. A. & J. R. MCDONOUGH. 1969. Stress testing in screening for cardiovascular disease. Bull. N.Y. Acad. Med. **45:** 1288–1301.
18. HOLLENBERG, M., R. BUDGE, J. A. WISNESKI & E. W. GERTZ. 1980. Treadmill score quantifies electrocardiographic response to exercise and improves test accuracy and reproducibility. Circulation **61:** 276–285.
19. PUPITA, G., J. C. KASKI, A. R. GALASSI, M. J. VEJAR, F. CREA & A. MASERI. 1989. Long-term variability of angina pectoris and electrocardiographic signs of ischemia in syndrome x. Am. J. Cardiol. **64:** 139–143.
20. GAZES, P. C., E. M. MOBLEY, M. H. FARIS, JR., R. C. DUNCAN & G. B. HUMPHRIES. 1973. Preinfarctional (unstable) angina: a prospective study. Ten-year follow-up. Circulation **48:** 331–336.
21. Multiple Risk Factor Intervention Trial Research Group. 1982. Multiple risk factor intervention trial. Risk factor changes and mortality results. J. Am. Med. Assoc. **248:** 1465–1474.
22. WEINER, D. A., T. J. RYAN, C. H. MCCABE, S. LUK, B. R. CHAITMAN, T. SHEFFIELD, F. TRISTANI & L. D. FISHER. 1987. Significance of silent myocardial ischemia during exercise testing in patients with coronary artery disease. Am. J. Cardiol. **59:** 725–729.

Echocardiography as an Aid in Understanding the Electrocardiographic Changes of Left Ventricular Hypertrophy, Ischemia, and Infarction[a]

JAMES L. WEISS

Cardiology Division
Department of Medicine
The Johns Hopkins
Medical Institutions
Baltimore, Maryland 21205

INTRODUCTION

This review will focus upon two subjects in which quantitative echocardiography has been particularly useful as a noninvasive technique in the understanding of left ventricular size, shape, and function. First, we will address the ability of echocardiography to determine left ventricular mass in an accurate fashion. Second, we will address the issue of the ability of the echocardiogram to assess regional myocardial function, and the limitations of echocardiography, particularly as regards infarct sizing.

ECHOCARDIOGRAPHY AND THE DETERMINATION OF LEFT VENTRICULAR MASS

Accurate noninvasive determination of left ventricular (LV) volume and mass is important to the evaluation and management of a variety of cardiovascular disorders. The introduction of echocardiography opened the possibility of repeated noninvasive measurements of volume and mass.[1-4] Important advances in noninvasive determination of LV mass were made years ago with M-mode echocardiographic studies. The seminal work of Reichek and Devereux[5,6] provided critical methodology for determining LV mass noninvasively (they termed this the "Penn" convention). These methods were found to be relatively accurate in humans when compared to necropsy studies. But the geometric assumptions required for M-mode methods introduced the potential for broad variability in mass determination and the possibility of significant error.

Two-dimensional echocardiographic techniques require fewer geometric assumptions and are potentially considerably more accurate than M-mode techniques.[7] Using standard two-dimensional (2D) echo cross-sectional views, in the absence of precise localization of each view, several investigators have reported increased accuracy in mass determination using multiple cross-sectional short axis views[8] or a combination of

[a]Supported in part by National Heart, Lung and Blood Institute, Ischemic Heart Disease SCOR grant 2P50-HL-17655-14, and RO1-HL-33385

one short axis and one long axis or longitudinal dimension.[7] Particularly useful and favored because of its simplicity is the oft-used "bullet" formula for left ventricular mass or volume determination (5/6th area × length). Such studies use 2D echo algorithms for mass calculation based on the subtraction of endocardial cavity volume from total epicardial volume, resulting in a residual myocardial volume. Schiller and colleagues have reported a method for accurate estimation in LV mass in dogs using a truncated ellipsoid model and report constancy of mass between end-diastole and end-systole.[9] Although these techniques are all more accurate than M-mode echocardiographic techniques, they may be hampered by even the more limited geometric assumptions employed by the 2D methods when ventricular shape is deformed or the architecture is irregular, as it may be in various disease states, including infarction, left ventricular aneurysm, or certain congenital malformations.

THREE-DIMENSIONAL RECONSTRUCTION OF 2D ECHOCARDIOGRAMS

Accurate determination of volume or mass in intact animals and in patients using multiple parallel views, a method that would eliminate the need for major geometric assumptions, would be impractical owing to the high probability of being unable to obtain such views. On the other hand, fewer views would introduce the requirement of major geometric assumptions for echocardiographic mass determination, most of which have uncertain validity in dysfunctional or misshaped hearts. In order to determine mass accurately in hearts with regional myocardial dysfunction, especially in intact patients, techniques need to be developed that would allow free angulation of the echocardiographic transducer with continuous recordings of the three-dimensional (3D) coordinates of each image without imposing restraints on transducer orientation. This step awaited development of a system for locating the position of the echo transducer, fixing the spatial registration of the echo image at any instant, and synchronizing the transducer location data with the echocardiographic data stored on videotape. We developed a transducer locating system for determining LV volume and mass with high degree of accuracy, but few assumptions of geometry.[10,11] This system consists of a series of spark gaps affixed to the echo transducer, a series of fixed microphones that receive the spark gap sonic signals, and digital electronics designed to convert the sonic signals into specific range data that give the 3D coordinates, in both position and angle, of the transducer in free 3D space. Individual echocardiographic contours for 3D reconstruction are generated using a computer-aided contouring system developed in our laboratory.[12] We have recently validated 3D reconstruction techniques in cardiac transplant patients, from echocardiographic studies taken prior to transplantation *in vivo*.[11] Preliminary data suggest that this method is extremely accurate for LV mass determination when compared to directly measured *ex vivo* LV weight: mean error for 3D echocardiographic LV mass determination is about 2.5 ± 6% standard deviation (SD). It should be noted that the explanted hearts that formed the basis for this study were all severely deformed, and it would be anticipated that LV mass determination using standard geometric assumptions, such as the "bullet" formula, would have limited applicability. In fact, the error introduced by applying such assumptions was severalfold greater than that encountered with the three-dimensional reconstruction technique using multiple (15–20) randomly oriented views. Thus, one important aspect of these data is the ability to obtain accurate indices even in the presence of major disturbances in ventricular architecture. If further validation studies on a larger patient population confirm the preliminary accuracy level, the method holds promise for highly accurate noninvasive estimation of LV mass, which could serve as a standard for comparison to other techniques. One drawback in the three-dimensional reconstruction technique is the cumbersome nature of this approach. At present, there are no commercially available systems that utilize such technology, and LV mass determination using this method is currently a laborious process, for both image acquisition, which requires multiple views, and image contouring, which is highly labor intensive. If these disadvantages could be eliminated, the method could have wide applicability.

ECHOCARDIOGRAPHIC REGIONAL CONTRACTION ABNORMALITIES FOR ESTIMATION OF INFARCT SIZE

Two-dimensional echocardiography is proven to be valuable in the identification of the functional and structural changes caused by myocardial infarction and its complications. One potential major utility has been the possibility of infarct size estimation by the extent of dysfunction, measured as either endocardial wall motion abnormalities or impaired segmental ability to thicken during systole. However, intrinsic characteristics of ultrasound technology, the dynamic nature of the beating heart, and the complex relationship between regional infarction and myocardial function have limited the usefulness of this technique in the accurate quantification of size and transmurality of infarction in man. This review addresses the assessment of regional myocardial function by echocardiography and its limitations, particularly as regards infarct sizing.

The advent of two-dimensional echocardiography was followed by repeated efforts to quantify infarct size experimentally, and, despite the technical difficulties and challenges intrinsic to such investigations, several studies have produced useful information on myocardial function during ischemic injury or infarction. Some years ago, we studied regional myocardial function with two-dimensional echocardiography in the dog 10 days after myocardial infarction.[13] Cross-sectional echocardiographic images were obtained at each centimeter along the long axis of the ventricle after thoracotomy. The images were quantified with the aid of a computer assisted contouring system, the extent of dysfunction compared with the extent of infarction determined by histology. Two indices of systolic myocardial function were studied: regional percentage of radial endocardial motion towards a centroid fixed at end-diastole, and percent systolic thickening obtained at 16 equidistant points around the endocardial cavity area. In this model, both motion and thickening were able to separate infarcted from noninfarcted myocardium distant from the ischemic border. Thickening, however, proved to be significantly better than wall motion in discriminating infarcted from noninfarcted zones. Indeed, the center of the infarcted region thinned during systole, whereas by contrast myocardium located remote from the ischemic border maintained preserved thickening. Significantly greater overlap of infarcted and noninfarcted myocardium was seen when wall motion was used as an index of myocardial function, compared to thickening. But it was in the noninfarcted zones adjacent to infarction that both echocardiographic wall motion and thickening provided confounding results. These zones showed intermediate levels of performance, regardless of the index used. Such a phenomenon had been identified previously with M-mode echocardiography[14] and epicardial strain gauges[15] during ischemia, and has been confirmed in several other studies utilizing both echocardiography and sonomicrometry.[16–22] Although the correlation between echocardiographic dysfunction, particularly dyskinesis, and necrosis in the canine model has been found to be good by several investigators, some degree of overestimation has consistently been present.[20,22]

As a first approximation to infarct sizing, our study addressed accuracy of percentage systolic thickening in determining the extent of transmural involvement in the infarct.[13] This study showed that even a small degree of transmural involvement resulted in an abrupt deterioration of systolic thickening. Further, segments containing greater than 20% transmural extent of infarction thinned during systole. Moreover, as the extent of transmural damage increased, there was no greater increase in the magnitude of systolic thinning. This "threshold phenomenon" thus precludes accurate determination of the degree of infarct transmurality by two-dimensional echocardiography.

The fact that the presence of *any* systolic thickening indicates less than 20% transmural extent of infarction does, however, have important implications; if systolic thickening *excludes* significant transmural infarction, echocardiography can potentially identify noninfarcted muscle, or muscle capable of "salvage."

The overestimation of infarction by regional dysfunction has received a great deal of attention in recent years. The quantification of infarct size in humans by techniques that measure myocardial dysfunction noninvasively is hampered by the difficulty in measuring myocardial necrosis and regional myocardial blood flow noninvasively in a reliable and reproducible way. One means of addressing this issue is by comparing echocardiographically determined dysfunction with necrosis pathologically at autopsy. While the temporal and technical limitations are clear, such studies have added to our understanding of the interplay between dysfunction and infarction in man. In one study, the relationship between wall motion abnormalities by echocardiography and morphologic evidence of infarction was evaluated in 20 autopsied patients.[23] Wall motion abnormalities were assessed by visual analysis using a scoring system to grade the degree of dysfunction. These were compared on a segment-by-segment basis with postmortem pathological results. In essence, it was found that while wall motion abnormalities were present in the vast majority of pathologically infarcted segments, infarct extent was overestimated in that almost half of morphologically normal segments also demonstrated wall motion abnormalities. Most of these segments were directly adjacent to scar. While all transmurally infarcted segments were seen to be akinetic or dyskinetic, the motion of subendocardially infarcted segments was unpredictable. However, and most importantly, normal wall motion excluded transmural infarction. This study also sought to compare the circumferential extent of wall motion abnormalities with the circumferential extent of transmural infarction. Here, the correlation between percentage of left ventricular circumference demonstrating morphologic infarction and the percentage of end-diastolic circumference showing regional akinesis or dyskinesis was excellent; but wall motion abnormalities tended to exceed the amount of myocardial circumference involved by injury by about 14%. Other studies comparing echocardiographic dysfunction with necrosis at autopsy have shown similar infarct overestimation.[24] In summary, regional myocardial function in the presence of transmural infarction is markedly depressed at the center of the infarcted area, and preserved or even increased in regions located distant from the injured segments of the left ventricular wall. Variable but consistent overestimation of infarct size by wall motion abnormalities has been reported repeatedly for both experimental and human studies, even when dyskinesis or systolic thinning are used as a *sine qua non* criterion for dysfunction. The absence of a predictable or, in some cases, even reliable relationship between either the extent of infarction and dysfunction indicates that echocardiography is imprecise in sizing myocardial infarction by the extent or degree of wall motion abnormalities.

The clinical application of infarct size quantification by echocardiography is further confounded by the common clinical practice of therapeutic reperfusion. In that setting, stunned myocardium cannot be distinguished readily from ischemic, infarcted, or even merely overloaded left ventricular segments, rendering the correlation between systolic dysfunction and infarct mass even more complex and unreliable. True distinction between infarcted and contiguous uninfarcted myocardium will in all likelihood ultimately require methods independent of regional wall motion as an index of the extent of transmural injury. What is still clear, and most encouraging about the use of echocardiography as a standard for comparison to other techniques (such as electrocardiography), is that while it is not possible to determine the exact size of a myocardial infarction by echocardiography, it is possible to determine its location, the approximate degree of its extent, and most importantly, to exclude transmural infarction by virtue of normal wall motion. A normal echocardiogram thus eliminates or greatly minimizes the possibility of a transmural infarction. A schema[25] for relating echocardiographic wall motion abnormalities with the presence and transmurality of myocardial infarction would be as follows: (1) Although akinesis usually means transmural infarction, a significant percentage of akinetic segments is not transmurally infarcted, some segments being histologically normal. (2) Hypokinesis cannot distinguish infarcted from noninfarcted tissue. (3) Normal wall motion excludes transmural infarction. This schema should provide useful information when comparing echocardiographic with electrocardiographic data in the evaluation of ischemic heart disease.

REFERENCES

1. TEICHOLZ, L. E., T. KREULEN, M. F. HERMAN & R. GORLIN. 1976. Problems in echocardiographic volume determinations: echocardiographic-angiographic correlations in the presence or absence of asynergy. Am. J. Cardiol. 37: 7–11.
2. LINHART, J. W., G. S. MINTZ, B. L. SEGAL, N. KAWAI & N. M. COTLER. 1975. Left ventricular volume measurements by echocardiography: fact or fiction? Am. J. Cardiol. 36: 114–118.
3. SCHILLER, N. B., H. ACQUATELLA, T. A. PORTS, et al. 1979. Left ventricular volume from paried biplane two-dimensional echocardiography. Circulation 60: 547–555.
4. FOLLAND, E. D., A. PARISI, P. F. MOYNIHAN, D. R. JONES, C. L. FELDMAN & D. E. TOW. 1979. Assessment of left ventricular ejection fraction and volume by real-time two-dimensional echocardiography. Circulation 60: 760–766.
5. DEVEREUX, R. B. & N. REICHEK. 1977. Echocardiographic determination of left ventricular mass in man. Circulation 55: 613–618.
6. REICHEK, N. & R. B. DEVEREUX. 1981. Left ventricular hypertrophy: relationship of anatomic, echocardiographic and electrocardiographic findings. Circulation 63: 1391–1398.
7. REICHEK, N., J. HELAK, T. PLAPPERT, M. ST. JOHN SUTTON & K. T. WEBER. 1983. Anatomic validation of left ventricular mass estimates from clinical two-dimensional echocardiography: initial results. Circulation 67: 348–352.
8. HELAK, J. W. & N. REICHEK. 1981. Quantitation of human left ventricular mass and volume by two-dimensional echocardiography: in vitro anatomic validation. Circulation 63: 1398–1407.
9. SCHILLER, N. B., C. G. SKIOLDEBRAND, E. J. SCHILLER, et al. 1983. Canine left ventricular mass estimation by two-dimensional echocardiography: in vitro anatomic validation. Circulation 68: 210–216.
10. WEISS, J. L., M. MCGAUGHEY & W. H. GUIER. 1987. Geometric considerations in determination of left ventricular mass by two-dimensional echocardiography. Hypertension 9(Suppl. II): II-85–II-89.
11. MCGAUGHEY, M. D., W. H. GUIER, M. J. HAUSKNECHT, A. HERSKOWITZ, B. WALTERS & J. L. WEISS. 1984. Three-dimensional echo reconstruction of the left ventricle in cardiac transplant patients: direct validation of mass determination. Circulation 70(Suppl. II): 397.
12. GARRISON, J. B., J. L. WEISS, W. L. MAUGHAN, O. M. TUCK, W. J. GUIER & N. J. FORTUIN. 1977. Quantifying regional wall motion and thickening in two-dimensional echocardiography with a computer-aided contouring system. In Computers in Cardiology: 25–35. IEEE. Long Beach, Calif.

13. LIEBERMAN, A. N., J. L. WEISS, B. I. JUGDUTT, L. C. BECKER, B. H. BULKLEY, J. B. GARRISON, G. M. HUTCHINS, C. A. KALLMAN & M. L. WEISFELDT. 1981. Two-dimensional echocardiography and infarct size: relationship of regional wall motion and thickening to the extent of myocardial infarction in the dog. Circulation **63:** 739–746.

14. KERBER, R. E., M. L. MARCUS, J. EHRHARDT, R. WILSON & F. M. ABBOUD. 1975. Correlation between echocardiography demonstrated segmental dyskinesis and regional myocardial perfusion. Circulation **71:** 1038–1047.

15. WYATT, H. L., J. S. FORRESTER, P. L. DA LUZ, G. A. DIAMON, R. CHAGRASULIS & H. J. C. SWAN. 1976. Functional abnormalities in nonoccluded regions of myocardium after experimental coronary occlusion. Am. J. Cardiol. **37:** 366–372.

16. HOMANS, D. C., R. ASINGER, J. ELSPERGER, D. ERLIEN, E. SUBLETT, F. MIKELL, et al. 1985. Regional function and perfusion at the lateral border of ischemic myocardium. Circulation **71:** 1083–1047.

17. SAKAI, K., K. WATANABE & R. W. MILLARD, 1985. Defining the mechanical border zone: a study in the pig heart. Am. J. Physiol. **249:** H88–H94.

18. MARINO, P. N., D. A. KASS, J. A. C. LIMA, W. L. MAUGHAN, W. GRAVES & J. L. WEISS. 1988. Influence of site of regional ischemia on left ventricular cavity shape change in dogs. Am. J. Physiol. **254:** H547–H557.

19. FORCE, T., A. KEMPER, L. PERKINS, M. GILFOIL, C. COHEN & A. F. PARISI. 1986. Overestimation of infarct size by quantitative two-dimensional echocardiography: the role of tethering and of analytic procedures. Circulation **73:** 1360–1368.

20. PANDIAN, N. G., S. KOYANAGI, D. J. SKORTON, S. M. COLLINS, C. L. EASTHAM, R. A. KIESO, et al. 1983. Relations between two-dimensional echocardiographic wall thickening abnormalities, myocardial infarct size and coronary risk area in normal and hypertrophied myocardium in dogs. Am. J. Cardiol. **52:** 1318–1325.

21. GALLAGHER, K. P., R. A. GERREN, M. C. STIRLING, M. CHOY, R. C. DYSKO, S. P. McMANIMON, et al. 1986. The distribution of functional impairment across the lateral border of acutely ischemic myocardium. Circ. Res. **58:** 570–583.

22. BUDA, A. J., R. J. ZOTZ & K. P. GALLAGHER. 1986. Characterization of the functional border zone around regionally ischemic myocardium using circumferential flow-function maps. J. Am. Coll. Cardiol. **8:** 150–158.

23. WEISS, J. L., B. H. BULKLEY, G. M. HUTCHINS & S. J. MASON. 1981. Two-dimensional echocardiographic recognition of myocardial injury in man: comparison with postmortem studies. Circulation **63:** 401–408.

24. HEGER, J. J., A. E. WEYMAN, L. S. WANN, J. C. DILLON & H. FEIGENBAUM. 1979. Cross-sectional echocardiography in acute myocardial infarction: detection and localization of regional left ventricular asynergy. **60:** 531–538.

25. LIMA, J. A. C. & J. L. WEISS. Use of echocardiographic regional contraction abnormalities for the estimation of infarct size. Am. J. Cardiac Imaging. (In press.)

The Predictive Accuracy of the Electrocardiogram in Identifying the Presence and Location of Myocardial Infarction and Coronary Artery Disease

EDWARD M. DWYER, JR.

Division of Cardiology
Department of Medicine
St. Luke's-Roosevelt Hospital Center
Amsterdam Avenue at 114th Street
New York, New York 10025

In the period between 1920 and 1950, pathologists and clinical physicians established the theoretical framework and empirical basis for the association between myocardial necrosis and a Q wave on the electrocardiogram (ECG).[1-4] The ECG continues to be an important tool in the diagnosis and management of ischemic heart disease. The relatively low cost of the ECG and our ability to perform it quickly and simply magnifies its value. The ECG's initial use in diagnosing an acute or chronic infarction has now been extended to the determination of infarct location, determination of the responsible coronary artery, and estimation of ventricular function and prognosis.

In correlation studies, different methods have been used to identify myocardial damage. These methods include pathologic study from autopsies; coronary angiographic and ventriculographic data obtained during cardiac catheterization; and more recently ventricular images from two-dimensional echocardiograms or radionuclide studies.

In necropsy studies, the correlation between the electrocardiogram and anatomy was usually approached from the pathologist's point of view. The pathologist's approach was to determine how sensitive the ECG is in the diagnosis of an infarction identified at autopsy. Most pathologic studies have demonstrated a relatively poor performance of the ECG in this correlation process.[5-9] Unfortunately, the pathologic-autopsy approach has an intrinsic bias. All patients have died and most patients have multiple infarctions and multivessel disease. The presence of extensive disease can confound electrocardiographic analysis. The occurrence of conduction abnormalities, such as left anterior hemiblock or left bundle branch block, and infarction on opposite sides of the left ventricle are more common in advanced coronary artery disease and can obscure abnormal Q waves.[10,11] Correlation analyses of the ECG with pathologic observations also frequently suffer from a lack of concurrent ECGs.

With the development and wide dispersal of coronary angiography and ventriculography in the 1960s, concurrent ECGs, ventriculograms, and coronary anatomy could be obtained in a larger number of patients in a prospective fashion.[12-19] The larger number of patients available for study also permitted subgroup analyses, such as in patients with single vessel disease[20] or specific electrocardiographic or myocardial contraction patterns.[13,21] These research advances were enhanced further by the development of echocardiographic and radionuclide imaging techniques which permitted a "noninvasive" correlation between left ventricular anatomy and electrocardio-

TABLE 1. Studies That Describe the Ability of the Electrocardiogram to Diagnose Myocardial Infarction

Author	Year	Method of Infarct Determination	Number of Patients	Percent Predicted
Woods[5]	1959	Autopsy	112	48
Gunnar[9]	1967	Autopsy	53	54
Horan[7]	1971	Autopsy	416	61
Miller[13]	1974	Catheterization	84	87
Hamby[14]	1974	Catheterization	2	80
Bodenheimer[15]	1975	Catheterization	119	51
Howard[16]	1976	Catheterization	156	49
Sullivan[8]	1978	Autopsy	50	88
Arkin[17]	1979	Catheterization	152	51
Viewig[18]	1980	Catheterization	245	36

graphic abnormalities.[22,23] Noninvasive imaging has been particularly useful in detailing ventricular abnormalities during acute ischemic syndromes.

More recently, treatment of acute coronary artery disease by thrombolysis and treatment of chronic coronary disease by angioplasty have resulted in more focused studies of the relationship between the ECG and the occluded coronary artery.[24,25]

SENSITIVITY OF THE ECG IN DETECTION OF MYOCARDIAL INFARCTION

An important aspect of the electrocardiographic–cardiac anatomy correlation is the ability of the ECG to detect ventricular infarction. In studies of patients in high prevalence populations, the sensitivity of the ECG in the detection of an infarction ranges between 30% and 88% (TABLE 1), with a mean value of approximately 50%. This is not an unexpected finding when the factors that affect the sensitivity of the ECG are analyzed.

The factors that most influence the ability of the ECG to identify an infarction are listed in TABLE 2. A significant number of infarctions occur without the development of a Q wave. In a recent multicenter postinfarction trial,[26] the incidence of non–Q wave infarction in a group of 2500 patients with documented infarction was approximately 25%. In this trial, entry into the study only required enzymatic abnormalities, therefore the electrocardiographic findings should accurately reflect the incidence of Q waves in survivors of an infarction. Infarctions without Q waves tend to be smaller (by enzyme or ventriculographic analysis) and have less severe contraction abnormalities. The most important pathophysiologic mechanisms that influence the development of a non–Q wave infarction appear to be early perfusion of an occluded coronary artery,[27] preexisting collateral connections,[28] or occlusion of smaller branch arteries.

Even when Q waves do occur, regression of an established Q wave following acute

TABLE 2. Factors Influencing Ability of ECG to Identify Infarction

1. Non–Q wave infarction
2. Q wave regression
3. Multiple infarctions
4. Conduction disorders

infarction is not unusual. Regression has been shown to occur in 10%–20% of patients over a 1–2 year period.[29,30] These regressive changes are equally distributed between anterior and inferior infarctions. Patients who lose their Q waves generally have smaller infarcts, higher ejection fraction, and fewer wall motion abnormalities. However, the degree of coronary arterial narrowing has not been found to be significantly different from patients who retain their Q wave.

Existing Q waves may also be obscured by subsequent damage to the ventricle. Such damage may produce conduction abnormalities such as left anterior hemiblock or left bundle branch block. Left anterior hemiblock, occurring in approximately 30% of patients with anterior infarction, is relatively common in patients with coronary artery disease. This conduction abnormality will frequently mask inferior wall Q wave infarction.[31] The occurrence of anterior Q wave infarction and posterolateral infarction (tall RV_1–V_2) will frequently have, as an end result, normal precordial complexes.[32] The exact incidence of obscuration of Q waves is presently unknown.

The frequency of the above-described factors that affect the sensitivity of the ECG is relatively fixed and will not likely change. However, one factor that influences the sensitivity of the ECG, i.e., criteria for infarction diagnosis (Q wave), is under physician control. Borderline abnormalities, such as seen with "poor R wave progression" or those "near diagnostic" Q waves, need closer study. It may be useful to evaluate the

TABLE 3. Factors Influencing Ability of ECG Q Wave to Detect Infarction Location and Coronary Artery

1. Early reperfusion following acute MI (thrombolytic therapy)
2. "False-positive" Q waves
LVH
Myocardial disorders
3. Single plane imaging
4. Normal variation in coronary anatomy
5. Collateral dependency

predictive value of more "liberal criteria" for abnormal Q waves in patient populations with already documented coronary disease.

PREDICTIVE ABILITY OF ELECTROCARDIOGRAPHIC Q WAVES IN IDENTIFICATION OF THE PRESENCE AND LOCATION OF A MYOCARDIAL INFARCTION

A more clinically relevant and realistic question is, How effectively does the presence of an abnormal Q wave or a Q wave equivalent predict the presence and location of an infarction? There are several factors, listed in TABLE 3, that affect the ability of a Q wave to predict the presence of an infarction.

The first factor is early reperfusion of a coronary artery. Although spontaneous early reperfusion is frequently associated with a non–Q wave infarction,[27] early reperfusion from thrombolytic therapy often results in normal wall motion with Q wave abnormalities.[33] The latter occurrence seems feasible as a spontaneous event, but little evidence exists in the literature to document and quantitate its incidence.

Other causes of "false-positive Q waves" may be found in patients with left ventricular hypertrophy, acute cor pulmonale, and in myocardial disorders.[34] Finally, a less common cause for a Q wave occurring without asynergy is the limited number of views by which our imaging techniques evaluate the left ventricle. For example, single plane ventriculography is usually employed during cardiac catheterization to establish the presence of an infarction. This may, on occasion, result in failure to demonstrate an asynergic region in a patient with an isolated lateral myocardial infarction.

ABILITY OF ELECTROCARDIOGRAPHIC Q WAVES IN PREDICTION OF THE CORONARY ARTERY RESPONSIBLE FOR INFARCTION

The ability of the Q wave to predict the responsible or "culprit" artery also has its pitfalls. The normal variation in coronary artery anatomy and the variable location (within a given artery) of an occlusion account for the wide variation in the location and extent of an infarction. This, in turn, influences the location of abnormalities on the ECG. All three major coronary arteries demonstrate significant variations in their distribution. The left anterior descending (LAD) artery has a variable length which may either just reach the apex of the heart or "wrap around," supplying up to one-third of the distal inferior surface. In the inferior and posterolateral surface, right coronary

TABLE 4. Studies That Describe the Ability of Electrocardiogram Q Waves to Detect and Localize Myocardial Infarction

Author	Year	Infarct Determination	Number of Patients	Percent Predicted
Gunnar[9]	1967	Autopsy	46	63
Horan[7]	1971	Autopsy	339	75
Williams[12]	1973	Catheterization	225	82
Hamby[14]	1974	Catheterization	110	86
Miller[13]	1974	Catheterization	73	94
Bodenheimer[15]	1975	Catheterization	64	95
Arkin[17]	1979	Catheterization	84	93
Veiwig[18]	1980	Catheterization	245	84

artery (RCA) and circumflex artery play complimentary roles in the supply of those regions. Either artery may assume a dominant role in that arterial supply.

The location of the occlusion within the artery, of course, also plays a major role in the site and extent of an infarction. Proximal occlusions produce more widespread damage which results in more extensive abnormalities on the ECG. The reverse is true for distal or branch occlusions.[13,35]

ANTERIOR Q WAVES: ABILITY TO PREDICT INFARCTION LOCATION AND RESPONSIBLE ARTERY

Definite evidence of chronic anterior wall infarction is generally accepted as a Q wave found in leads V_2-V_4. An anterior wall infarction may have associated Q waves in electrocardiographic "lateral" leads V_5-V_6 and/or I, AVL as well.

We reviewed studies with data obtained from cardiac catheterization and echocardiography in patients with healed infarcts[8,12-15,18,36] (TABLE 4) as well as from catheterization studies in patients with acute occlusion or unstable angina.[23,24] Investigators, in these catheterization and echocardiogram studies of patients with chronic infarction, examined over 1000 patients which included approximately 500 patients with anterior infarction. The presence of Q waves in precordial leads V_1-V_4 was usually associated with asynergy of the anterior wall and/or the apex. The predictive accuracy ranged between 75% and 100% in eight of these correlation studies.

Reversed R wave progression (RRWP) and "poor R wave progression" (PRWP) were not specifically addressed in any of the studies described above. However, in a study by Zema et al., these electrocardiographic findings were frequently associated with nontransmural infarctions,[37] which contrasts with Q wave anterior infarctions which are usually transmural. In a subsequent study, Zema et al. confirmed the low incidence (38%) of contraction abnormalities found with RRWP and PRWP.[21] In their experience, the incidence of anterior infarction in all patients presenting with RRWP and PRWP was 34%. In patients with this ECG pattern, predictive accuracy can be enhanced by excluding patients with right ventricular hypertrophy or left ventricular hypertrophy, and by including patients with coincident ST elevation or T wave inversion in the anterior precordial leads.

Although most authors attribute Q waves in the anterior precordial leads to obstruction of the LAD artery, data have not usually been analyzed in a manner that confirms and quantitates this correlation. In one of the few studies that addresses this question, Fuchs et al. examined the artery-electrocardiogram correlation in patients with single vessel coronary artery disease.[20] Anterior Q waves V_1-V_3 were found in 25 patients, and all had a diseased LAD artery. None of the 31 patients with right coronary or circumflex artery disease had Q waves in the right precordial leads (V_1-V_3). This suggests a very strong correlation between anterior Q waves and LAD artery obstruction.

Acute occlusion of the LAD artery during angioplasty has provided an opportunity to study associated electrocardiographic changes.[23,24] With LAD artery occlusion, ST elevation is most commonly (85%) found in lead V_2 and adjacent precordial leads. In addition to adjacent precordial leads, ST elevation was also recorded in V_5 (25%) and AVL (40%).

INFERIOR Q WAVES: ABILITY TO PREDICT INFARCTION LOCATION AND RESPONSIBLE ARTERY

Infarction of the inferior and/or posterior surface of the left ventricle results in characteristic Q waves in leads 2, 3, AVF. Catheterization studies and echocardiography uniformly show that the presence of Q waves in leads 2, 3, AVF reflects asynergy in the inferior region of the left ventricle. The predictive accuracy, in the eight studies reviewed, varied from 76% to 97%.

Predicting which artery is responsible for inferior electrocardiographic changes is more problematic. The inferior/posterior ventricular region may be supplied by the RCA, circumflex artery, or both. In addition, a large "wrap-around" LAD artery may, on occasion, supply the distal inferior wall. In the catheterization study by Fuchs et al., isolated disease of the RCA was responsible for Q waves in 83% of patients studied.[20] In the remaining patients, inferior Q waves were due to the circumflex artery in 14% and LAD artery in 3%. A similar observation was made by Dwyer et al. in an analysis of coronary artery disease associated with Q waves in the inferior leads.[19] Supporting evidence of this correlation was observed in patients undergoing angioplasty. The RCA (but not LAD artery) occlusion was associated with echocardiographic inferior wall asynergy[23] and inferior lead electrocardiographics ischemic changes.[24]

The determination of which coronary artery is responsible for an inferior infarction is often aided by other findings in the electrocardiogram. Bough and associates (23 patients),[22] Fuchs et al. (25 patients),[20] and Bairy et al. (41 patients)[38] showed that

RCA occlusions tend to produce electrocardiographic changes that are confined to the inferior leads. Although on occasion, a large occluded RCA, extending to the postero-lateral wall or apex, may produce Q waves in lead V_6 or tall R waves in V_1–V_2, this is the exception rather than the rule. The presence of a right ventricular infarction provides further assistance in the determination of the responsible artery. Right ventricular infarction is usually associated with an RCA occlusion and can be best documented on the ECG by lead V_4R. When ST elevation in V_4R is present, it predicts, with high likelihood, that the RCA is the artery responsible for the inferior infarction.[39] On the other hand, the studies by Bairey et al.[38] and Dunn and associates[35] demon-strated that inferior infarction, associated with lateral lead Q waves in I, V_5, V_6 and tall R waves in V_1–V_2, is usually secondary to circumflex artery occlusion.

LATERAL LEAD Q WAVES: ABILITY TO PREDICT PRESENCE AND LOCATION OF INFARCTION

Lateral wall infarction, since its early description by Wood et al. in 1938,[40] has been the subject of considerable investigation and debate. "Lateral" leads (I, AVL, V_5–V_6) in electrocardiographic nomenclature have carried the implication that Q waves in these leads represent anatomic changes in the lateral wall of the left ventricle due to disease of certain branches of the circumflex artery. Considerable evidence now exists that indicates that this perception is in error.

Recent studies have shown that changes (Q, elevated ST) in I/AVL occur from either occlusion of the LAD or circumflex artery. However, changes in I and AVL are, in fact, most often due to LAD artery disease with anterolateral infarction. A recent report by Takatsu et al., in abstract form, showed that an isolated Q in I, AVL in 29 patients was primarily due to occlusion of the diagonal branches of the LAD artery.[41] In the investigation by Fuchs et al., Q waves in I and AVL were only associated with disease in the LAD artery.[20] From these studies, it appears that changes in I, AVL are only rarely due to circumflex artery disease. A Q wave or ST elevation in V_5–V_6 may occur due to LAD, RCA, or circumflex artery disease. Huey et al. concluded that ST elevation and a Q in V_5 is more likely to be LAD artery disease while ST elevation or a Q in V_6 is more likely to be associated with circumflex artery disease.[42] Necropsy data[7,8,43] suggest that changes in V_5–V_6 represent anteroapical or lateral-apical infarc-tions. When considered separately, the number of patients with changes isolated to the lateral leads is quite small. Review of the limited number of patients with lateral lead changes suggests that the predictive accuracy of Q wave abnormalities in those leads is similar to anterior and inferior Q waves.

ANTERIOR TALL R WAVE: ABILITY TO PREDICT INFARCTION LOCATION AND RESPONSIBLE ARTERY

Prominent right precordial R waves have been known since 1944 to represent myocardial infarction. Because of different electrocardiographic labels such as "true posterior," "lateral," "posterolateral" and "inferoposterior" among others, the ana-tomic location of the infarction has been controversial. Bough et al. concluded, from a study directed at correlation of left ventricular anatomy with these electrocardio-graphic changes, that basal lateral asynergy correlates best with the prominent right precordial R waves.[22] They demonstrated a 91% positive predictive value of the tall R wave precordial pattern. The sensitivity of this ECG abnormality in detecting infarc-tion, in their study, varied from 36% to 61% dependent on the strictness of the electrocardiographic criteria. Several early autopsy studies confirmed,[6] in a qualitative fashion, the association between lateral infarction and these precordial ECG findings. In their pathologic studies, Ward *et al.* demonstrated that 50% of patients with lateral wall infarction had an associated tall RV_1–V_2 pattern.[44] In their study of patients with isolated circumflex disease, Dunn and associates found Q waves or RV (tall RV_1–V_2) patterns in 68 patients and S-T changes in 19 others.[35] The RV pattern was found in 50% of the total group. They concluded that circumflex artery disease can produce ECG abnormalities in the three lead regions (inferior, lateral, and anterior). Q waves in lateral leads I, AVL, as noted earlier, are extremely uncommon, although occasionally seen. The hallmark finding of lateral infarction and circumflex disease, from the evidence of these highly focused studies, is the presence of tall or prominent R and T waves in the anterior precordial leads.

SUMMARY

In summary, the electrocardiogram is limited in its ability to detect a myocardial infarction. Its sensitivity is compromised seriously by a substantial number of patients

TABLE 5. Summary of Relationship between Electrocardiogram, Infarction Site, and Coronary Artery[a]

Electrocardiographic Leads	Site of Infarction	Responsible Coronary Artery
Q V_1–V_4	Anterior	LAD
Q 2, 3 AVF	Inferior/posterior	RCA/CIRC
Q I, AVL	Anterolateral	LAD/CIRC
Q V_5–V_6	Apical/lateral	LAD/CIRC/RCA
Tall R V_1–V_2	Lateral	CIRC

[a]Abbreviations: left anterior descending artery = LAD; right coronary artery = RCA; circumflex artery = CIRC.

with non-Q wave infarction or regression of Q waves. Once a Q wave occurs, the predictive accuracy of those changes, in delineating the location of the infarction, is quite high. The ability of Q waves or ST segment elevation to predict or identify the "culprit artery" is less strong, primarily due to the variation in coronary anatomy commonly found.

The relationship between anterior or inferior lead changes and anterior or inferior myocardial damage is close. However, lateral lead changes may more accurately represent anterolateral (I, AVL) or apical (V_5–V_6) infarction. Tall R waves in anterior precordial leads is most often associated with posterolateral infarction (TABLE 5).

ACKNOWLEDGMENT

The author wishes to express his thanks to Ms. Kristin Summers for her expert assistance in the preparation of this manuscript.

REFERENCES

1. PARDEE, H. E. 1930. The significance of an electrocardiogram with a large Q wave in lead 3. Arch. Intern. Med. **46:** 470–481.

2. BARNES, A. R. 1935. Electrocardiogram in myocardial infarction. Review of one hundred and seven clinical cases and one hundred and eight cases proved at necropsy. Arch. Intern. Med. **55:** 457–483.
3. GOLDBERGER, E. 1945. The differentiation of normal from abnormal Q waves. Am. Heart J. **30:** 341–365.
4. FELL, H., E. H. CUSHING & J. T. HARDESLY. 1938. Accuracy in diagnosis and localization of myocardial infarction. Am. Heart J. **15:** 721–738.
5. WOODS, J. D., W. LAURIE & W. G. SMITH. 1963. The reliability of the electrocardiogram in myocardial infarction. Lancet **2:** 265–269.
6. DUNN, W. J., J. E. EDWARDS & R. D. PRUITT. 1956. The electrocardiogram in infarction of the lateral wall of the left ventricle. Circulation **14:** 540–555.
7. HORAN, L. G., N. C. FLOWERS & J. C. JOHNSON. 1971. Significance of the diagnostic Q wave of myocardial infarction. Circulation **43:** 428–436.
8. SULLIVAN, W., Z. VLODAVER, N. TUNA, L. LONG & J. E. EDWARDS. 1978. Correlation of electrocardiographic and pathologic findings in healed myocardial infarction. Am. J. Cardiol. **42:** 724–732.
9. GUNNAR, R. M., R. J. PIETRAS, J. BLACKALLER, S. E. DADMUN, P. B. SZANTO & J. R. TOBIN, JR. 1967. Correlation of vectorcardiographic criteria for myocardial infarction with autopsy findings. Circulation **35:** 158–171.
10. RAUNIO, H., V. RISSANEN, T. ROMPPANEN, Y. JOKINEN, S. REHNBERG, M. HELIN & K. PYORALA. 1979. Changes in QRS complex and ST segment in transmural and subendocardial myocardial infarction. A clinicopathologic study. Am. Heart J. **98:** 176–184.
11. DOUCET, P., T. J. WALSH & E. MASSIE. 1966. A vectorcardiographic and electrocardiographic study of left bundle branch block with myocardial infarction. Am. J. Cardiol. **17:** 171–179.
12. WILLIAMS, R. A., P. F. COHN, P. S. VOKONAS, E. YOUNG, M. V. HERMAN & R. GORLIN. 1973. Electrocardiographic, arteriographic and ventriculographic correlations in transmural myocardial infarction. Am. J. Cardiol. **31:** 595–599.
13. MILLER, R. R., E. A. AMSTERDAM, H. G. BOGREN, R. A. MASSUMI, R. ZELIS & D. T. MASON. 1974. Electrocardiographic and cineangiographic correlations in assessment of the location, nature and extent of abnormal left ventricular segmental contraction in coronary artery disease. Circulation **49:** 447–454.
14. HAMBY, R. I., I. HOFFMAN, J. HILSENRATH, A. AINTABLIAN, S. SHANIES & V. S. PADMANABHAN. 1974. Clinical, hemodynamic and angiographic aspects of inferior and anterior myocardial infarctions in patients with angina pectoris. Am. J. Cardiol. **34:** 513–519.
15. BODENHEIMER, M. M., V. S. BANKA & R. H. HELFANT. 1975. Q waves and ventricular asynergy: predictive value and hemodynamic significance of anatomic localization. Am. J. Cardiol. **35:** 615–618.
16. HOWARD, P. F., A. BENCHIMOL, K. B. DESSER, F. D. REICH & C. GRAVES. 1976. Correlation of electrocardiogram and vectorcardiogram with coronary occlusion and myocardial contraction abnormality. Am. J. Cardiol. **38:** 582–587.
17. ARKIN, B. M., D. C. HUETER & T. J. RYAN. 1979. Predictive value of electrocardiographic patterns in localizing left ventricular asynergy in coronary artery disease. Am. Heart J. **97:** 453–459.
18. VIEWEG, W. V. R., J. S. ALPERT, A. D. JOHNSON, G. W. DENNISH, D. P. NELSON, S. E. WARREN & A. D. HAGAN. 1980. Electrocardiographic and left ventriculographic correlations in 245 patients with coronary artery disease. Comput. Biomed. Res. **13:** 105–119.
19. DWYER, E. M., S. COQUIA, H. GREENBERG & B. H. PINKERNELL. 1975. Inferior myocardial infarction and right coronary artery occlusive disease. A correlative study. Br. Heart J. **37:** 464–470.
20. FUCHS, R. M., S. C. ACHUFF, L. GRUNWALD, F. C. P. YIN & L. S. C. GRIFFITH. 1982. Electrocardiographic localization of coronary artery narrowings: studies during myocardial ischemia and infarction in patients with one-vessel disease. Circulation **66:** 1168–1176.
21. ZEMA, M. J. & P. KLIGFIELD. 1979. Electrocardiographic poor R wave progression II: correlation with angiography. J. Electrocardiol. **12:** 11–15.

22. BOUGH, E. W., W. E. BODEN, K. S. KORR & E. J. GANDSMAN. 1984. Left ventricular asynergy in electrocardiographic "posterior" myocardial infarction. J. Am. Coll. Cardiol. 4: 209–215.

23. HAUSER, A. M., V. GANGADHARAN, R. G. RAMOS, S. GORDON & G. C. TIMMIS. 1985. Sequence of mechanical, electrocardiographic and clinical effects of repeated coronary artery occlusion in human beings: echocardiographic observations during coronary angioplasty. J. Am. Coll. Cardiol. 5: 193–197.

24. COHEN, M., S. J. SCHARPF & K. P. RENTROP. 1987. Prospective analysis of electrocardiographic variables as markers for extent and location of acute wall motion abnormalities observed during coronary angioplasty in human subjects. J. Am. Coll. Cardiol. 10: 17–24.

25. HIASA, Y., T. WADA, K. HAMAI, Y. NAKAYA & H. MORI. 1988. ST-segment depression in inferior ECG leads during percutaneous transluminal coronary angioplasty for left anterior descending artery. Clin. Cardiol. 11: 614–618.

26. Multicenter Diltiazem Postinfarction Research Group. 1988. The effect of diltiazem on mortality and reinfarction after myocardial infarction. N. Engl. J. Med. 319: 385–392.

27. DEWOOD, M. A., W. F. STIFTER, C. S. SIMPSON, J. SPORES CRNA, G. S. EUGSTER, T. P. JUDGE & M. L. HINNEN. 1986. Coronary arteriographic findings soon after non-q-wave myocardial infarction. N. Engl. J. Med. 315: 417–423.

28. HANSEN, J. F. 1989. Coronary collateral circulation: clinical significance and influence on survival in patients with coronary artery occlusion. Am. Heart J. 117: 290–295.

29. BURNS COX, C. J. 1967. Return to normal of the electrocardiogram after myocardial infarction. Lancet 1: 1194–1197.

30. COLL, S., A. BETRIU, T. DE FLORES, E. ROIG, G. SANZ, L. MONT, J. MAGRINA, A. SERRA & F. N. LOPEZ. 1988. Significance of Q-wave regression after transmural acute myocardial infarction. Am. J. Cardiol. 61: 739–742.

31. WARNER, R. A., N. E. HILL, S. MOOKHERJEE & H. SMULYAN. 1983. Electrocardiographic criteria for the diagnosis of combined inferior myocardial infarction and left anterior hemiblock. Am. J. Cardiol. 51: 718–722.

32. MASSIE, E. & T. J. WALSH. 1960. Miscellaneous cardiac abnormalities. In Clinical Vectorcardiography and Electrocardiography. 1st edit.: 317–338. Year Book Publishers. Chicago, Ill.

33. RENTROP, P., H. BLANKE, K. R. KARSCH, H. KAISER, H. KOSTERING & K. LEITZ. 1981. Selective intracoronary thrombolysis in acute myocardial infarction and unstable angina pectoris. Circulation 63: 307–317.

34. HILSENRATH, J., R. I. HAMBY, E. GLASSMAN & I. HOFFMAN. 1972. Pitfalls in prediction of coronary arterial obstruction from patterns of anterior infarction on electrocardiogram and vectorcardiogram. Am. J. Cardiol. 29: 164–170.

35. DUNN, R. F., H. N. NEWMAN, L. BERNSTEIN, P. J. HARRIS, G. S. ROUBIN, J. MORRIS & D. T. KELLY. 1984. The clinical features of isolated left circumflex coronary artery disease. Circulation 69: 477–484.

36. HEIKKILA, J. & M. NIEMINEN. 1975. Echoventriculographic detection, localization, and quantification of left ventricular asynergy in acute myocardial infarction. A correlative echo- and electrocardiographic study. Br. Heart J. 37: 46–59.

37. ZEMA, M. J., M. COLLINS, D. R. ALONSO & P. KLIGFIELD. 1981. Electrocardiographic poor R-wave progression. Correlation with postmortem findings. Chest 79: 195–200.

38. BAIREY, C. N., P. K. SHAH, A. S. LEW & S. HULSE. 1987. Electrocardiographic differentiation of occlusion of the left circumflex versus the right coronary artery as a cause of inferior acute myocardial infarction. Am. J. Cardiol. 60: 456–459.

39. BRAAT, S. H., P. BRUGADA, C. DE ZWAAN, J. M. COENEGRACHT & H. J. J. WELLENS. 1983. Value of electrocardiogram in diagnosing right ventricular involvement in patients with an acute inferior wall myocardial infarction. Br. Heart J. 49: 368–372.

40. WOOD, F. C., C. C. WOLFERTH & S. BELLET. 1938. Infarction of the lateral wall of the left ventricle: electrocardiographic characteristics. Am. Heart J. 16: 387–410.

41. TAKATSU, F., T. NAGAYA & J. OSUGI. 1988. Relationship between abnormal Q waves in lead aVL and angiographic findings: a study to redefine "high lateral" infarction. J. Electrocardiol. 22: 271.

42. HUEY, B. L., G. A. BELLER, D. L. KAISER & R. S. GIBSON. 1988. A comprehensive analysis

of myocardial infarction due to left circumflex occlusion: comparison with infarction due to right coronary artery and left anterior descending artery occlusion. J. Am. Coll. Cardiol. **12**: 1156–1166.

43. SAVAGE, R. M., G. S. WAGNER, R. E. IDEKER, S. A. PODOLSKY & D. B. HACKEL. 1977. Correlation of postmortem anatomic findings with electrocardiographic changes in patients with myocardial infarction. Retrospective study of patients with typical anterior and posterior infarcts. Circulation **55**: 279–285.

44. WARD, R. M., R. D. WHITE & R. E. IDEKER. 1984. Evaluation of a QRS scoring system for estimating myocardial infarct size. IV. Correlation with quantitative anatomic finds for posterolateral infarcts. Am. J. Cardiol. **53**: 706–714.

Positron Emission Tomography as an Aid in Understanding Electrocardiographic Changes of Ischemia, Infarction, and Cardiomyopathy[a]

MALEAH GROVER-McKAY

Departments of Internal Medicine and Radiology
The University of Iowa
Iowa City, Iowa 52242

INTRODUCTION

Electrocardiographic identification of infarction and ischemia is the oldest and least expensive method of diagnosis. However, localization of infarction and ischemia by the electrocardiogram (ECG) is not always accurate[1] and in some patients Q-waves disappear.[2,3] Therefore, as described elsewhere in this volume, other methods have been utilized for confirmation of the presence of myocardial infarction, such as evaluation of wall motion, myocardial blood flow, and tissue characterization including metabolism. The advantage of the positron emission tomography (PET) technique is that combined evaluation of myocardial blood flow and metabolism is possible, thereby enabling differentiation of infarcted and viable myocardium. The positron-emitting tracers used in the studies cited are briefly discussed. The reader is referred to more in-depth reviews for a more detailed discussion of PET.[4,5]

POSITRON-EMITTING TRACERS OF MYOCARDIAL BLOOD FLOW

To date, the three most important positron-emitting tracers of myocardial blood flow are ^{13}N-ammonia, ^{82}rubidium, and ^{15}O-water.

^{13}N-Ammonia

The advantages of ^{13}N-ammonia include rapid clearance from blood and high myocardial extraction (80–90%) and retention (82%), which results in high contrast myocardial images.[6,7] A linear relationship was observed between microspheres and ^{13}N-ammonia for myocardial blood flow between 44 and 200 ml/minute per 100 g of myocardium.[8] Potential disadvantages of ^{13}N-ammonia include the fact that it is probably retained in the myocardium by metabolic trapping mainly by the glutamic acid–glutamine pathway, and therefore, may not accurately reflect blood flow during conditions such as extremely low pH or reduced intracellular ATP.[9–11] In addition, a recent study indicates that after intravenous injection, ^{13}N-ammonia is rapidly converted to metabolic intermediates.[12]

[a]Supported in part by grants IA 89-G-13 American Heart Association, Iowa Affiliate and Radiological Society of North America Seed Grant Award.

77

$^{82}Rubidium$

The advantages of ^{82}Rb include that it is available from a generator, hence is continuously available, and that its short half-life (76 seconds) enables repeat studies at 7.5 minutes. A preliminary study using a two-compartment tracer kinetic model demonstrated a good correlation between microspheres and ^{82}Rb for myocardial blood flow between 48 and 457 ml/minute per 100 g.[13] Disadvantages include the following: (1) the high energy of the ^{82}Rb positron (3.15 MeV 82.8%) means that the positron travels farther from the site of emission to the site of annihilation than positrons from other positron-emitting nuclides, hence, localization of the site of emission is less accurate; (2) the short half-life requires high-efficiency tomographs for adequate statistical information; (3) myocardial extraction is only 50%–70%[14–16] and appears to vary with ischemia and reperfusion; although this characteristic may be turned to advantage for assessment of cell viability.[17–19]

$^{15}O\text{-}Water$

Advantages of the diffusible tracer ^{15}O-water include that it is least susceptible to metabolic alterations, that it has an extraction fraction of 80%–99%,[20] and that its short-half life (2 minutes) enables repeat studies in 10 minutes. A good correlation exists between microspheres and ^{15}O-water for MBF between 12 and 238 ml/minute per 100 g.[20] Disadvantages are that the short half-life requires high-efficiency tomographs and that high activity in blood and lungs makes accurate measurement of myocardial blood flow difficult. Quantitation of regional myocardial blood flow has recently been described in humans.[53]

POSITRON-EMITTING TRACERS OF MYOCARDIAL METABOLISM

Utilization of substrates by the heart is in part dependent on substrate availability.[21,22] During fasting when arterial levels of fatty acids are high, the heart preferentially uses fatty acids. During ischemia when fatty acid beta-oxidation is impaired, the heart switches to anaerobic metabolism of glucose.[23] Therefore, investigation of myocardial metabolism enables differentiation of normal, ischemic but viable, and infarcted myocardium.

$^{11}C\text{-}Palmitate$

The positron-emitting carbon is placed in the C1 position, and therefore, it is cleaved when the palmitate undergoes beta-oxidation. Evaluation of ^{11}C-palmitate time-activity curves (FIGURE 1) demonstrates biexponential clearance with an early rapid clearance phase and a subsequent slow clearance phase; the area under the early rapid phase correlates with the amount of beta-oxidation.[24] If beta-oxidation does not occur, as during ischemia, the ^{11}C-palmitate is retained in the myocardium, possibly by deposition in endogenous lipid pools (FIGURES 1 and 2).[25] Therefore, images obtained early after tracer injection reflect myocardial^{11}C-palmitate uptake which is related to blood flow, although in ischemic myocardium some ^{11}C-palmitate rapidly diffuses out of the myocardium.[26] Images obtained approximately 30 minutes after tracer injection reflect clearance of the ^{11}C label from normally perfused myocardium and retention of the ^{11}C label in myocardium able to take up ^{11}C-palmitate (i.e., not infarcted) but unable to perform beta-oxidation (i.e., ischemic). Thus, infarcted myocardium demonstrates decreased ^{11}C-palmitate uptake on both early and late images. Ischemic myocardium demonstrates normal or somewhat decreased ^{11}C-palmitate uptake on early images and increased activity compared with normal myocardium on delayed images (FIGURE 2). An experimental study demonstrated that a 20 minute coronary artery occlusion with subsequent reperfusion resulted in abnormal ^{11}C-palmitate kinetics for up to 3 hours in viable myocardium; the metabolic recovery occurred along with recovery of regional myocardial function.[27]

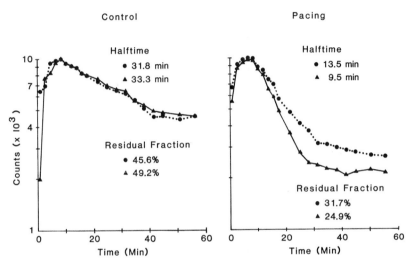

FIGURE 1. Effect of pacing on regional myocardial ^{11}C-palmitate time-activity curves in the patient whose images are shown in FIGURE 2. The lateral wall of the myocardium is supplied by a normal circumflex coronary artery and is represented by triangles. The septum and anterior walls are supplied by a significantly stenosed left anterior descending coronary artery and are represented by circles. At control, the ^{11}C-palmitate time-activity curves in the two areas of myocardium are similar. During pacing, a greater amount of the ^{11}C label clears more rapidly from the lateral than the anteroseptal myocardium suggesting impaired fatty acid oxidation in myocardium supplied by significantly stenosed coronary artery. (Reproduced from Reference 41 with permission of the American Heart Association.)

^{18}F 2-Fluoro-2-deoxy-D-glucose

^{18}F 2-Fluoro-2-deoxy-D-glucose (FDG) is a glucose analogue which is taken up by a cell via facilitated transport, undergoes phosphorylation, but does not undergo further glycolysis, glycogenolysis, nor does it readily undergo dephosphorylation or diffuse out of the cell, hence it is "trapped" in the cell.[28] Therefore, FDG is a tracer of exogenous glucose uptake and phosphorylation. In the experimental study of coronary artery occlusion with subsequent reperfusion cited above, the lack of myocardial FDG uptake at 24 hours correlated with histologic infarction whereas the presence of myocardial FDG uptake identified viable myocardium in which function subsequently recovered.[29]

C - 11 PALMITIC ACID
Control   Pacing

8 min

40 min

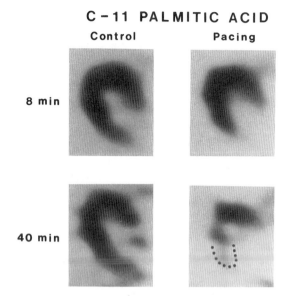

FIGURE 2. Tomographic images at two midventricular levels of myocardial ^{11}C-palmitate at control (on left) and during pacing (on right). The images are oriented with the septum at the upper right, the anterior wall at the upper left, the lateral wall at the lower left, and the mitral valve plane at the lower right. The 8-minute images (on top) reflect myocardial uptake of ^{11}C-palmitate and the 40-minute images (on bottom) reflect ^{11}C-palmitate clearance from the myocardium. Myocardial clearance of ^{11}C-palmitate which was homogeneous at control became heterogeneous during pacing when ^{11}C-palmitate cleared more rapidly from the normally perfused lateral wall than from the septum and anterior wall which were supplied by a left anterior descending coronary artery with a 90% proximal stenosis. Persistence of ^{11}C activity in the septum and anterior wall on the 40-minute images reflects a relative impairment in fatty acid oxidation during pacing in myocardium supplied by a stenotic coronary artery. (Reproduced from Reference 41 with permission of the American Heart Association.)

CLINICAL STUDIES

Patients with Myocardial Infarction

Acute Myocardial Infarction

To investigate the effect of myocardial infarction (see TABLE 1) on myocardial blood flow and exogenous glucose uptake, Marshall and colleagues[30] performed PET studies at rest in 15 patients with 17 recent and 2 remote myocardial infarctions. Electrocardiographic infarct location was possible in 13 infarctions. Studies were performed an average of 2.9 weeks (range 2 days to 13 weeks) after either Q- or non–Q wave acute myocardial infarction. Nine patients had postinfarction angina at rest, five of whom had transient ST-T wave changes during angina and two of whom had elevation of pulmonary artery wedge pressure. Patients with angina were studied an average of 20.2 hours after an episode of pain (range 2 to 56 hours). Myocardial blood flow was evaluated with ^{13}N-ammonia, and glucose was given orally prior to FDG injection. Results in patients were compared with studies obtained in 10 normal volunteers. Three PET patterns were identified: (1) normal myocardial uptake of ^{13}N-ammonia and FDG, defined as normal myocardium; (2) concordantly decreased myocardial uptake of ^{13}N-ammonia and FDG (2 standard deviations below values obtained in normal volunteers in at least two contiguous 30° myocardial segments), defined as PET infarction; and (3) decreased myocardial uptake of ^{13}N-ammonia yet normal or relatively increased FDG uptake, described as PET "mismatch" and thought to reflect ischemic glucose utilization in viable myocardium (PET ischemia or viability). Of the 19 documented clinical infarctions, 14 were classified as PET infarction. ECG localization of infarction was possible in 13 patients; PET and ECG location of infarction corresponded in all 13. Of the 5 patients in whom PET infarction was not detected, 2 had recent inferior infarctions and 3 had non–Q wave infarctions. However, the 3 patients with non–Q wave infarctions had PET studies that demonstrated PET viability. PET studies in 10 patients identified 11 myocardial regions with PET viability. Eight of these 10 patients had angina at rest and 1 had exertional angina; the patient without angina had right ventricular PET viability. Seven of the 8 patients with angina at rest had ECG or hemodynamic changes during angina. In the 9 patients in whom ECG localization of the infarct was possible, PET viability was present in the distribution of the coronary artery supplying the infarcted myocardium in 5 and in another coronary artery in 3; 1 patient had PET viability in both infarcted and remote myocardium.

To investigate acute myocardial infarction PET studies as described above were performed in 13 patients an average of 54 ± 12 hours after the onset of symptoms.[31] In 12 patients electrocardiographic Q waves developed, 10 anteriorly, 1 inferiorly, and 1 inferoposteriorly; in the 13th patient left bundle branch block (LBBB) precluded electrocardiographic infarct localization. Two patients had ECG evidence of prior inferior infarction. PET infarct or ischemia was identified in all patients in the anatomic regions of acute infarction identified by the ECG. One of the prior inferior infarctions was not identified by PET. However, PET enabled identification of involvement of the septal, apical, and lateral myocardium in patients with acute anterior myocardial infarction by ECG. Patients in whom wall motion subsequently improved all had areas of FDG uptake.

To investigate "reciprocal" ST segment depression during acute myocardial infarction, Billadello and colleagues obtained ^{11}C-palmitate images starting at least 3 minutes after injection in 20 patients an average of 9 ± 7 hours (range 3.5 to 27) after the onset of symptoms.[32] Repeat studies were performed an average of 14 ± 7 days (range 5 to 30) later. None of the 7 patients with anterior infarction had ST depression in the inferior leads. Nine of the 13 (69%) patients with inferior infarction had ST

TABLE 1. PET as an Aid to Understanding the Electrocardiogram: Acute Myocardial Infarction

	Number of Pts	Number of MIs	Number of MIs by ECG	Number of MI by PET	MI not detected by PET	Comments
Marshall[30]	15	19	13	14	2 inferior 3 non-Q	3 non-Q-wave 1 LBBB
Schwaiger[31]	13	15	12	14	1 inferior	12 Q-wave 1 LBBB
Geltman[34]	24 non-Q	24	22	23	1 anterolateral	3 PET & ECG different
	22 Q	22	22	22		

depression in the anterior precordial leads. Myocardial damage tended to be larger in patients with inferior infarction and anterior ST segment depression than in those without as evaluated by magnitude of inferior ST segment elevation, peak plasma MB creatine kinase activity, and estimated infarct size by PET. Three of the 9 patients with inferior infarction and anterior ST segment depression demonstrated decreased ^{11}C-palmitate uptake anteriorly, and in two of these patients partial improvement was seen on the repeat study. However, all 3 patients had left anterior descending coronary artery disease ≥50% (one was completely occluded) and all 3 had an anterior wall motion abnormality. Therefore, the decreased ^{11}C-palmitate uptake anteriorly may have reflected decreased blood flow. A second set of ^{11}C-palmitate images obtained at a later time (e.g., 40 minutes after injection) would have enabled evaluation of the presence or absence of ischemia.

To investigate acute subendocardial infarction nine patients were studied with ^{13}N-ammonia and evaluation of wall motion.[33] In the five patients with lateral subendocardial infarction by ECG, three had decreased blood flow in the posterolateral and two in the anteroseptal myocardium; all wall motion abnormalities were in the location identified by PET. In the three patients with anteroseptal subendocardial infarction by ECG, two had decreased blood flow in the posterolateral and one in the anteroseptal myocardium; concordant wall motion abnormalities were present in the former two and absent in the latter patient. The patient with inferior subendocardial infarction by ECG had concordant decrease in blood flow and wall motion in the posterolateral myocardium. Thus, the location of ECG changes did not always predict the site of decreased PET blood flow.

[11]C-Palmitate images were obtained in 24 patients with non-Q and 22 patients with Q wave infarction an average of 31 days (range 3–46) after non–Q wave infarction and an average of 42 days (range 2–175) after Q wave infarction.[34] The PET area of infarction was defined as myocardium that contained <50% of the maximal myocardial radioactivity. PET infarction was detected in all patients with Q wave infarction and in 23 of 24 (96%) of patients with non–Q wave infarction. The electrocardiographic site of non–Q wave infarction was indeterminate in two patients in whom PET identified the site, and in three patients PET identified a different area than the ECG.

Remote Myocardial Infarction

Early ^{11}C-palmitate imaging was performed as described above in 10 normals and 12 patients 3–12 months after Q-wave myocardial infarction.[35] Infarction was anterior in 6, lateral in 4, and posteroinferior in 2. Myocardial ^{11}C-palmitate uptake was homogeneous in normals. Areas of decreased ^{11}C-palmitate uptake were reported to correspond to the electrocardiographic site of infarction.

[13]N-Ammonia and FDG were injected at rest after oral glucose in 20 patients with prior Q wave myocardial infarction.[36] Patients were studied an average of 20.6 months (range 1 to 96 months) after their most recent infarction. Four ECG infarct regions were defined: septal, anterior, lateral, and inferior. Twenty-eight Q wave regions were identified on the stricter criteria for correlation of the ECG and PET regions. Of these 28 regions, 13 (46%) demonstrated PET infarction, 7 (25%) demonstrated PET viability (FIGURE 3), and 8 (29%) were normal by PET criteria. The only distinguishing clinical characteristic between patients with and without PET viability was the greater prevalence of three-vessel coronary artery disease in patients with PET viability (7/10 vs. 1/9; $p < 0.01$). Therefore, PET identifies viable myocardium in some regions identified as infarcted by the presence of Q waves on the ECG.

Myocardial blood flow was evaluated both at rest and during exercise, and FDG images were obtained at rest after fasting in 22 patients an average of 20 weeks (range 5 to 80) after anterior myocardial infarction determined by ECG and enzymes (TABLE 2).[37] ^{13}N-Ammonia was evaluated by circumferential profile analysis, and FDG images were interpreted visually. Decreased ^{13}N-ammonia uptake was observed in myocardium corresponding to the infarct site in 19 of 22 (86%) patients. PET infarction was

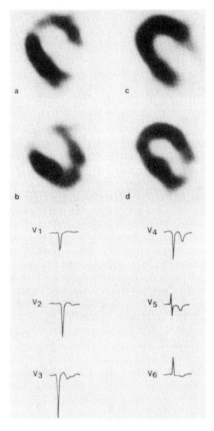

FIGURE 3. Precordial electrocardiographic leads (on bottom) and PET images at two myocardial levels (on top with the ^{13}N-ammonia images on the left and the [18]F 2-fluoro-2-deoxy-D-glucose images on the right) in a patient with a prior anterior myocardial infarction. QS waves are seen in leads V_{1-4}. Decreased ^{13}N-ammonia uptake is present anteriorly, but FDG uptake is present indicating the presence of viable myocardium. (Reproduced from Reference 36 with permission of the American Heart Association.)

not identified in 3 patients with non–Q wave infarction. During exercise the area of decreased ^{13}N-ammonia uptake became larger in 16 of 22 (73%) patients. Twelve of these 16 patients complained of angina and had ischemic electrocardiographic changes. Eighteen patients had PET viability, in 6 patients this occurred at the edges of the hypoperfused myocardium, and in 12 patients the entire area of hypoperfused myocar-

TABLE 2. PET as an Aid to Understanding the Electrocardiogram: Remote Myocardial Infarction

	Number of Pts	Defect on Resting 13 N-ammonia	Defect on Exercise 13 N-ammonia	Increased Resting FDG	Comments
Fudo[37]	22	19	16	10	All anterior
Hashimoto[38]	11 Q	11	22	4	19 anterior
					3 lateral
	11 non-Q	5	8	10	

dium demonstrated relatively increased FDG uptake. In general, the wall motion was less abnormal in patients with larger areas of FDG uptake.

Hashimoto and colleagues performed PET studies as described for the above study in 22 patients, 11 with prior Q wave and 11 with prior non–Q wave anterior (19) or lateral (3) myocardial infarction.[38] Patients were studied 1 to 24 months after their most recent infarction. All patients were taking nitrates and calcium channel blocking medication at the time of the PET study. All Q wave infarctions were anterior, and all these patients had decreased ^{13}N-ammonia uptake anteriorly both at rest and during exercise whereas only 4 (36%) patients had PET viability. In the 11 patients with non–Q wave infarctions, decreased ^{13}N-ammonia uptake in the regions of ECG abnormality was demonstrated in 5 patients (45%) at rest and 8 patients (73%) during exercise; PET viability was demonstrated in 10 patients (91%). Therefore, more viable myocardium was identified in patients with non–Q than Q wave myocardial infarction.

Yonekura and colleagues performed PET studies as described above in 26 patients.[39] They studied nine patients with a total of 10 remote myocardial infarctions (>3 months), two patients with remote and recent myocardial infarction (within 4–12 weeks), eight patients with recent myocardial infarction (one non–Q wave), and seven patients with effort angina. Of the 8 remote inferior and the 4 remote anterior myocardial infarctions, 2 in each group demonstrated some viable myocardium by PET. All patients with recent myocardial infarction demonstrated PET viability as did two patients with effort angina. The remaining five patients with effort angina had normal FDG uptake.

Preliminary data on Q wave septal infarction were obtained in 11 patients who underwent rest ^{13}N-ammonia and FDG studies after oral glucose.[40] Six of eight patients with visible collateral vessels on coronary arteriography had normal PET studies. In the three patients without visible collaterals, two had PET infarct and 1 had a normal PET study despite septal akinesis. Thus, the presence of septal collaterals may have a beneficial effect on myocardial viability.

Stress Studies

To evaluate the metabolic effects of pacing at a subanginal threshold, Grover-McKay and colleagues studied 10 patients with single vessel coronary artery disease with ^{11}C-palmitate time-activity curves obtained at rest and during pacing[41] (FIGURE 4). Two patients had a prior Q wave anterior myocardial infarction. Decreased uptake of ^{13}N-ammonia and ^{11}C-palmitate was seen in these 2 patients (FIGURE 5). None of the patients experienced angina during pacing for the ^{11}C-palmitate imaging, and only 2 of the 10 patients developed ≤2 mm flat or downsloping ST depression. Myocardium supplied by either normal or by stenosed coronary arteries demonstrated similar

[11]C-palmitate time-activity curves at rest. However, during pacing, visual evaluation of myocardium supplied by a stenosed coronary artery revealed retention of ^{11}C-palmitate activity on the later images in 6 patients (FIGURES 2 and 5) and abnormal ^{11}C-palmitate time-activity curves (FIGURE 1); these findings are consistent with impairment of beta oxidation during pacing-induced ischemia.

To investigate the effect of exercise in patients with coronary artery disease on myocardial blood flow and exogenous glucose uptake, Camici and colleagues investigated rest and exercise myocardial blood flow with [82]Rb and FDG uptake 6 to 15 minutes after exercise when all variables, including myocardial blood flow, had returned to control values in 12 patients with coronary artery disease.[42] Results were compared with studies obtained in 10 normal volunteers. In the patients, the initial electrocardiograms were normal in 5, demonstrated prior inferior infarction in 4, prior anterior infarction in 1, and poor R wave progression in the precordial leads in 2. All 8 patients who exercised had angina, ischemic electrocardiographic changes, and reduced regional myocardial [82]Rb uptake. The regional myocardial [82]Rb uptake returned to control values within 5 to 14 minutes after the end of exercise. In 7 of 8 patients who performed exercise, [18]F 2-deoxyglucose uptake was increased in myocardial regions demonstrating reduced [82]Rb uptake, identifying ischemic glucose utilization in patients with exercise-induced ischemia.

To investigate exercise-induced ST segment elevation, Fudo and colleagues studied 27 patients with prior Q wave anterior myocardial infarction,[43] 13 of whom developed exercise-induced ST segment elevation. Patients were studied with rest and exercise ^{13}N-ammonia and at rest with FDG. A greater number of patients with ST segment elevation had not only exercise-induced decreases in regional ^{13}N-ammonia uptake but

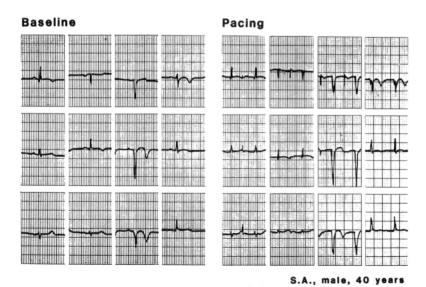

Baseline   **Pacing**

S.A., male, 40 years

FIGURE 4. Electrocardiograms at control (on left) and during pacing at a subanginal threshold in a patient with a prior Q wave anterior myocardial infarction as confirmed by the QS and inverted T waves in leads V_{1-4}. The patient had a residual 90% proximal stenosis of the left anterior descending coronary artery. During pacing the T wave became upright in lead V_2 but no ST segment depression or angina occurred.

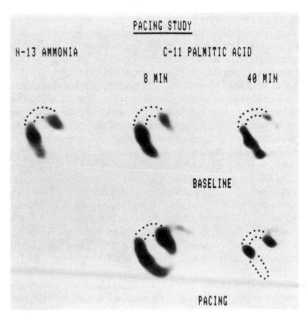

FIGURE 5. ^{13}N-ammonia and ^{11}C-palmitate images from the patient whose ECGs are seen in FIGURE 4. The images are displayed as in FIGURE 2. The dots delineate the infarcted myocardium anteriorly which has markedly decreased ^{13}N-ammonia and ^{11}C-palmitate uptake. During pacing, the 40-minute images demonstrate delayed ^{11}C-palmitate clearance in myocardium adjacent to the infarcted myocardium. (Reproduced from Reference 41 with permission of the American Heart Association.)

also increased regional FDG uptake indicating the presence of viable myocardium in patients who develop exercise-induced ST segment elevation.

To investigate ^{13}N-glutamate uptake at maximal exercise and compare its uptake with that of thallium-201 (^{201}Tl) Zimmermann and colleagues obtained images using a gamma camera in 25 patients with single vessel left anterior descending coronary artery disease, 14 of whom had prior myocardial infarction.[44] Eighteen of 25 (72%) patients exercised to angina and/or 1.5 mm horizontal or downsloping ST segment depression. The images in patients with prior myocardial infarction demonstrated a concordant decrease in ^{201}Tl and ^{13}N-glutamate; the decreased uptake was more severe in the 6 patients with Q wave than in the 8 patients with non–Q wave infarction. However, in patients without prior infarction, an inverse correlation existed between decreased ^{201}Tl and increased ^{13}N-glutamate uptake, consistent with the presence of viable myocardium.

Silent Ischemia

Deanfield and colleagues investigated 30 patients with stable angina (at least five times a week) and a positive exercise test.[45] Ambulatory ST segment monitoring was performed for four consecutive days in all patients, and technically adequate PET studies using ^{82}Rb during exercise, cold pressor testing, and during painless ST segment depression were obtained in 19 patients (FIGURE 6). During exercise until the onset of angina, all patients developed ST segment depression and reversibly decreased regional myocardial [82]Rb uptake. During cold pressor testing in 18 patients, 7 had a negative test and 2 developed ST segment depression (1 associated with angina); both of the latter patients had decreased regional myocardial [82]Rb uptake. In the other 9 patients, decreased regional myocardial [82]Rb uptake occurred without angina or ST segment depression. A spontaneous episode of transient ST segment depression developed in 3 patients, two of which were painless; all three episodes were associated with regional myocardial [82]Rb uptake. Therefore, abnormalities of myocardial blood flow could be detected by PET imaging with [82]Rb even in the absence of symptoms and/or electrocardiographic changes.

Shea and colleagues performed [82]Rb PET studies in 35 patients and 10 normals during cold pressor stimulation and during exercise.[46] During cold pressor stimulation, 24 of 35 patients developed decreased regional myocardial [82]Rb uptake although only 9 developed ST segment depression and only 7 experienced angina. All 29 patients who

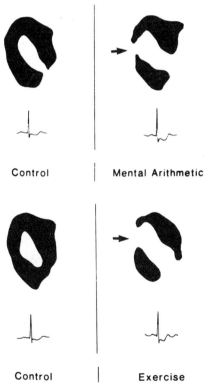

FIGURE 6. [82]Rubidium images and a single Holter ECG lead are shown at a single myocardial level at control and during mental arithmetic (on top) and during exercise (on bottom). At control, myocardial uptake of [82]Rb is homogeneous. Performance of mental arithmetic results in no symptoms, ST segment depression, and a regional decrease of [82]Rb uptake. Angina, in addition to similar ST segment depression and regional decrease of [82]Rb uptake, occurs during exercise. (Reproduced from Reference 17 with permission of the *American Journal of Cardiology*.)

performed exercise developed decreased regional myocardial ^{82}Rb uptake, 27 developed ST segment depression, and 25 experienced angina. Therefore, cold pressor testing produced more frequent asymptomatic episodes of decreased regional myocardial ^{82}Rb uptake than exercise.

Cardiomyopathy

Perloff and colleagues studied 15 boys with Duchenne muscular dystrophy.[47] All had electrocardiographic abnormalities consisting of increased right precordial R waves and increased R/S (13), abnormally deep Q waves in leads I, aVL, and V_{5-6} (9), and abnormal Q waves in leads II, III, and aVF (1) (FIGURE 7). In 13 of the 15 patients ^{13}N-ammonia was decreased in the posterior, posterolateral, or inferolateral left ventricular myocardium (FIGURE 8). Twelve FDG studies were adequate, and exogenous glucose uptake was increased in the areas of decreased ^{13}N-ammonia uptake in 11. Therefore, in patients with Duchenne muscular dystrophy, PET identifies abnormal blood flow and glucose utilization in areas identified as abnormal by the electrocardiogram.

Grover-McKay and colleagues studied patients with hypertrophic cardiomyopathy using ^{13}N-ammonia, ^{11}C-palmitate, and FDG.[48] Electrocardiograms in 2 of the 10 patients did not demonstrate left ventricular hypertrophy, 6 patents had deep Q waves in leads V_{3-6}, and two patients had an R/S ratio of 0.2 in V_1 (FIGURE 9). One patient, who also had coronary artery disease, had first degree atrioventricular block and right bundle branch block. Although ^{11}C-palmitate kinetics were similar in the hypertrophied septum compared to the lateral wall, ^{13}N-ammonia and FDG uptake in the septum compared with the lateral wall were decreased (FIGURE 10).

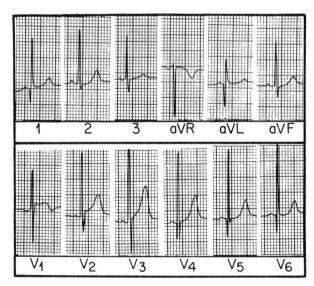

FIGURE 7. Electrocardiogram from a boy with Duchenne muscular dystrophy with deep Q waves in leads I, aVL, and V_{4-6} and a prominent R wave in V_1. (Reproduced from Reference 47 with permission of the American Heart Association.)

A   B

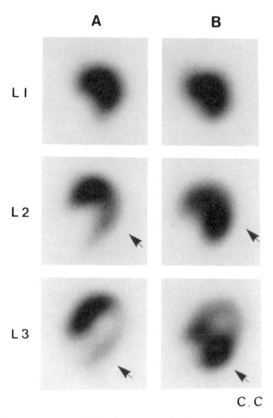

L 1

L 2

L 3

C . C

FIGURE 8. PET images in a boy with Duchenne muscular dystrophy. The myocardial levels are shown with the more cranial images at the top; ^{13}N-ammonia images are on the left and the [18]F 2-fluoro-2-deoxy-D-glucose images are on the right. Decreased ^{13}N-ammonia uptake is seen in the inferolateral wall (arrows); the corresponding FDG images demonstrate relatively increased uptake. (Reproduced from Reference 51 with permission of G. K. Hall Publishers.)

FUTURE DIRECTIONS

In conclusion, PET and ECG location of infarction correspond. However, PET viable myocardium can be demonstrated in some patients with Q wave and many patients with non–Q wave infarction. The presence of PET viable myocardium may identify patients in whom wall motion may subsequently improve, either spontaneously after acute myocardial infarction, or after intervention such as coronary artery bypass surgery. PET viability is also demonstrated in patients with exercise-induced ischemia by ECG.

Work is currently being performed to validate quantitation of regional myocardial blood flow with positron-emitting tracers.[13,49,50,52,53] When quantitation is possible, several important questions can be addressed. For example, at what absolute level of reduction in myocardial blood flow during exercise does the myocardium switch from aerobic to anaerobic metabolism and how does the severity of coronary artery disease

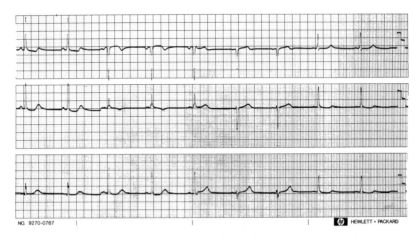

NO. 9270-0767   HEWLETT · PACKARD

FIGURE 9. Electrocardiogram from a patient with hereditary classic hypertrophic cardiomyopathy demonstrating left ventricular hypertrophy and an increased R wave in V_1 (note that precordial leads are recorded at half standard).

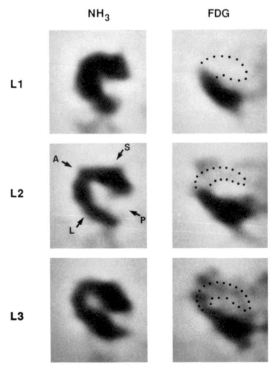

FIGURE 10. PET images acquired at rest in the patient whose electrocardiogram is shown in FIGURE 9. ^{13}N-ammonia images are on the left and the ^{18}F 2-fluoro-2-deoxy-D-glucose images are on the right. The septum (S), anterior (A) and lateral (L) walls, and posterior mitral valve (P) are indicated. Septal FDG uptake is decreased compared with septal ^{13}N-ammonia uptake. (Reproduced from Reference 48 with permission of the *Journal of the American College of Cardiology*.)

in different vascular territories affect this value? When does this switch occur relative to electrocardiographic evidence of ischemia? Other questions may not require a quantitative approach, such as, what factors help determine which patients may have residual viable myocardium both in Q wave and non–Q wave myocardial infarction? Can changes in blood flow and metabolism be detected in patients with hypertrophy or different types of cardiomyopathy, and, if so, how do these changes relate to electrocardiographic changes? Although PET has already shed new light on the pathophysiology underlying electrocardiographic changes, many more questions remain to be formulated and answered in order to answer basic scientific questions and to improve patient care.

REFERENCES

1. SULLIVAN, W., Z. VLODAVER, N. TUNA, L. LONG & J. E. EDWARDS. 1978. Correlation of electrocardiographic and pathologic findings in healed myocardial infarction. Am. J. Cardiol. **42:** 724–732.
2. WILLEMS, J., J. DRAULANS & H. DeGEEST. 1970. An appraisal of the Minnesota code in "inferior" myocardial infarction. J. Electrocardiol. **3:** 147.
3. PYOALA, K. & E. KENTALA. 1974. Disappearance of Minnesota Code Q-QS patterns in the first year after myocardial infarction. Ann. Clin. Res. **6:** 137–141.
4. SCHELBERT, H. R. & M. SCHWAIGER. 1986. PET studies of the heart. *In* Positron Emission Tomography and Autoradiography: Principles and Applications for the Brain and Heart. M. Phelps, J. Mazziotta, H. Schelbert, Eds.: 581–661. Raven Press. New York, N.Y.
5. GROVER-McKAY, M. 1988. Clinical applications of positron emission tomography in cardiology. *In* Cardiovascular Nuclear Medicine. K. P. Lyons, Ed.: 293–318. Appleton & Lange. Norwalk, Conn.
6. SCHELBERT, H. R., M. E. PHELPS, E. J. HOFFMAN, S. C. HUANG, C. E. SELIN & D. E. KUHL. 1979. Regional myocardial perfusion assessed with N-13 labeled ammonia and positron emission computerized axial tomography. Am. J. Cardiol. **43:** 209–218.
7. SCHELBERT, H. R., M. E. PHELPS, S. C. HUANG, N. S. MacDONALD, H. HANSEN, C. SELIN & D. E. KUHL. 1981. N-13 ammonia as an indicator of myocardial blood flow. Circulation **63:** 1259–1272.
8. SHAH, A., H. R. SCHELBERT, M. SCHWAIGER, E. HENZE, H. HANSEN, C. SELIN & S. C. HUANG. 1985. Measurement of regional myocardial blood flow with N-13 ammonia and positron-emission tomography in intact dogs. J. Am. Coll. Cardiol. **5:** 92–100.
9. BERGMANN, S. R., S. HACK, T. TEWSON, M. J. WELCH & B. E. SOBEL. 1980. The dependence of accumulation of $^{13}NH_3$ by myocardium on metabolic factors and its implications for quantitative assessment of perfusion. Circulation **61:** 34–43.
10. KRIVOKAPICH, J., S. C. HUANG, M. E. PHELPS, N. S. MacDONALD & K. I. SHINE. 1982. Dependence of $^{13}NH_3$ myocardial extraction and clearance on flow and metabolism. Am. J. Physiol. **242:** H536–H542.
11. RAUCH, B., F. HELUS, M. GRUNZE, E. BRAUNWELL, G. MALL, W. HASSELBACH & W. KÜBLER. 1985. Kinetics of ^{13}N-ammonia uptake in myocardial single cells indicating potential limitations in its applicability as a marker of myocardial blood flow. Circulation **71:** 387–393.
12. ROSENSPIRE, K. C., M. SCHWAIGER, T. J. MANGNER, G. D. HUTCHINS, A. SUTORIK & D. E. KUHL. 1990. Metabolic fate of [^{13}N] ammonia in human and canine blood. J. Nucl. Med. **31:** 163–167.
13. GROVER-McKAY, M., S. C. HUANG, E. J. HOFFMAN, M. E. PHELPS & H. R. SCHELBERT. 1986. Noninvasive quantification of myocardial blood flow in dogs with rubidium-82 and PET. J. Nucl. Med. **27:** 976 (abstr.).
14. MULLANI, N. A., R. A. GOLDSTEIN, K. L. GOULD, S. K. MARANI, D. J. FISHER, H. A. A. O'BRIEN, JR. & M. D. LOBERG. 1983. Perfusion imaging with rubidium-82: I. Measurement of extraction and flow with external detectors. J. Nucl. Med. **24:** 898–906.
15. GOLDSTEIN, R. A., N. A. MULLANI, S. K. MARANI, D. J. FISHER, K. L. GOULD & H. A. O'BRIEN, JR. 1983. Perfusion imaging with rubidium-82: II. Effects of pharmacologic interventions on flow and extraction. J. Nucl. Med. **24:** 907–915.

16. GROVER, M., M. H. SCHWAIGER, C. SELIN & H. R. SCHELBERT. 1984. Coronary artery occlusion and reperfusion alters rubidium-82 extraction fraction. Circulation 70: II-148 (abstr.).
17. SELWYN, A. P., R. M. ALLAN, A. L'ABBATE, P. HORLOCK, P. CAMICI, J. CLARK, H. A. O'BRIEN & P. M. GRANT. 1982. Relation between regional myocardial uptake of rubidium-82 and perfusion. Absolute reduction of cation uptake in ischemia. Am. J. Cardiol. 50: 112-121.
18. GOLDSTEIN, R. A. 1985. Kinetics of rubidium-82 after coronary occlusion and reperfusion. J. Clin. Invest. 75: 1131-1137.
19. GOLDSTEIN, R. A. 1986. Rubidium-82 kinetics after coronary occlusion: temporal relation of net myocardial accumulation and viability in open-chested dogs. J. Nucl. Med. 27: 1456-1461.
20. BERGMANN, S. R., K. A. A. FOX, A. L. RAND, M. D. MCELVANY, M. J. WELCH, J. MARKHAM & B. E. SOBEL. 1984. Quantification of regional myocardial blood flow in vivo with $H_2^{15}O$. Circulation 70: 724-733.
21. NEELY, J. R., M. J. ROVETTO & J. F. ORAM. 1972. Myocardial utilization of carbohydrate and lipids. Prog. Cardiovasc. Dis. 15: 289-329.
22. TAEGTMEYER, H. 1986. Myocardial metabolism. In Positron Emission Tomography and Autoradiography: Principles and Applications for the Brain and Heart. M. Phelps, J. Mazziotta, & H. Schelbert, Eds.: 149-195. Raven Press. New York, N.Y.
23. LIEDTKE, A. J. 1981. Alterations of carbohydrate and lipid metabolism in the acutely ischemic heart. Prog. Cardiovasc. Dis. 23: 321-336.
24. SCHON, H. R., H. R. SCHELBERT, G. ROBINSON, A. NAJAFI, S-C. HUANG, H. HANSEN, J. BARRIO, D. E. KUHL & M. E. PHELPS. 1982. C-11 labeled palmitic acid for the noninvasive evaluation of regional myocardial fatty acid metabolism with positron-computed tomography. I. Kinetics of C-11 palmitic acid in normal myocardium. Am. Heart J. 103: 532-547.
25. SCHON, H. R., H. R. SCHELBERT, A. NAJAFI, H. HANSEN, H. HUANG, J. BARRIO & M. E. PHELPS. 1982. C-11 labeled palmitic acid for the noninvasive evaluation of regional myocardial fatty acid metabolism with positron-computed tomography. II. Kinetics of C-11 palmitic acid in acutely ischemic myocardium. Am. Heart J. 103: 548-561.
26. FOX, K. A. A., D. R. ABENDSCHEIN, H. D. AMBOS, B. E. SOBEL & S. R. BERGMANN. 1985. Efflux of metabolized and nonmetabolized fatty acid from canine myocardium. Implications for quantifying myocardial metabolism tomographically. Circ. Res. 57: 232-243.
27. SCHWAIGER, M., H. R. SCHELBERT, R. KEEN, J. VINTEN-JOHANSEN, H. HANSEN, C. SELIN, J. BARRIO, S. C. HUANG & M. E. PHELPS. 1985. Retention and clearance of C-11 palmitic acid in ischemic and reperfused canine myocardium. J. Am. Coll. Cardiol. 6: 311-320.
28. SOKOLOFF, L., M. REIVICH, C. KENNEDY, M. H. DES ROSIERS, C. S. PATLAK, K. D. PETTIGREW, O. SAKURADA & M. SHINOBARA. 1977. The (^{14}C)-deoxyglucose method for the measurement of local cerebral glucose utilization: theory, procedure and normal values in the conscious and anesthetized albino rat. J. Neurochem. 28: 897-916.
29. SCHWAIGER, M., H. R. SCHELBERT, D. ELLISON, H. HANSEN, L. YEATMAN, J. VINTEN-JOHANSEN, C. SELIN, J. BARRIO & M. E. PHELPS. 1985. Sustained regional abnormalities in cardiac metabolism after transient ischemia in the chronic dog model. J. Am. Coll. Cardiol. 6: 336-347.
30. MARSHALL, R. C., J. H. TILLISCH, M. E. PHELPS, S. C. HUANG, R. CARSON, E. HENZE & H. R. SCHELBERT. 1983. Identification and differentiation of resting myocardial ischemia and infarction in man with positron computed tomography, ^{18}F-labeled fluorodeoxyglucose and N-13 ammonia. Circulation 67: 766-778.
31. SCHWAIGER, M., R. BRUNKEN, M. GROVER-MCKAY, J. KRIVOKAPICH, J. CHILD, J. H. TILLISCH, M. E. PHELPS & H. R. SCHELBERT. 1986. Regional myocardial metabolism in patients with acute myocardial infarction assessed by positron emission tomography. J. Am. Coll. Cardiol. 8: 800-808.
32. BILLADELLO, J. J., J. L. SMITH, P. A. LUDBROOK, A. J. TIEFENBRUNN, A. S. JAFFE, B. E. SOBEL & E. M. GELTMAN. 1983. Implications of "reciprocal" ST segment depression associated with acute myocardial infarction identified by positron tomography. J. Am. Coll. Cardiol. 2: 616-624.

33. PARODI, O., M. SCHWAIGER, J. KRIVOKAPICH & H. R. SCHELBERT. 1984. Regional myocardial blood flow and wall motion study in patients with designated acute "subendocardial infarction." J. Am. Coll. Cardiol. 3: 552 (abstr.).

34. GELTMAN, E. M., D. BIELLO, M. J. WELCH, M. M. TER-POGOSSIAN, R. ROBERTS & B. E. SOBEL. 1982. Characterization of nontransmural myocardial infarction by positron-emission tomography. Circulation 65: 747–755.

35. SOBEL, B. E., E. S. WEISS, M. J. WELCH, B. A. SIEGEL & M. M. TER-POGOSSIAN. 1977. Detection of remote myocardial infarction in patients with positron emission transaxial tomography and intravenous ^{11}C-palmitate. Circulation 55: 853–857.

36. BRUNKEN, R., J. TILLISCH, M. SCHWAIGER, J. S. CHILD, R. MARSHALL, M. MANDELKERN, M. E. PHELPS & H. R. SCHELBERT. 1986. Regional perfusion, glucose metabolism, and wall motion in patients with chronic electrocardiographic Q wave infarctions: evidence for persistence of viable tissue in some infarct regions by positron emission tomography. Circulation 73: 951–963.

37. FUDO, T., H. KAMBARA, T. HASHIMOTO, M. HAYASHI, R. NOHARA, N. TAMAKI, Y. YONEKURA, M. SENDA, J. KONISHI & C. KAWAI. 1988. F-18 deoxyglucose and stress N-13 ammonia positron emission tomography in anterior wall healed myocardial infarction. Am. J. Cardiol. 61: 1191–1197.

38. HASHIMOTO, T., H. KAMBARA, T. FUDO, M. HAYASHI, S. TAMAKI, S. TOKUNAGA, N. TAMAKI, Y. YONEKURA, J. KONISHI & C. KAWAI. 1988. Non-Q wave versus Q wave myocardial infarction: regional myocardial metabolism and blood flow assessed by positron emission tomography. J. Am. Coll. Cardiol. 12: 88–93.

39. YONEKURA, Y., N. TAMAKI, H. KAMBARA, M. SENDA, H. SAJI, T. BAN, C. KAWAI & J. KONISHI. 1988. Detection of metabolic alterations in ischemic myocardium by F-18 fluorodeoxyglucose uptake with positron emission tomography. Am. J. Cardiac Imaging 2: 122–132.

40. BRUNKEN, R., M. SCHWAIGER, J. CHILD, J. TILLISCH, R. MARSHALL & H. R. SCHELBERT. 1985. Septal metabolism, wall motion and collateral blood flow in ECG septal infarcts. J. Am. Coll. Cardiol. 5: 386 (abstr.).

41. GROVER-MCKAY, M., H. R. SCHELBERT, M. SCHWAIGER, H. SOCHOR, P. M. GUZY, J. KRIVOKAPICH, J. S. CHILD & M. E. PHELPS. 1986. Identification of impaired metabolic reserve by atrial pacing in patients with significant coronary artery disease. Circulation 74: 281–292.

42. CAMICI, P., L. I. ARAUJO, T. SPINKS, A. A. LAMMERTSMA, J. C. KASKI, M. J. SHEA, A. P. SELWYN, T. JONES & A. MASERI. 1986. Increased uptake of ^{18}F-fluorodeoxyglucose in postischemic myocardium of patients with exercise-induced angina. Circulation 74: 81–88.

43. FUDO, T., H. KAMBARA, M. HAYASHI, T. HASHIMOTO, R. NOHARA, N. TAMAKI, K. YAMASHITA, J. KONISHI & C. KAWAI. 1989. Significance of exercise-induced ST-segment elevation in patients with Q wave anterior myocardial infarction: evaluation by positron emission tomography. J. Am. Coll. Cardiol. 13: 203A (abstr.).

44. ZIMMERMAN, R., H. TILLMANNS, W. H. KNAPP, F. HELUS, P. GEORGI, B. RAUCH, F. J. NEUMANN, S. GIRGENSOHN, W. MAIER-BORST & W. KÜBLER. 1988. Regional myocardial nitrogen-13 glutamate uptake in patients with coronary artery disease: inverse post-stress relation to thallium-201 uptake in ischemia. J. Am. Coll. Cardiol. 11: 549–556.

45. DEANFIELD, J. E., A. P. SELWYN, S. CHIERCHIA, A. MASERI, P. RIBEIRO, S. KRIKLER & M. MORGAN. 1983. Myocardial ischaemia during daily life in patients with stable angina: its relation to symptoms and heart rate changes. Lancet 2: 753–758.

46. SHEA, M. J., J. E. DEANFIELD, C. M. DELANDSHEERE, R. A. WILSON, M. KENSETT & A. P. SELWYN. 1987. Asymptomatic myocardial ischemia following cold provocation. Am. Heart J. 114: 469–476.

47. PERLOFF, J. K., E. HENZE & H. R. SCHELBERT. 1984. Alterations in regional myocardial metabolism, perfusion and wall motion in Duchenne's muscular dystrophy studied by radionuclide imaging. Circulation 69: 33–42.

48. GROVER-MCKAY, M., M. SCHWAIGER, J. KRIVOKAPICH, P. K. PERLOFF, M. E. PHELPS & H. R. SCHELBERT. 1989. Regional myocardial blood flow and metabolism at rest in mildly

symptomatic patients with hypertrophic cardiomyopathy. J. Am. Coll. Cardiol. **13:** 317–324.

49. KRIVOKAPICH, J., G. T. SMITH, S. C. HUANG, E. J. HOFFMAN, O. RATIB, M. E. PHELPS & H. R. SCHELBERT. 1989. [13]N ammonia myocardial imaging at rest and with exercise in normal volunteers: quantification of absolute myocardial perfusion with dynamic positron emission tomography. Circulation **80:** 1328–1337.

50. ARAUJO, L., E. O. MCFALLS, A. LAMMERTSMA, T. JONES, G. PUPITA & A. MASERI. 1989. Quantitative measurement of myocardial blood flow and coronary flow reserve in patients with CAD employing O-15 water and positron emission tomography (PET). J. Am. Coll. Cardiol. **13:** 97A (abstr.).

51. GROVER, M. & H. R. SCHELBERT. 1985. Assessment of regional myocardial substrate metabolism with positron emission tomography. *In* New Concepts in Cardiac Imaging: 158–182. G. K. Hall Medical Publishers. Boston, Mass.

52. GAMBIR, S. S., M. SCHWAIGER, S. C. HUANG, J. KRIVOKAPICH, H. R. SCHELBERT, C. A. NIENABER & M. E. PHELPS. 1989. Simple noninvasive quantification method for measuring myocardial glucose utilization in humans employing positron emission tomography and fluorine-18 deoxyglucose. J. Nucl. Med. **30:** 359–366.

53. BERGMANN, S. R., P. HERRERO, J. MARKHAM, C. J. WEINHEIMER & M. N. WALSH. 1989. Noninvasive quantitation of myocardial blood flow in human subjects with oxygen-15 labeled water and positron emission tomography. J. Am.Coll. Cardiol. **14:** 639–652.

Magnetic Resonance Imaging as a Noninvasive Standard for the Quantitative Evaluation of Left Ventricular Mass, Ischemia, and Infarction[a]

JAMES L. WEISS, EDWARD P. SHAPIRO,
MAURICE B. BUCHALTER, AND RAFAEL BEYAR[b]

Cardiology Division
Department of Medicine
The Johns Hopkins
Medical Institutions
Baltimore, Maryland 21205

INTRODUCTION

Magnetic resonance imaging (MRI) acquires data in a spatially unambiguous manner, and the three-dimensional interrelationships of one image plane to another are easily ascertained in a manner much less cumbersome than with other imaging techniques, including echocardiography. There are far fewer technical restrictions imposed on this method than on other imaging techniques. In addition, the quality of images, so frequently limited in echocardiography, is more uniformly high with MRI. MRI is thus well suited to the highly accurate quantification of both global and regional left ventricular (LV) size and function, and might thereby be used as a standard for comparison to other techniques, such as electrocardiography, once validated. Nonetheless, accurate assessment of regional function and structure in all regions of the left ventricle requires solution to a series of problems inherent in any tomographic imaging approach. The three-dimensional nature of MRI acquisition permits a possible solution to these problems by the use of several interlocking but differing methodologies, which we will review below. This review will take a tripartite approach. We will first address the capability of magnetic resonance imaging to determine left ventricular mass in normal hearts, and in hearts distorted by severe transmural myocardial infarction, with a degree of accuracy previously unavailable by noninvasive techniques. The second subject for review will be improved quantification of regional wall thickening by a three-dimensional (3D) volume element approach. This approach to regional wall thickening accounts for a three-dimensional geometric characteristic of the left ventricle in a reconstructed volume element, rather than depending simply on the thickening of a single planar slice. Finally, we will review a new MRI method designed to improve quantification of regional left ventricular function, myocardial tissue tagging, which, in essence, is an MRI electronic marker

[a]Supported in part by National Heart, Lung and Blood Institute, Ischemic Heart Disease SCOR grant 2P50-HL-17655-14, and RO1-HL-33385.
[b]Present affiliation: Technion—Israel Institute of Technology, Department of Biomedical Engineering, Haifa 32 000, Israel.

applied to the myocardium, riding with it and persisting through ejection, which enables tracking of specific areas of the myocardium through the cardiac cycle.

LEFT VENTRICULAR MASS DETERMINATION BY MAGNETIC RESONANCE IMAGING

A number of noninvasive techniques have played important roles in the accurate determination of left ventricular mass in both man and experimental animals. Of these methods, echocardiography is the most widely available; both M-mode[1] and two-dimensional[2,3] techniques have been found to be accurate when compared against actual measurements of LV mass. However, most of these studies have used model systems that depend heavily on geometric assumptions. These assumptions may not always be accurate, especially in hearts distorted by disease processes such as infarction or congenital malformations. Specialized techniques utilizing three-dimensional reconstruction methodologies obviate the need for using such geometric assumptions.[4,5] However, these methods are cumbersome and, like all echocardiographic studies, are ultimately limited by image quality which is not uniformly high in all patient groups. Prior studies[6-8] have demonstrated the accuracy of MRI in determining LV mass in normally shaped, noninfarcted hearts, but not in hearts that have undergone deformation by ischemic or other processes. Because of the inherent three-dimensionality of MR image acquisition, as well as the known three-dimensional interrelations of one image plane to another, MRI seemed suitable for measuring LV mass in abnormally shaped hearts distorted by acute myocardial infarction. We determined the accuracy of MRI measurements of left ventricular mass in *in vivo* canine hearts with shape abnormalities induced by acute myocardial infarction.[9] Gated MRI was performed in 15 dogs before and after acute myocardial infarction. The LV mass of each dog was calculated by a Simpson's reconstruction approach from 5 short axis images acquired at end-systole, when shape distortion is greatest, and at end-diastole, and also from slices at varying phases of the cycle with a multiphase mode requiring only one acquisition. Correlation was excellent between actual (weighed) mass and end-systolic mass before infarction ($r = 0.98, p = < 0.001$, standard error of the estimate [SEE] = 5.1 g) and after infarction ($r = 0.97, p = < 0.001$, SEE = 6.6 g). Likewise, values correlated closely at end-diastole before ($r = 0.96, p < 0.001$, SEE = 6.7 g) and after infarction ($r = 0.094, p = 0.001$, SEE = 8.7 g). Surprisingly, measurements of mass by a multiphase image acquisition mode were also highly accurate both before and after infarction. An example of regression plots of LV mass by actual weight and by magnetic resonance imaging (multislice acquisition) is seen in FIGURE 1. At the same phase and at multiple phases of the cardiac cycle, MRI thus permits highly accurate determination of LV mass, even in severely deformed hearts. Significant distortion was produced in many cases by injecting a biologically inert polymer (dental rubber) into the left anterior descending coronary artery. This viscous polymer occluded antegrade and retrograde collateral flow into the risk region and resulted in dense transmural infarction.[10] The extent of left ventricular shape distortion was profound in these hearts, as verified at postmortem examination. Despite this profound change in LV shape, MRI mass calculations were nonetheless accurate. Using the multislice mode, MR imaging for this purpose can be performed in a relatively brief period of time, approximately 15 minutes. Calculations of LV mass by this technique are simple and accomplished easily on either the MRI measurement software or on a personal computer. Because of its high degree of accuracy, MRI may become a noninvasive standard for comparison to other techniques seeking to quantify left ventricular mass.

MRI IN THE QUANTITATIVE ASSESSMENT OF ISCHEMIA AND INFARCTION

Three-Dimensional Volume Element Approach to the Quantification of Left Ventricular Wall Thickening

Previous studies using echocardiography have shown that regional LV dysfunction can be detected based on wall motion abnormalities or regional LV wall thickening.[11,12] The latter has been shown to be more precise than the former in detecting infarcted regions.[12] However, the typical echocardiographic window may be limited to views not optimal for evaluation of wall thickening. In addition, epicardial borders, which are essential for thickening measurements, are not always detectable. A further limitation in the measurement of thickness or thickening by echocardiography, as well as with other planar imaging methods, is the oblique course of the plane of the cross-sectional image through the LV wall, especially near the apex. This obliquity results in

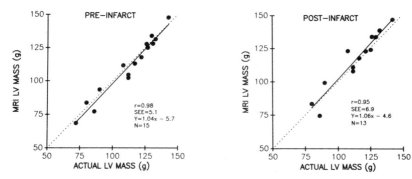

FIGURE 1. Regression plots of left ventricular (LV) mass by actual weight and by magnetic resonance image (MRI) calculation with multislice acquisition. Each slice is acquired at a different phase of the cardiac cycle. Preinfarction and postinfarction data are shown. The dotted line represents the line of identity. (Reproduced from Reference 9 by permission.)

overestimation of wall thickness by "in plane" analysis methods. Furthermore, any change in the tilt of the LV wall with regard to the image plane between end-diastole and end-systole will affect the accuracy of thickening measurements considerably.

The potential of magnetic resonance imaging for detecting regions of wall thickening abnormalities in patients has been demonstrated previously.[13–15] In these studies, several potential sources of error were not assessed, including the above-described "in-plane" analysis problem. To overcome these limitations, we have developed a method to quantify and map regional wall thickening throughout the LV with magnetic resonance imaging. In contrast to those methods that measure planar wall thickness and thickening, this method uses the three-dimensional geometry of the LV to calculate the "perpendicular" thickness of the wall.[16] FIGURE 2 shows a schematic representation of a three-dimensional volume element between two imaging planes. With this technique, the average perpendicular thickness may be computed from any two adjacent planar images (FIGURE 2). We tested this method at three levels of increasing complexity using (1) phantom studies, (2) in vivo experiments in dogs with normal cardiac function, and (3) in vivo studies in dogs during acute ischemia.

Image plane 1

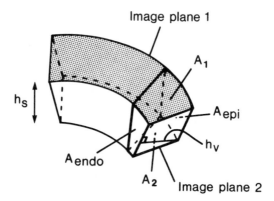

FIGURE 2. Schematic representation of a three-dimensional volume element between two image planes. Image planes 1 and 2 represent any two adjacent cross-sectional image planes. The average perpendicular thickness (h_v) is computed by dividing its volume by the mean of the endocardial and epicardial areas (A_{endo} A_{epi}). h_s, distance between imaging planes. Actual calculations of endocardial and epicardial segment lengths are based on linear approximations of curved edges. A_1 and A_2, areas of the top and bottom of the volume element, respectively. Image planes 1 and 2 represent any two adjacent cross-sectional image planes. (Reproduced from Reference 16 by permission.)

Experiments were conducted in 15 open-chest dogs imaged on a 0.38 T iron core magnet. Five short axis images in end-diastole and end-systole were obtained with the spin echo technique by use of the QRS as a trigger for end-diastole and the second heart sound, S_2, to time end-systole. After acquisition of preischemic images, acute ischemia was induced by either coronary artery ligation or intracoronary dental rubber injection which, as described previously, produces severe transmural ischemia. By computer-aided contouring of the endo- and epicardial borders, each cross-sectional image was divided into 16 segments with radial lines originating from the mid-wall centroid. A 3D volume element was defined as that generated by connecting two matched planar segments in two adjacent image planes (FIGURE 2). This defined 64 volume elements comprising the entire LV. Thickness and thickening before and during ischemia were then calculated by using the planar segments and the 3D volume elements.

In phantom studies, the 3D method was accurate, and independent of the angle of inclination of the image to the phantom wall, whereas the planar method showed considerable overestimation of the thickness when the image plane was oblique to the phantom wall (FIGURE 3). In the dogs before induction of ischemia, the 3D method demonstrated the well-established normal taper in end-diastolic wall thickness from 1.10 ± 0.02 cm at the base to 1.05 ± 0.11 cm at the apex ($p < 0.01$). By contrast, the planar method did not detect the decrease in thickness toward the apex (1.13 ± 0.07 cm at the base vs. 1.16 ± 0.14 cm at the apex, $p = NS$). During acute ischemia, thickening was calculated by both methods at the center of the ischemic zone defined by Monastral blue nonstaining and compared with the preischemic values. There was no overlap between the baseline and ischemic values of percent thickening with 3D method ($38.7 \pm 14.1\%$ [range, 17%–85%] vs. $-12.8 \pm 13.0\%$ [range, -40 to $+13\%$], $p < 0.001$), whereas there was considerable overlap (34 of 80 regions) with the planar method (FIGURE 4).

Without the three-dimensional volume element approach to regional wall thickness and thickening, planar methods thus overestimate perpendicular thickness, especially when the image plane is oblique to the structure being imaged, such as the left ventricular apex. Prior existing imaging methods of calculating wall thickness and thickening have based their calculations on measurements made in the plane of the image. Although this problem is amplified toward the apex and may not be apparent at the midventricular level for the normal heart, it may nonetheless introduce significant error if the image plane is not strictly perpendicular to the wall or if the heart is distorted by a disease process such as a transmural infarct, ventricular aneurysm, or certain congenital malformations. Therefore, a method of measuring thickness that is independent of the angle between the image plane and the LV wall should enhance significantly the accuracy of thickness measurements. The method described is designed to overcome this limitation by being independent of the angle between the measured structure and the image plane. The three-dimensional volume element approach to the quantification of wall thickness and thickening results in less variability of normal thickening, and better discrimination of ischemic from nonischemic zones in a model of acute ischemia. Future validation studies will be undertaken to determine whether the volume element approach allows a clearer distinction between infarcted and noninfarcted myocardium. If so validated, this method could serve as a useful standard for comparison to other noninvasive techniques of assessing ischemia and infarction.

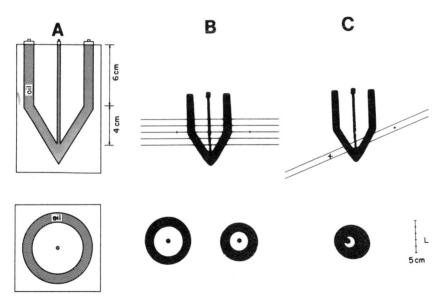

FIGURE 3. Schematic representation of an oil-filled cylindrical/conical phantom simulating the left ventricle and used for validation of wall thickness measurements in relation to the image planes. Panel A: Diagram of the phantom (1 cm constant thickness). Panel B: Magnetic resonance images of long (top) and short (bottom) axis. The planar images through the conical ("apical") portion overestimate wall thickness (bottom right). Panel C: Apparent circumferential thickness asymmetry generated by an oblique plane traversing the conical ("apical") portion of the phantom. (Reproduced from Reference 16 by permission.)

MRI Myocardial Tissue Tagging

Myocardial tissue tagging is a new magnetic resonance imaging technique, and unavailable with other imaging modalities.[17] Tagging labels specific regions of myocardium just prior to image acquisition. FIGURE 5 shows two images of the heart of an anesthetized dog (1.5 T GE scanner). These cross-sectional images show eight equidistant tags emanating from the left ventricular cavity. Myocardial tags traverse the heart and surrounding fixed structures which serve as a stable reference to enable tracking of the heart itself. We hypothesized that tags could be used to quantify rigid body motion, deformation, and torsion noninvasively and that, furthermore, such quantification would improve measures of regional function without contamination by different

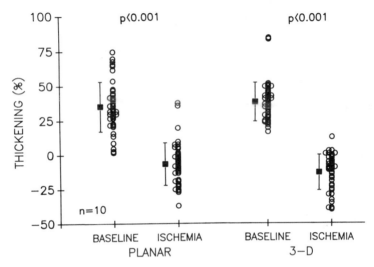

FIGURE 4. Plot of thickening in the center of the ischemic zone (1 slice, 4 segments) versus baseline thickening (same zone) in 10 dogs by the three-dimensional volume element and planar methods. The 3D method resulted in no overlap between the preschemic and ischemic values of percent thickening ($38.7 \pm 14.1\%$ [range, 17% to 85%] versus $-12.8 \pm 13.0\%$ [range, -40% to $+13\%$], $p < 0.001$), whereas there was considerable overlap (34 of 80 regions) with the planar method ($35.5 \pm 18\%$ [range, 3%–75%] versus $-6.3 \pm 15.6\%$ [range, -35% to $+40\%$], $p < 0.001$). (Reproduced from Reference 16 by permission.)

segments of myocardium through the cardiac cycle. Rather, we would be comparing identical segments. Tagging is achieved by selective radiofrequency saturation of thin planes intersecting the myocardium perpendicular to the cross-sectional image (FIGURE 6). In the tagged regions, protons are in a different state of magnetization from surrounding tissues. This produces a contrasting signal (FIGURE 5) which appears as a contrasting stripe embedded or inscribed in the myocardium and surrounding stationary structures. Applied at end-diastole, tags persist for up to 500 mseconds, thus enabling tracking of tags throughout ejection. It is thus possible to track any intervening displacement or deformation of the tag lines as a change in the tag position or shape relative to their end-diastolic positions. We can thus compare where the tags *were at* end-diastole to where they *are* at end-systole. Thus, as seen in FIGURE 5, nonuniform counterclockwise rotation of a cross-sectional slice of myocardium is evident. Regional

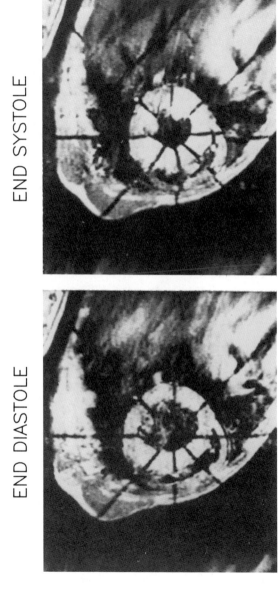

END DIASTOLE   END SYSTOLE

FIGURE 5. End-diastolic and end-systolic magnetic resonance images, cross-sectional views (GE Signa scanner, 1.5 T). Mid–left ventricular views, showing 8 equidistant tags (dark stripes) emanating from the left ventricular cavity. The tags traverse the heart and the surrounding fixed structures which serve as a stable reference to enable tracking of the heart itself. The myocardial tags, appearing as contrasting stripes, are actually embedded or inscribed in the myocardium and surrounding stationary structures. Tagging in this example shows counterclockwise rotation when comparing the end-systolic position of the myocardial tags, particularly in the inferoseptal region, to the position of the corresponding tag lines as they traverse fixed extracardiac structures. A small oil-filled balloon, seen as a bright dot sewn to the epicardium at approximately 2 o'clock, bears a constant relationship to the underlying tag line.

counterclockwise rotation is seen when comparing the end-diastolic position of the myocardial tags in the inferoseptal region to the position of the corresponding tags as they traverse the fixed noncardiac structures.

It has been postulated previously that rotation of the LV apex with respect to the base is a component of normal systolic function,[18] but until now it has not been possible to measure it noninvasively. Myocardial tissue tagging provides the means to quantify such torsion. A diagrammatic representation of the cross section of the left ventricular base and any lower cross section is depicted in FIGURE 7. This diagram defines what we mean by LV torsion. It is the angular rotation (α) of a tag line with respect to its fixed counterpart at the base of the left ventricle. Thus, torsion is a regional, nonuniform effect, not just rigid body rotation of the heart in its entirety. Eight normal volunteers were imaged in a resistive iron core magnet.[19,20] Five short-axis LV images were obtained at end-systole. Four equiangular tags were applied at end-diastole, intersecting the myocardium at eight locations. We calculated the difference in angular displacement of each endo- and epicardial tag point at end-systole from the systolic position of the corresponding tag point in the basal plane (FIGURE 8). This value was called the torsion angle. The mean torsion angles on the apical slice relative to the mean torsion angles of the base for the endocardial and epicardial points are seen in FIGURE 8. Mean endocardial torsion was 19.1 ± 2.0° (counterclockwise), and exceeded mean epicardial torsion (also counterclockwise, 11.0 ± 1.3°). From base to apex, endocardial torsion exceeded epicardial torsion at each cross-sectional level, and both endo- and epicardial torsion increased progressively from base to apex, the base remaining stationary through the cardiac cycle, and the apex showing the greatest degree of counterclockwise torsion. Furthermore, torsion in the anterolateral region exceeded that in the posteroseptal region for both endocardium and epicardium.

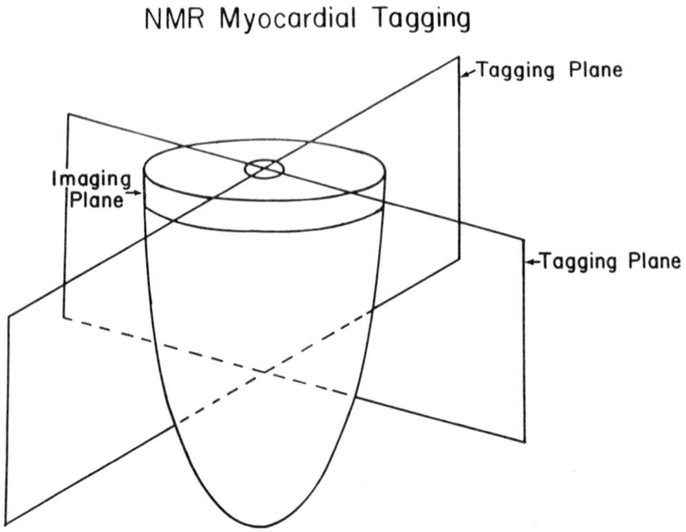

FIGURE 6. Simplified diagram of two myocardial tag planes. Tagging is achieved by selective radiofrequency saturation of thin planes intersecting the myocardium perpendicular to the cross-sectional slice, in this case at the base of the left ventricle. Here, only two planes are shown for simplification. Usually, 4 to 6 equidistant tag planes are used, producing 8–12 equidistant tag lines.

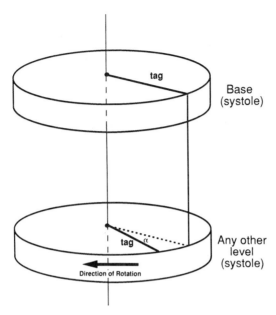

FIGURE 7. Diagram defining left ventricular torsion. This is a representation of a cross section of the base of the left ventricle and any lower cross section, at end-systole. Torsion is depicted as the angular rotation (α) of the tag line at the lower cross section with respect to the corresponding tag line at the base of the LV. Torsion is thus a regional effect, not simply rigid body rotation of the heart in its entirety.

We have recently sought to characterize the hemodynamic determinants of torsion in the anesthetized dog, and have found in-plane and through-plane heterogeneity, with progressively increasing degrees of counterclockwise torsion towards the apex with respect to the fixed base, much as in the normal human studies. Furthermore, we have found that torsion increases with increasing inotropy and with decreased load; increases slightly with higher heart rates; and diminishes markedly or reverses with regional ischemia.[21,22]

Thus, we can conclude that regional myocardial torsion is measurable noninvasively in humans, as documented by tagging, and that its undetected presence could confound measures of regional function, such as wall thickening. We feel we have the means to explore the precise approaches to quantification of regional left ventricular function and wall thickening by magnetic resonance, using the combined methodologies described. These methods may eventually serve as standards for comparison to other noninvasive techniques in the assessment of myocardial ischemia and infarction.

SUMMARY

Because magnetic resonance imaging (MRI) acquires data in a spatially unambiguous fashion and the three-dimensional interrelationships of one image plane to another are easily ascertained, there are far fewer technical restrictions imposed on this method than on other imaging techniques. Furthermore, the multiplanar nature of MRI image acquisition, in any plane desired, is a feature unique to this imaging technology. MRI is thus well suited to the highly accurate quantification of global and regional left ventricular (LV) size and function, and can be used as a standard for comparison to other techniques, once validated. Because the determination of LV mass by MRI requires no assumptions about ventricular shape, it should be well suited to the evaluation of both normal hearts and those distorted by infarction. We performed gated MRI on 15 dogs before and after myocardial infarction. LV mass was calculated with 5 short axis planes. The correlation was excellent between actual mass before infarction and after MI. Accuracy was similar for both end-diastole and end-systole. Thus, MRI accurately determines LV mass in both distorted and normal hearts. We have also developed a method for quantification and mapping of regional wall thickening throughout the LV as an index of regional ischemia by utilizing the 3D geometry to calculate the perpendicular wall thickness of a 3D volume element of

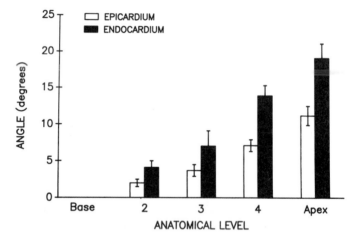

FIGURE 8. Mean torsion angles of the epicardium and endocardium of 5 cross-sectional LV slices (± standard error). Through-plane inhomogeneity of torsion is seen. With respect to the fixed base, progressive increase in torsion, in the counterclockwise direction, is seen at each succeeding level towards the apex, being greatest there. Further, at each level, endocardial exceeds epicardial torsion. The difference in torsion angle between slices is significant both for epicardium ($p < 0.001$) and endocardium ($p < 0.001$). Endocardial torsion angles are greater than epicardial ($p < 0.001$). ANOVA. (Reproduced from Reference 19 by permission.)

tissue. This 3D volume element results in less variability of normal wall thickening and provides a better discriminator of ischemic from nonischemic zones in a canine model of acute ischemia, whereas there is considerably greater overlap between ischemic and normal zones with standard planar MRI techniques. The 3D method is more accurate than planar methods in avoiding biases resulting from the oblique course of an image plane through the LV wall, resulting in better distinction of ischemic from nonischemic tissue. Finally, the accurate assessment of regional LV function for the identification of ischemic or infarcted myocardium has been enhanced greatly by a new technique, myocardial tissue tagging, in which an electronic marker is applied to the myocardium which persists through ejection, enabling the accurate tracking of specific areas of the heart as they move and rotate through the cardiac cycle.

REFERENCES

1. DEVEREUX, R. B. & N. REICHEK. 1977. Echocardiographic determination of left ventricular mass in man. Circulation 55: 613–618.
2. REICHEK, N., J. HELAK, T. PLAPPERT, M. ST. JOHN SUTTON & K. T. WEBER. 1983. Anatomic validation of left ventricular mass estimates from clinical two-dimensional echocardiography: initial results. Circulation 67: 348–352.
3. SCHILLER, N. B., C. D. SKIOLDERBRAND, E. J. SCHILLER, C. C. MAVROUDIS, N. H. SILVERMAN, S. H. RAHIMTOOLA & M. J. LIPTON. 1983. Canine left ventricular mass estimation by two-dimensional echocardiography. Circulation 68: 210–216.
4. MCGAUGHEY, M., W. H. GUIER, M. HAUSKNECHT, A. HERSKOWITZ, B. WALTERS & J. L. WEISS. 1984. Three-dimensional echo reconstruction of the left ventricle in cardiac transplant patients: direct validation of mass determination. Circulation 70(Suppl. III): III-397.
5. WEISS, J. L., M. MCGAUGHEY & W. H. GUIER. 1987. Geometric considerations in determination of left ventricular mass by two-dimensional echocardiography. Hypertension 9(Suppl. II): 85–89.
6. KELLER, A. M., R. M. PESHOCK, C. R. MALLOY, C. P. FITZGERALD, L. M. BUJA, R. L. NUNNALLY, R. W. PARKEY & J. T. WILLERSON. 1985. In vivo measurement of myocardial mass using MRI. Circulation 72(Suppl. III): III-123.
7. FLORENTINE, M. S., C. L. GROSSKRUTZ, W. CHANGE, J. A. HARTNETT, V. D. DUNN, J. C. EHRHARDT, S. R. FLEAGLE, S. M. COLLINS, M. L. MARCUS, & D. J. SKORTON. 1986. Measurement of left ventricular mass in vivo using gated nuclear magnetic resonance imaging. J. Am. Coll. Cardiol. 8: 107–112.
8. KELLER, A. M., R. M. PESHOCK, C. R. MALLOY, L. M. BUJA, R. NUNNALLY, R. W. PARKEY & J. T. WILLERSON. 1986. In vivo measurement of myocardial mass using nuclear magnetic resonance imaging. J. Am. Coll. Cardiol. 8: 113–117.
9. SHAPIRO, E. P., W. J. ROGERS, R. BEYAR, R. L. SOULEN, E. A. ZERHOUNI, J. A. C. LIMA & J. L. WEISS. 1989. Determination of left ventricular mass by magnetic resonance imaging in hearts deformed by acute infarction. Circulation 79: 706–711.
10. EATON, L. W. & B. H. BULKLEY. 1981. Expansion of acute myocardial infarction: its relationship to infarct morphology in a canine model. Circ. Res. 49: 80–88.
11. KERBER, R. E., M. L. MARCUS, J. EHRHARDT, R. WILSON & F. M. ABBOUD. 1975. Correlation between echocardiographically demonstrated segmental dyskinesis and regional myocardial perfusion. Circulation 52: 1097–1104.
12. LIEBERMAN, A. N., J. L. WEISS, B. I. JUGDUTT, L. C. BECKER, B. H. BULKLEY, J. B. GARRISON, G. M. HUTCHINS, C. A. KALLMAN & M. L. WEISFELDT. 1981. Two-dimensional echocardiography and infarct size: relationship of regional wall motion and thickening to the extent of myocardial infarction in the dog. Circulation 63: 739–746.
13. ROGERS, W. J. 1987. Cine MR imaging: potential for the evaluation of cardiovascular function. Am. J. Roentgenol. 148: 239–246.
14. FISHER, M. R., G. K. VON SCHULTHESS & C. B. HIGGINS. 1985. Multiphasic cardiac magnetic resonance imaging: normal left ventricular wall thickening. Am. J. Roentgenol. 145: 27–30.
15. SECHTEM, U., B. A. SOMMERHOFF, W. MARKIEWICZ, R. D. WHITE, M. D. CHEITLIN & C. B. HIGGINS. 1987. Regional left ventricular wall thickening by magnetic resonance imaging: evaluation in normal persons and patients with global and regional dysfunction. Am. J. Cardiol. 59: 145–151.
16. BEYAR, R., E. P. SHAPIRO, W. L. GRAVES, W. J. ROGERS, W. H. GUIER, G. A. CAREY, R. L. SOULEN, E. A. ZERHOUNI, M. L. WEISFELDT & J. L. WEISS. 1990. Quantification and validation of left ventricular wall thickening by a three-dimensional volume element magnetic resonance imaging approach. Circulation 81: 297–307.
17. ZERHOUNI, E. A., D. M. PARISH, W. J. ROGERS, A. YANG & E. P. SHAPIRO. 1988. Human heart: tagging with MR imaging—a method for non-invasive assessment of myocardial motion. Radiology 169: 59–63.
18. BEYAR, R., F. C. P. YIN, M. HAUSKNECHT & M. L. WEISFELDT. 1989. Dependence of left ventricular twist-radial shortening relations on cardiac cycle phase. Am. J. Physiol. 26: H1119–H1126.

19. BUCHALTER, M. B., J. L. WEISS, W. J. ROGERS, E. A. ZERHOUNI, M. L. WEISFELDT & E. P. SHAPIRO. 1988. Human myocardial twist and shear. Circulation 78:(Suppl. II): 524.
20. BUCHALTER, M. B., J. L. WEISS, W. J. ROGERS, E. A. ZERHOUNI, M. L. WEISFELDT, R. BEYAR & E. P. SHAPIRO. Noninvasive quantification of left ventricular twist rotational deformation in normal humans using magnetic resonance myocardial tagging. Circulation. (In press.)
21. SHAPIRO, E. P., M. B. BUCHALTER, W. J. ROGERS, E. A. ZERHOUNI, W. H. GUIER & J. L. WEISS. 1988. LV twist is greater with inotropic stimulation and less with regional ischemia. Circulation 78(Suppl. II): 466.
22. BUCHALTER, M. B., W. J. ROGERS, J. L. WEISS, J. A. C. LIMA, F. E. RADEMAKERS, E. A. ZERHOUNI & E. P. SHAPIRO. 1989. Inotropic stimulation increases and disrupts the pattern of left ventricular circumferential shear. Clin. Res. 37: 249A.

Myocardial Perfusion Scintigraphy as an Aid in Understanding Electrocardiographic Changes of Ischemia and Infarction

BARRY L. ZARET AND FRANS J. TH. WACKERS

Cardiology Section
Department of Internal Medicine
and Nuclear Medicine Section
Department of Diagnostic Radiology
Yale University School of Medicine
333 Cedar Street
New Haven, Connecticut 06510

INTRODUCTION

It has been apparent for at least a decade that myocardial perfusion scintigraphy with thallium-201, and more recently with the technetium-99m isonitriles, provides significant incremental information to that obtained from the electrocardiogram alone in clinical states of ischemia and infarction.[1] This incremental value of perfusion scintigraphy is demonstrable in a number of ways including correlation with coronary arteriography, clinical parameters, and patient outcome. This review will focus on specific issues relevant to myocardial infarction and exercise-induced myocardial ischemia, and will indicate the interaction between electrocardiographic and scintigraphic data. In addition, new concepts related to the onset of the thrombolytic era also will be discussed.

ACUTE MYOCARDIAL INFARCTION

Clinical Recognition

The electrocardiogram has long been the hallmark for clinical characterization of patients hospitalized with suspected acute myocardial infarction. However, it is well recognized that electrocardiographic criteria utilized diagnostically are far from perfect. The MILIS study evaluated the clinical utility of electrocardiographic criteria for recognition of acute myocardial infarction at the time of admission.[2] This analysis was based upon 3697 patients. The criteria employed included one or more of the following abnormalities: (1) new or presumably new Q waves of sufficient width and depth in at least two diaphragmatic leads, two precordial leads, or in leads I and aVL, (2) new or presumably new ST segment elevation or depression of greater than or equal to 0.1 mV in one of the same lead combinations, (3) left bundle branch block. The diagnostic sensitivity of the electrocardiographic criteria was 81%, the diagnostic specificity 69%, and the predictive value was 72%. More specifically, ST elevation had a sensitivity of 46% and specificity of 91%, ST elevation or depression a sensitivity of 75%, and specificity of 77%.

In the thrombolytic era the diagnosis of acute infarction based upon electrocardiographic criteria is of even greater consequence, since immediate decisions concerning the administration of thrombolytic therapy must be made. A recent study by Lee *et al.* demonstrated that for every eight patients with true positive diagnostic results treated with thrombolytic therapy based on interpretation of a single electrocardiogram, one to two false-positive results will also be encountered.[3] That is, using electrocardiographic criteria alone a significant number of patients may be subjected to unnecessary risk and expense.

The utility of perfusion scintigraphy for early detection of acute infarction was first demonstrated in 1976.[4] This study demonstrated quite clearly that resting thallium-201 scintigraphy was an extremely sensitive and reliable means of infarct detection (FIGURE 1). In addition, it was noted that the temporal sequence of imaging was quite important. In that study of 200 patients with acute myocardial infarction, all 44 patients studied within six hours of the onset of chest pain had abnormal scintigraphic images. Of 52 patients imaged between 6 and 24 hours of the onset of chest pain, 88% had demonstrable perfusion defects. Of 104 patients studied later than 24 hours after the onset of pain, only 72% had scintigraphic defects. In addition, serial imaging in selected patients frequently demonstrated a decrease in infarct size over time. Changes in size tended to occur more frequently in individuals with small infarcts as opposed to those with larger infarction. These data were obtained in the prethrombolytic era. It is likely that at least a subset of patients demonstrating a temporal decrease in perfusion deficits experienced spontaneous thrombolysis.

Comparable temporal data also have been obtained in an experimental infarct model involving sequential thallium imaging.[5] In addition, it has been demonstrated in animal models that the minimal mass of hypoperfused myocardium detectable on scintigraphic studies is 4.9 g.[6] Finally, postmortem data have demonstrated a good correlation between scintigraphically measured infarct defect size and infarct size obtained at the time of necropsy. Such measurements have been obtained in both experimental animals and man.[7,8]

Risk Stratification following Infarction

Major prognostic impact can be obtained from thallium-201 scintigraphic data in patients with acute infarction. Silverman *et al.* utilizing a quantitative measure of perfusion defect size at rest demonstrated that patients with larger defects had a poorer prognosis than patients with small defects.[9] This remained the case following adjustment for all clinical data, including electrocardiographic variables. Thallium data provided the single best prognostic index. Gibson *et al.* demonstrated the predictive power of exercise thallium-201 scintigraphy for defining cardiac events after uncomplicated myocardial infarction.[10] Their study involved 140 consecutive patients who were evaluated with submaximal exercise treadmill testing, thallium scintigraphy, and coronary angiography. High-risk thallium scintigraphy involved either perfusion defects in more than one discrete vascular region, the presence of redistribution, or increased lung uptake. Exercise testing was considered abnormal if either greater or equal to 1 mm of ST segment depression or angina occurred; coronary angiography was considered high risk if multivessel disease was demonstrated. Within a mean follow-up of 15 months, 50 patients experienced a cardiac event. When all events were combined, scintigraphy identified 94% of high-risk patients, whereas exercise testing abnormalities identified only 56% ($p < 0.001$) (FIGURE 2). The overall sensitivity of high-risk coronary angiography with respect to predicting cardiac events was also lower than that of scintigraphy (71% vs. 94%, $p < 0.01$). In addition, scintigraphy predicted low-risk status better than either exercise testing or angiography. These data, combined with comparable prognostic benefit of thallium imaging in patients

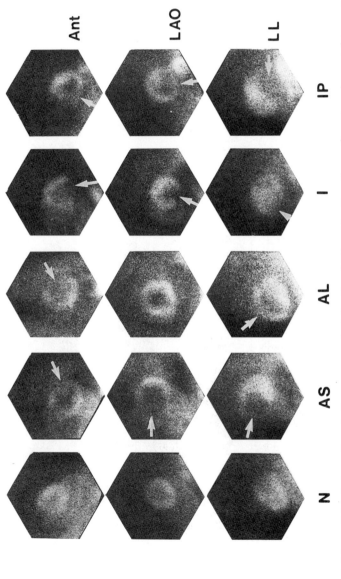

FIGURE 1. Myocardial perfusion patterns in Q wave myocardial infarction of different locations. Images from three views are shown: anterior (Ant), left anterior oblique (LAO), and left lateral (LL). Patterns are shown for normal (N) anteroseptal (AS), anterolateral infarction (AL), inferior (I) and inferoposterior (IP) infarction. The site of perfusion defect is indicated by the white arrow. (From Reference 4, with permission.)

with stable coronary artery disease (see below), clearly highlight the incremental prognostic value of perfusion scintigraphy in comparison to the electrocardiogram alone.

Thrombolysis

In addition to the ability for identifying infarction prior to administration of thrombolytic therapy, it is exceedingly important to define perfusion status in a simple,

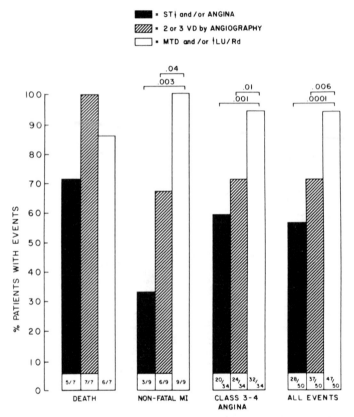

FIGURE 2. Sensitivity of exercise test, angiography, and thallium-201 perfusion imaging findings for identifying postinfarction patients who either died, experienced reinfarction, or developed unstable angina. As is noted, perfusion imaging was most sensitive for identifying high-risk patients. (MTD = multiple thallium defects, LU = lung uptake and Rd = redistribution.) (From Reference 10, with permission.)

practical, and noninvasive manner following intravenous thrombolysis. Califf *et al.* assessed the efficacy of clinical measurements for predicting perfusion status in a group of 386 patients treated with tissue plasminogen activator (rt-PA) who also underwent coronary arteriography 90 minutes after initiation of therapy to determine perfusion status.[11] It was noted that 96% of patients with complete resolution of ST segment elevation and 84% of those with partial improvement in the ST segment showed reperfusion on coronary arteriography. However, these ST segment changes occurred in only a minority of individuals with reperfusion: namely, 6% and 38% of patients respectively. Furthermore, arrhythmias occurring in the first 90 minutes of therapy bore no relationship to patency rate. In addition, when complete resolution of chest pain occurred prior to angiography, 84% of patients showed reperfusion. However, this finding too occurred in only 29% of patients. A logistic regression model involving clinical variables identified 25% of patients with 90% or greater probability of patency; but 64% of patients with no ST segment resolution or symptom resolution also had patent arteries at the time of angiography. Thus, simple electrocardiographic assessment appears inadequate and insensitive for defining the occurrence of infarct artery reperfusion and salvage of viable myocardium. These findings were confirmed by Kircher et al. who also noted that ST segment improvement occurred in only 44% of patients treated with thrombolytic therapy, but was associated with an 84% probability of reperfusion when present.[12]

Bren et al. also noted, on the basis of literature review as well as their own data, that accurate diagnosis of successful reperfusion based on monitoring of a single ECG lead was quite difficult.[13] This results primarily from the fact that there is only a small magnitude of change in the presence of a large degree of intrinsic variation. This results in extensive overlap between groups with and without successful reperfusion. When large numbers of patients are analyzed, small but significant declines in ST segment elevation are noted in those successfully reperfused in comparison to those who are not. However, the differences are small and of limited value in individual patients. Although comparisons of single electrocardiograms before and after therapy may not be helpful, it is conceivable that continuous monitoring of ST segments to determine "time to steady state ST elevation" may be of greater value in predicting postthrombolytic patency.[13] Bren also noted that while R and Q wave amplitude might be of value in distinguishing large group differences, these findings were of limited value in individual patients. The electrocardiogram was also felt not to be helpful for identification of patients with initially incomplete coronary occlusion who would not require thrombolytic therapy.[13]

The intrinsic limitations of electrocardiographic and other clinical indices for defining both perfusion status of the infarct artery in the early stages of thrombolytic therapy and long-term thrombolytic efficacy has led to the application of perfusion scintigraphy as a potential solution to this problem. Perhaps the most exciting of the new approaches involves the use of technetium-99m isonitrile perfusion imaging to define both prethrombolysis risk zone and subsequent reperfusion. The isonitriles represent a new class of radioisotope-labeled myocardial perfusion agents with interesting and unique biological properties.[14] Much like thallium-201 and other potassium analogue perfusion agents, the isonitriles accumulate in the myocardium according to regional blood flow. However, unlike thallium-201, this radiopharmaceutical does not demonstrate kinetic changes that result in significant redistribution over time. Rather, it remains bound stably to myocardial cytosolic protein. Because of this property, the myocardial perfusion pattern at the time of injection is reflected in images obtained several hours thereafter. Thus, this radiopharmaceutical allows serial noninvasive imaging that yields quantification of initial area at risk as well as identification of the occurrence of reperfusion following thrombolysis. An initial study can be obtained with injection of the radioisotope in the emergency room setting prior to thrombolysis. Imaging can then be performed several hours thereafter when the patient has been stabilized in the coronary care unit. This imaging sequence results in no delay for the critical administration of thrombolytic therapy. The perfusion defect defined in this initial study will demonstrate the initial prethrombolysis *risk zone*. A subsequent comparative study obtained with a repeat injection will identify the zone of hypoperfusion that represents the *final infarct*. Quantitative comparison of these two image sets will therefore allow definition of the extent of improvement of myocardial perfusion following thrombolysis (FIGURE 3).

We recently employed this strategy in a study of 30 patients with a first acute

THROMBOLYSIS

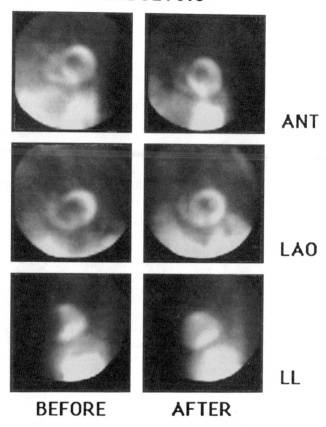

BEFORE   AFTER

FIGURE 3. Isonitrile perfusion images before and after thrombolytic therapy in a patient with an anteroseptal infarct. Images are shown for the anterior (ANT), left anterior oblique (LAO), and left lateral (LL) views. Note the perfusion defect involving the septum and inferoapical wall in the LAO view and anteroapical wall in the LL view present before thrombolysis, and the significant reperfusion noted following the administration of therapy. (From Reference 15, with permission.)

myocardial infarction, 23 of whom received thrombolytic therapy with recombinant tissue plasminogen activator.[15] All patients showed ST segment elevation in two or more leads of at least one millimeter in magnitude. All perfusion defects were quantified in an objective manner using techniques developed in our laboratory.[16] There was wide variation in the size of the risk zone measured in the patients.

Furthermore, there was no apparent relationship between the number of arteries involved or the presence of collateral circulation and the size of the risk zone. The serial imaging data revealed that there was a highly significant difference in the change in defect size noted in patients with patent as opposed to those with occluded infarct arteries. A relative change in defect size of ≥30% on serial studies best separated those with and without reperfusion. Additional comparisons were made between final isonitrile defect size and defect size on redistribution thallium images. In general, there was an excellent agreement between the two studies demonstrating that improved uptake of isonitrile noted on serial studies more than likely represents salvage of viable tissue rather than reperfusion of nonviable myocardium.

This pilot study demonstrates the feasibility of performing serial quantitative planar isonitrile imaging studies in patients receiving thrombolysis while not interfering with the time-dependent initiation of therapy. This study also indicates the potential power of this approach for both defining risk zones accurately and demonstrating therapeutic efficacy. It should be noted that in this particular study the second images were obtained several days later. Approaches using split dose techniques should allow performance of both images within several hours, thereby providing data that might be utilized for urgent intervention.[17] In addition to providing information concerning individual patients, this approach may offer major investigative potential with respect to appropriate categorization of patients undergoing thrombolysis. As has been noted in experimental animal studies, it is extremely important to define accurately the magnitude of the risk zone involved in order to assess infarct salvage and therapeutic thrombolytic benefit.[18]

A number of other investigators have utilized planar thallium-201 scintigraphy at rest or with exercise for evaluating thrombolytic therapy. One approach has employed intracoronary administration of thallium-201 before and after intracoronary thrombolytic therapy.[19] New regional uptake of thallium following therapy correlated with recovery of regional function. However, it should be noted that the temporal sequence of radioisotope administration is critical in this instance. If thallium is administered too early after reperfusion, uptake may occur in the setting of reactive hyperemia, thereby resulting in artifactual excessive accumulation of the tracer in reperfused myocardium destined for subsequent necrosis.[20] Other clinical studies involving intravenous administration of thallium have demonstrated progressive improvement of myocardial uptake of the tracer in patients with angiographically demonstrable infarct artery reperfusion.[21,22] However, these thallium-201 studies are hampered by logistic problems attendant with the need both to administer tracer and to image prior to the onset of therapy. The practical limitations of this particular approach are self-evident. It is for this reason that isonitrile imaging appears particularly effective and offers great potential. Nevertheless, predischarge stress thallium scintigraphy also can play a significant role currently in identifying residual viable myocardium at risk following thrombolysis and can be of particular value in assessing efficacy in large populations of patients. This has been demonstrated in several studies employing both planar and tomographic techniques.[23,24]

CHRONIC CORONARY ARTERY DISEASE

Identifying Ischemia

As stated above, perfusion scintigraphy adds significantly to the ECG evaluation of the postinfarction patient. In addition to the data of Gibson *et al.,* several other studies have demonstrated the efficacy of thallium scintigraphy with respect to incremental information concerning patient outcome and the presence of multivessel coronary artery disease. Comparable data can also be obtained in the postinfarction patient using dypridamole thallium scintigraphy. Leppo *et al.* have demonstrated the prognostic value of this particular evaluation.[25] In all studies where direct comparisons have been made, perfusion scintigraphy, using appropriate criteria, has added to conventional electrocardiographic assessment of ischemia.[26]

In the presence of stable coronary artery disease the addition of thallium-201 scintigraphy likewise adds incremental value to exercise ECG analysis for detection of myocardial ischemia. Although there may be significant selection bias involved in direct diagnostic comparisons, it is clear from pooled data that the exercise ECG has, at best, a sensitivity of approximately 70% and a specificity of approximately 80% for the recognition of individuals with angiographic evidence of significant coronary stenosis.[27] In addition there are numerous situations in which the ECG will not be of diagnostic help. These include clinical circumstances involving administration of drugs such as digitalis, the presence of baseline electrocardiogram abnormalities such as bundle branch block, Wolff-Parkinson-White syndrome, nonspecific ST and T wave changes, or ventricular hypertrophy. It is also clear that the exercise electrocardiogram has a greater tendency for abnormality in patients with multivessel as opposed to single or double vessel disease.[27,28]

A cumulative sensitivity and specificity for planar exercise thallium-201 scintigraphy approximates 84% and 90% respectively.[27] These data were obtained primarily with qualitative techniques. It is clear that the addition of quantification of planar data[16] as well as the application of single photon emission computed tomography (SPECT) has further improved both sensitivity (90%) and specificity 95%.[1] It appears that SPECT may have a major role in defining multivessel perfusion abnormalities with a higher degree of accuracy than planar studies.[29] It is also anticipated that the introduction of technetium-99m isonitrile imaging, with attendant increasing photon flux and better counting statistics as well as a better imaging energy, will result in higher resolution and, hence, more accurate SPECT studies than can be achieved currently with thallium-201.

There are several specific imaging circumstances that require further comment. Thallium scintigraphy appears to be somewhat less accurate in women than in men.[30] This is comparable to some of the exercise ECG data.[27] The reasons for this are not totally clear. One factor certainly involves the presence of breast imaging artifact.[1] Because of the relatively low energy of thallium-201, emanating radioactivity is easily attenuated by overlying structures such as breast tissue. Perfusion scintigraphy appears to be particularly beneficial diagnostically in individuals who are not capable of exercise to an appropriate heart rate approaching 85% of predicted maximum.[31] This has been demonstrated in several studies and now appears well established. Furthermore, in the presence of an inability to exercise due to lack of cooperation or a specific neurologic or musculoskeletal problem, the option of obtaining comparable data using dypyridamole pharmacologic stress rather than exercise stress remains an option.[1,27] In the presence of left bundle branch block, there is some dispute as to whether thallium scintigraphy will demonstrate abnormalities in the absence of coronary artery disease. Hirzel *et al.* have demonstrated reversible abnormality in such patients.[32] Perfusion defects have been attributed to compression of coronary flow as a result of the abnormal temporal sequence of contraction. Others have felt that findings may have been related more to ventricular dilation in the presence of a clinical or subclinical cardiomyopathy.[1] At the present time abnormal perfusion images associated with left bundle branch block must be interpreted with caution.

Questions have arisen concerning the occurrence of ischemia in patients with chest pain and angiographically normal coronary arteries. Such patients have been noted to have abnormal exercise perfusion scintigraphy with or without an abnormal exercise

ECG. Does this represent a false positive response or a new phenomenon? Legrand *et al.* demonstrated abnormal coronary flow reserve in a group of such patients with chest pain, perfusion defects, and angiographically normal coronaries.[33] The abnormal flow reserve was demonstrated using a digital subtraction angiographic technique. The coronary flow reserve in arterial distributions with abnormal perfusion was significantly lower than in distributions associated with normal radionuclide update. These data strongly support the idea that at least a portion of individuals with chest pain and angiographically normal coronary arteries without evidence of coronary spasm but with scintigraphic evidence of altered myocardial perfusion do have abnormal coronary flow reserve. One may hypothesize that the abnormality here resides in the smaller resistance vessels.

Prognosis

Myocardial perfusion scintigraphy provides substantial incremental prognostic information over the exercise electrocardiogram in patients with stable coronary artery disease. A number of specific factors have been evaluated. In a series of 525 patients followed for five years, increased lung thallium-201 uptake was the single best predictor of subsequent cardiac events.[34] Using a stepwise regression model, increased lung uptake had twice the relative risk of exercise ST segment depression in this patient cohort. In a grouping of the univariate predictors, severe ST segment depression ranked 14th; while increased lung uptake of thallium was 1st. In addition, the first four univariate predictors all involved imaging parameters (increased lung uptake, number of myocardial perfusion defects on initial imaging, presence of redistribution, number of segments with redistribution, respectively). In addition to abnormal lung uptake, the degree and extent of severity of myocardial hypoperfusion have also been determined to be independent risk factors. Ladenheim identified three specific factors on the exercise thallium study that were independent predictors: the number of regions with reversible hypoperfusion, the maximal magnitude of hypoperfusion, and the achieved heart rate.[35] An additional study by Weiss *et al.* identified transient ischemic dilation of the left ventricle on stress imaging as a marker of severe and extensive coronary disease.[36] In no study has the exercise ECG found to provide either comparable or stronger prognostic information than that contained in the perfusion imaging alone.

A final issue to consider involves late reversibility of thallium-201 perfusion defects. Recent observations have indicated that, independent of the baseline electrocardiogram, individuals may demonstrate reversibility on perfusion scintigraphy that requires delayed imaging at 24 hours (with or without a second injection of tracer).[37] This particular phenomenon has been associated with more severe coronary artery stenosis. In addition, those individuals showing late reversibility of thallium imaging have been noted to have improvement in regional function following a revascularization with either bypass surgery or coronary angioplasty.[37] The finding of late reversibility has also been associated with abnormal regional myocardial metabolism in a pattern consistent with viable but chronically ischemic myocardium.[38] This particular finding represents yet another instance in which imaging data have provided fresh insights that have expanded upon available electrocardiographic profiles.

SUMMARY

In summary, myocardial perfusion scintigraphy with either thallium or the isonitriles has added substantially to electrocardiographic definition of both myocardial infarction and acute and chronic myocardial ischemia. Using perfusion scintigraphy, one can define infarct zones, risk zones, and the presence of reperfusion following thrombolytic therapy. When perfusion scintigraphy is combined with physiologic or pharmacologic stress, myocardial ischemia can be documented, irrespective of electrocardiographic documentation of the phenomenon. Delayed imaging may be important for defining viability even in the presence of significant Q waves. Myocardial perfusion scintigraphy provides prognostic evaluation of patients with both acute and chronic coronary syndromes. When the current cumulative experience is looked at critically, it is clear that myocardial perfusion scintigraphy has helped in the development of an understanding of the limitations of electrocardiography in the diagnostic and functional categorization of patients with acute and chronic coronary disease.

REFERENCES

1. WACKERS, F. J. TH. 1988. Myocardial perfusion imaging. In Diagnostic Nuclear Medicine. A. Gottschalk, P. Hoffer & J. Potchen, Eds.: 291–354. Williams and Wilkins. Baltimore, Md.
2. RUDE, R. E., W. K. POOLE, J. E. MULLER, et al. 1983. Electrocardiographic and clinical criteria for recognition of acute myocardial infarction based on analysis of 3,697 patients. Am. J. Cardiol. 52: 936–941.
3. LEE, T. H., M. C. WEISBERG, D. A. BRAND, G. W. ROUAN & L. GOLDMAN. 1989. Candidates for thrombolysis among emergency room patients with acute chest pain. Ann. Intern. Med. 110: 957–962.
4. WACKERS, F. J. TH., E. RUSEMANN-SOKOLE, G. SAMSON, et al. 1976. Value and limitations of thallium-201 scintigraphy in the acute phase of myocardial infarction. N. Engl. J. Med. 295: 1–7.
5. UMBACH, R. E., R. C. LANGE, J. C. LEE & B. L. ZARET. 1978. Temporal changes in sequential quantitative thallium-201 imaging following myocardial infarction in dogs. Yale J. Biol. Med. 51: 597–602.
6. MUELLER, T. M., M. L. MARCUS, J. C. EHRHARDT, T. CHAUDHURI & F. M. ABBOUD. 1976. Limitations of thallium-201 myocardial perfusion scintigrams. Circulation 54: 640–651.
7. WACKERS, F. J. TH., A. E. BECKER, G. SAMSON, et al. 1977. Location and size of acute transmural myocardial infarction estimated from thallium-201 scintiscans. A clinicopathological study. Circulation 56: 71–79.
8. PRIGENT, F., J. MADDAHI, E. V. GARCIA, et al. 1986. Quantification of myocardial infarct size by thallium-201 single-photon emission computed tomography: experimental validation in the dog. Circulation 74: 852–861.
9. SILVERMAN, K. J., L. C. BECKER, B. H. BULKLEY, et al. 1980. Value of early thallium-201 scintigraphy for predicting mortality in patients with acute myocardial infarction. Circulation 61: 996–1003.
10. GIBSON, R. S., D. D. WATSON, G. B. CRADDOCK, et al. 1983. Prediction of cardiac events after uncomplicated myocardial infarction: a prospective study comparing predischarge exercise thallium-201 scintigraphy and coronary angiography. Circulation 68: 321–336.
11. CALIFF, R. M., W. O'NEIL, R. S. STACK, et al. 1988. Failure of simple clinical measurements to predict perfusion status after intravenous thrombolysis. Ann. Intern. Med. 108: 658–662.
12. KIRCHNER, B. J., E. J. TOPOL, W. W. O'NEIL & B. PITT. 1987. Prediction of infarct artery reconilization after intravenous thrombolytic therapy. Am. J. Cardiol. 59: 513–515.
13. BREN, G. B., A. G. WASSERMAN & A. M. ROSS. 1987. The electrocardiogram in patients undergoing thrombolysis for myocardial infarction. Circulation 76: II-18–II-24.
14. VERANI, M. S., M. O. JEROUDI, J. J. MAHMARIAN, et al. 1988. Quantification of myocardial infarction during coronary occlusion and myocardial salvage after reperfusion using cardiac imaging with technetium-99m hexakis 2-methoxyisobutyl isonitrile. J. Am. Coll. Cardiol. 12: 1573–1581.
15. WACKERS, F. J. TH., R. J. GIBBONS, M. S. VERANI, et al. 1989. Serial quantitative planar technetium-99m isonitrile imaging in acute infarction: efficacy for noninvasive assessment of thrombolytic therapy. J. Am. Coll. Cardiol. 14: 861–873.

16. WACKERS, R. J. TH., R. C. FETTERMAN, J. A. MATTERA & J. P. CLEMANS. 1985. Quantification planar thallium-201 stress scintigraphy: a critical evaluation of the method. Semin. Nucl. Med. **15:** 46–66.

17. OKADA, R. D., Y. L. LIM, J. ROTHENDLER, et al. 1983. Split dose thallium-201 dypridimole imaging: a new technique for obtaining thallium images before and immediately after an intervention. J. Am. Coll. Cardiol. **1:** 1302–1309.

18. SIMPSON, P. J., R. F. TODD, J. C. FANTONE, et al. 1988. Reduction of experimental canine myocardial reperfusion injury by a monoclonal antibody (Anti-MO$_1$, Anti-CD$_{11}$b) that inhibits leukocyte adhesion. J. Clin. Invest. **81:** 624–629.

19. MARKIS, J. E., M. MALAGOLD, J. A. PARKER, et al. 1981. Myocardial salvage after intracoronary thrombolysis with streptokinase in acute myocardial infarction: assessment by intracoronary thallium-201. N. Engl. J. Med. **305:** 777–782.

20. MELIN, J. A., L. C. BECKER & B. H. BULKELY. 1983. Differences in thallium-201 uptake in reperfused and nonreperfused myocardial infarction. Circ. Res. **53:** 414–419.

21. DECOSTER, P. M., J. A. MELIN, J. M. R. DETRY, et al. 1985. Coronary artery reperfusion in acute myocardial infarction: assessment by pre- and postintervention thallium-201 myocardial perfusion imaging. Am. J. Cardiol. **55:** 889–895.

22. MELIN, J. A., P. M. DECOSTER, J. RENKIN, et al. 1985. Effect of intracoronary thrombolytic therapy on exercise-induced ischemia after acute myocardial infarction. Am. J. Cardiol **56:** 705–711.

23. MAUBLANT, J. C., P. PEYCELON, J. C. CARDOT, et al. 1988. Value of myocardial defect size measured by thallium-201 SPECT: results of a multicenter trial comparing heparin and a new fibrinolytic agent. J. Nucl. Med. **29:** 1486–1491.

24. VAN DER WALL, E. E., J. C. J. RES, R. VAN DEN POL, et al. 1988. Improvement of myocardial perfusion after thrombolysis assessed by thallium-201 exercise scintigraphy. Eur. Heart J. **9:** 828–835.

25. LEPPO, J. A., J. O'BRIEN, J. A. ROTHENDLER, et al. 1984. Dipyridamole-thallium-201 scintigraphy in the prediction of future events after acute myocardial infarction. N. Engl. J. Med. **310:** 1014–1019.

26. SCHNEIDER, J. F. 1987. Radionuclide studies in the postmyocardial infarction patient. In Cardiac Nuclear Medicine. M. C. Gerson, Ed.: 247–308. McGraw Hill. New York, N.Y.

27. GERSON, M. C. 1987. Test accuracy, test selection and test result interpretation in chronic coronary artery disease. In Cardiac Nuclear Medicine. M. C. Gerson, Ed.: 309–347. McGraw-Hill. New York, N.Y.

28. ISKANDRIAN, A. S. & A. HAKKI. 1985. Thallium-201 myocardial scintigraphy. Am. Heart J. **109:** 113–129.

29. PASQUALE, E. E., A. C. NODY, E. G. DEPUEY, et al. 1988. Quantitative rotational thallium-201 tomography for identifying and localizing coronary artery disease. Circulation **77:** 316–327.

30. FRIEDMAN, T. D., A. C. GREENE, A. S. ISKANDRIAN, et al. 1982. Exercise thallium-201 myocardial scintigraphy in women: correlation with coronary arteriorgraphy. Am. J. Cardiol. **49:** 1632–1639.

31. ESQUIVEL, L., S. G. POLLOCK, G. A. BELLER, et al. 1989. Effect of the degree of effort on the sensitivity of the exercise thallium-201 stress test in symptomatic coronary artery disease. Am. J. Cardiol. **63:** 160–165.

32. HIRZEL, H. W., M. SENN, K. NUESCH, et al. 1984. Thallium-201 scintigraphy in left bundle branch block. Am. J. Cardiol. **53:** 764–771.

33. LEGRAND, V., J. M. HODGSON, E. R. BATES, et al. 1985. Abnormal coronary flow reserve and abnormal radionuclide exercise stress test results in patients with normal coronary angiograms. J. Am. Coll. Cardiol. **6:** 1245–1254.

34. GILL, J. B., T. D. RUDDY, J. B. NEWELL, et al. 1987. Prognostic importance of thallium uptake in the lungs during exercise in coronary artery disease. N. Engl. J. Med. **317:** 1485–1489.

35. LADENHEIM, M. L., B. H. POLLOCK, A. ROZANSKI, et al. 1986. Extent and severity of myocardial hypoperfusion as predictors of prognosis in patients with suspected coronary artery disease. J. Am. Coll. Cardiol. **7:** 464–471.

36. WEISS, A. T., D. S. BERMAN, A. S. LEW, et al. 1987. Transient ischemic dilation of the left

ventricle on stress thallium scintigraphy: a marker of severe and extensive coronary artery disease. J. Am. Coll. Cardiol. **9:** 752–759.

37. KIAT, H., D. S. BERMAN, J. MADDAHI, *et al.* 1988. Late reversibility of tomographic myocardial thallium-201 defects: an accurate marker of myocardial viability. J. Am. Coll. Cardiol. **12:** 1456–1463.

38. BRUNKEN, R., M. SCHWAIGER, M. GROVER-MCKAY, *et al.* 1987. Positron emission tomography detects tissue metabolic activity in myocardial segments with persistent thallium perfusion defects. J. Am. Coll. Cardiol. **10:** 557–567.

Endocardial Monophasic Action Potentials

Correlations with Intracellular Electrical Activity

S. B. OLSSON, P. BLOMSTRÖM,
C. BLOMSTRÖM-LUNDQVIST,
AND B. WOHLFART

*Department of Cardiology
University Hospital
S-221 85 Lund, Sweden*

INTRODUCTION

The exploration of the electrical activity of single myocardial cells began after the invention of the glass microelectrode 40 years ago.[1] With the advent of this technique, which allows an accurate recording of the actual transmembrane potential gradient during the entire electrical cardiac cycle, different types of action potentials from different cardiac structures were demonstrated. Thus, atrial and ventricular myocardial action potentials were characterized by a stable resting membrane potential, a rapid phase of depolarization, and a repolarization course that differed between the two types of myocardium.

The striking monophasic appearance of the action potential was however not a new finding. It was in fact concluded by 1879 that the current field arising from the electrical activity of the heart was of monophasic origin![2] It was also well recognized during the early days of electrocardiology that a monophasic signal could be recorded between an electrode terminal placed in contact with an injured part of the heart muscle and another electrode terminal at any other place apart from the injured region.[3]

The signal recorded by microelectrodes across the myocardial cellular membrane is referred to as an action potential (AP) while the corresponding signal recorded from an area of injured myocardium is called a monophasic action potential (MAP). It was early recognized that a MAP had a gross configuration that was very similar to that of an AP recorded in its immediate vicinity.[4,5]

The MAP signal in these studies was obtained by a suction electrode catheter technique. By applying a similar technique during routine cardiac catheterizations, Korsgren and coworkers recorded in 1966 MAPs from the intact human heart.[6] Successively, a simplification and refinement of the suction electrode technique for human MAP recordings was done.[7,8] A major step in the further improvement of the catheter method for recording of endocardial MAPs was the development of a contact catheter, thereby abolishing the need of endocardial suction.[9] Today, the contact electrode catheter principle for recording of endocardial MAPs is generally adopted.[10–12]

RELATION OF AP TO MAP

A MAP has a configuration that is similar to that of a myocardial AP recorded in its immediate vicinity. The MAP is however always of lower amplitude and has a slower depolarization phase than the AP.[13] Furthermore, the relation between MAP overshoot and signal level after complete repolarization differs from that of an AP. The MAP signal often reaches the same potential level as an AP at the end of depolarization but will only reach a fraction of the true resting membrane potential level. However, when a MAP is amplified and superimposed upon an AP, it becomes evident that the repolarization courses are very close. It was therefore already concluded by 1959 that the MAP is a "reliable index of the shape of the action potential during the entire phase of repolarization" and that the start of the upstroke of the MAP is a "reliable index of the time of arrival of excitation at the electrode."[4]

The close correspondence between MAP and AP signals has been repeatedly verified. Of special interest are two recent comparisons.[14,15] Both have analyzed the resemblance between APs and MAPs recorded with contact electrodes of the types used in human catheter studies. These studies have also incorporated different ways of modifying the appearance of the AP, by using different rates and rhythms or chemical interactions, including the production of automaticity and repolarization disturbances.

Franz and coworkers compared, in a rabbit ventricular myocardial preparation, MAPs using a 1.5 mm wide contact electrode with APs recorded from cells 0.1 to 1.0 mm distant from the edge of the MAP electrode.[14] With AP duration at 90% repolarization varying between 150 and 513 mseconds, the mean absolute difference ± standard deviation (SD) between the simultaneous AP and MAP recordings was 5.4 ± 11.3 mseconds and the relation was linear with a correlation coefficient $r = 0.96 \pm 0.03$. Similar good relations were found between the durations at 60% and 30% repolarization levels. FIGURE 1 gives an example of the similarities between AP and MAP, reproduced with permission from Franz et al.[14]

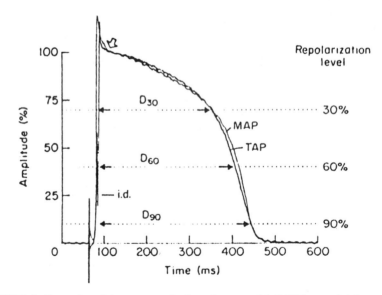

FIGURE 1. Comparison between monophasic action potential (MAP) recorded by contact electrode and transmembrane action potential (TAP). The signals were scaled so their respective plateau amplitudes matched (open arrow). Note the electrogram component of the upstroke of the MAP and the similarities between the repolarization courses of the signals. (Reproduced with permission from Franz et al.)[14]

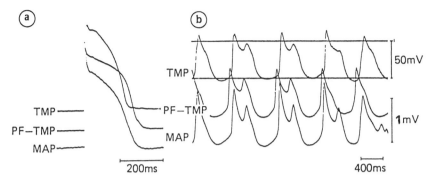

FIGURE 2. Transmembrane action potentials from ventricular myocardium (TMP) and Purkinje fiber (PF-TMP) together with monophasic action potential (MAP) recorded from the immediate vicinity of the TMP recording site. Panel a illustrates control recordings, panel b after addition of barium chloride to the preparation. Note the development of early afterdepolarization in all signals. (Reproduced with permission from Ino *et al.*)[15]

Ino *et al.* used isolated canine preparations and recorded multiple APs from the myocardial cell populations underlying the MAP contact electrode,[15] however not always simultaneously. The MAP recording was done from endocardial and epicardial surfaces as well as from free running Purkinje fibers. The mean AP duration at 50% and 90% repolarization was not significantly different from the MAP duration in any of the tissues studied. They also concluded that the MAP signal reflected more the myocardial AP repolarization than Purkinje repolarization when the recording was performed from an area with superficial Purkinje fibers covering myocardial tissue. Modifications of APs by tetrodoxin or barium chloride were accurately detected by the MAP recordings, as was the supression of automatic activity by verapamil. FIGURE 2 illustrates the similarities between APs from ventricular myocardium (TMP), Purkinje fibers (PF-TM), and the MAP from an endocardial area before (a) and during (b) the effect of barium chloride.

GENERATION OF MAP

Although the origin of the MAP has been extensively discussed,[4,5,9] no actual experiments have been performed to substantiate the generation of the MAP. At present, the only publication that gives information about this topic is a theoretical modeling study.[16] In this study, it was assumed that the electrode, used for MAP recording, induced ischemiclike changes in the cells immediately beneath the MAP electrode. This assumption was then applied in conventional field theory models. The excitation propagation was modeled in 50,000 single elements, representing the structure of the myocardium. Artificial MAPs could be modeled which were similar to MAPs recorded by the catheter technique, supposing a gradual change between completely depolarized cells and normal cells within a total area that was not more extensive than the electrode (FIGURE 3). The major determinants for influencing the MAP signal were (1) impulse propagation direction, (2) thickness of injured tissue, (3) unisotropy of sources, and (4) the ratio between longitudinal and transverse propagation velocity.

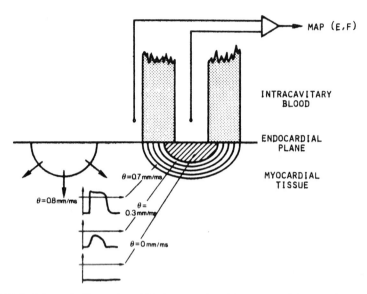

FIGURE 3. Schematic illustration of MAP generation theory successfully tested in modeling experiments by Hirsch *et al.*[16] It is assumed that there is a gradual depolarization of the cells immediately beneath the MAP electrode. (Reproduced with permission from the authors.)[16]

Although the modeling study gives a trustworthy explanation of the MAP generation, it still remains to be verified experimentally by concomitant MAP-AP recordings from the same place in the tissue, i.e., not separated as in earlier cited studies of AP-MAP resemblance.

Although suction and pressure (contact) are the most commonly used methods for obtaining a MAP signal, it can in fact be obtained in a wide variety of ways.[13] A MAP can thus easily be recorded from the surface of an exposed heart between a piece of cotton soaked with KCl and another piece of cotton soaked with NaCl beside the heart. The superficial myocardial cells will be depolarized because the transmembrane K gradient is reduced. The induced changes are principally identical to those presumed in the earlier cited modeling study, further supporting the concept that the MAP is created in the way that was successfully illustrated in the modeling study.

It should be stressed that the intentionally produced cellular injury, an important prerequisite for the MAP recording, is reversible, provided that the tissue damage is spatially and temporally limited.[13]

LIMITATIONS OF MAP RECORDINGS

In spite of the resemblance between APs and MAPs, several important differences are also present. Firstly, true maximal overshoot and resting membrane potential cannot be deduced from a MAP recording with the present knowledge of the generation of the MAP. Secondly, since the MAP is created from electrical phenomena of a large number of cells, the upstroke of a MAP is always of longer duration than that of the corresponding AP. MAP upstroke is furthermore mingled with the electrogram, making the interpretation of changes of phase 0 even more difficult. This phenomenon can be observed in FIGURE 1. It should be pointed out that the interpretation of AP recordings may be hampered by the same phenomenon.[17]

Another electrophysiological limitation of the MAP recording technique is linked to the bipolar recording principle. Thus, unless a careful control of the unipolar signal from the secondary electrode terminal is done, distorted MAP signals may be recorded when even this terminal has a firm contact with the myocardial structures.[13] Although this problem can be overcome by unipolar MAP recording technique, the improvement of signal quality by correctly applied bipolar technique[13] clearly makes this mode of recording preferable.

Further limitations of the MAP recording from the intact heart are caused by the

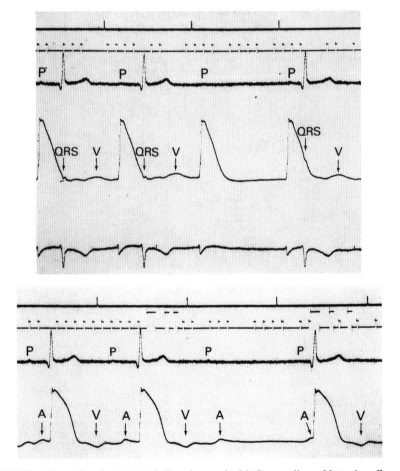

FIGURE 4. Example of mechanical disturbances in MAP recordings. Note the effect of mechanical atrial activity in the ventricular MAP recording and the effect of mechanical ventricular activity in the atrial MAP recording. The recordings also include electrogram superimposition in the MAP recording.

mechanical activity of the heart. Thus, a ventricular MAP recording is obviously influenced by the mechanical activity of the atrium as well as by that of the ventricle. Similarily, an atrial MAP recording can without any doubt be effected as well by the ventricular mechanical activity as that of the atrium itself. FIGURE 4 illustrates electrical and mechanical disturbances in a MAP recording. The phenomenon of artefacts of mechanical ventricular orgin in ventricular MAP recordings limits the interpretation of possible true pathoelectrophysiological phenomena concomitant with the mechanical ventricular activity, as for instance in patients with long QT syndrome (LQTS). Although signal stability and reproducibility at different recording sites are good indicators of true electrophysiological findings, no method is available today by which it is possible to distinctly separate genuine electrophysiological phenomena in the MAP signal from those artificially induced by the mechanical activity of the heart.

ENDOCARDIAL MAP RECORDING—APPLICATIONS IN MAN

As earlier pointed out, the MAP recording has major inherent limitations with respect to the study of myocardial cellular depolarization. Therefore, it is not surprising to find that procainamide, a class I antiarrhythmic drug, which is expected to slightly delay myocardial depolarization, causes insignificant changes of phase 0 of the MAP.[19]

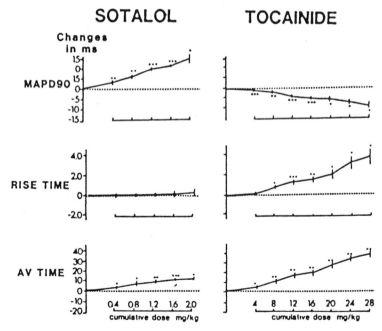

FIGURE 5. Effect of sotalol and tocainide, a class I antiarrhythmic drug, on duration of epicardially recorded monophasic action potential (MAPD90), rise time of the MAP, and AV conduction time. Epicardial contact electrodes were used for MAP recordings. Note that tocainide, but not sotalol, prolongs significantly the rise time of the ventricular MAP. (Reproduced with permission from Duker *et al.*)[20]

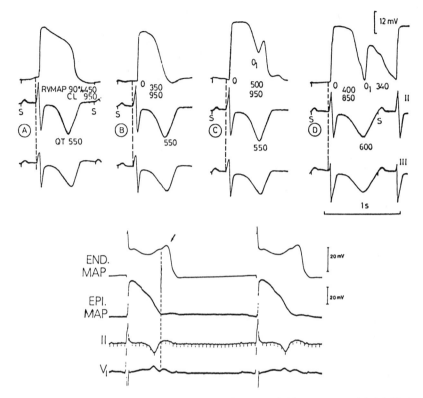

FIGURE 6. Endocardial monophasic action potentials recorded in a patient with LQTS (top panel) and from a dog with advanced, experimentally induced electrocardiographic QTU prolongation with polymorphic ventricular arrhythmias. Note the early afterdepolarization in both endocardial tracings. Note also the normal epicardial MAP, recorded in the dog. (Reproduced with permission from the authors.)[26,28]

We cannot exclude, however, that the method can be used for detection of real changes of depolarization, provided that the effects on phase 0 can be studied during a continuous MAP recording obtained during conditions that minimize the electrogram distortion of the rising phase of the MAP. Statistically significant slowing of phase 0 of epicardially recorded MAPs from guinea pigs was thus observed after administration of tocainide, a class I antiarrythmic drug,[20] as illustrated in FIGURE 5.

Repolarization changes are easily detected with the MAP recording method. Thus several class III antiarrythmic drugs prolong the MAP to an extent that can easily be documented by MAP recordings from the intact human heart.[21] Acceleration of ventricular myocardial repolarization, induced by ischemia[22–24] or by changes of rate[9,13] has also been documented by MAP recordings in man.

Using the MAP recording technique, prolongation of ventricular repolarization and increased dispersion of repolarization have been documented in patients with LQTS.[25,26] In addition a deviation from the traditionally smooth repolarization course has been documented, concomitant with deformations of the end of the T wave.

Recently, endocardial MAPs have been recorded in dogs with artificially induced extreme repolarization disturbances and even polymorphic ventricular tachycardia.[11,27,28]

These MAP recordings show bizarre afterdepolarizations, similar to some of the findings presented from MAP recordings in patients with LQTS and polymorphic ventricular tachycardia. These experimentally induced changes are neither uniform nor stable, but coincide distinctly with the repolarization abnormalities of the surface ECG. Consequently, these studies support some, but not all of the observations from MAP recordings in patients with LQTS.[25,26] FIGURE 6 illustrates selected findings from MAP recordings in patients with LQTS and dogs with experimentally induced repolarization disorder of similar electrocardiographic type.

SAFETY OF MAP RECORDINGS IN MAN

The recording of an endocardial MAP demands a catheter to be pressed and sometimes sucked against the endocardial wall. Consequently, there is a genuine risk with this method that the catheter will perforate the atrial or ventricular myocardial wall, leading to pericardial hemorrhage and tamponade. The MAP catheters, used by us for suction and contact MAP recordings,[8,10,18] have therefore been given a blunt end and a 7F size, in order to minimize the risk of perforation. We have performed 601 endocardial right heart MAP studies in total. Pericardial tamponade developed in one case but could be treated uneventfully by subxiphoid pericardial puncture and drainage. This patient had in addition to the MAP catheter a quadripolar 5F right ventricular apical catheter. It is unclear to us which one of these two catheters was responsible for the ventricular perforation.

Other possible side effects of the MAP recording techniques are similar to those of conventional hemodynamic cardiac catheterizations.

REFERENCES

1. LING, G. & R. W. GERARD. 1949. The normal potential of frog sartorius fibers. J. Cell. Comp. Physiol. 34: 383.
2. BURDON-SANDERSSON, J. & F. J. M. PAGE. 1979–80. On the time-relations of the excitatory process in the ventricle of the heart of the frog. J. Physiol. 2: 384.
3. SCHUTZ, E. 1931. Monophasische Aktionsströme vom in Situ durchbluteten Säugertierherzen. Klin. Wschr. 10: 1454.
4. HOFFMAN, B. F., P. F. CRANEFIELD, E. LEPESCHKIN, B. SURAWICZ & H. C. HERRLICH. 1959. Comparison of cardiac monophasic action potentials recorded by intracellular and suction electrodes. Am. J. Physiol. 196: 1297.
5. CHURNEY, L. & H. OHSHIMA. 1964. An improved suction electrode for recording from the dog heart in situ. J. Appl. Physiol. 19: 793.
6. KORSGREN, M., E. LESKINEN, U. SJOSTRAND & E. VARNAUSKAS. 1966. Intracardiac recording of monophasic action potentials in the human heart. Scand. J. Clin. Lab. Invest. 18: 561.
7. SHABETAI, R., B. SURAWICZ & W. HAMMILL. 1968. Monophasic action potentials in man. Circulation 38: 341.
8. OLSSON, S. B., E. VARNAUSKAS & M. KORSGREN. 1971. Further improved method for measuring monophasic action potentials of the intact human heart. J. Electrocardiology 4(1): 19–23.
9. FRANZ, M. 1983. Long-term recording of monophasic action potentials from human endocardium. Am. J. Cardiol. 51: 1629–1634.
10. OLSSON, S. B., N. EDVARDSSON, I. HIRSCH & P. BLOMSTROM. Methodological aspects on invasive evaluation of myocardial repolarization. (In press).
11. BEN-DAVID, J. & D. ZIPES. 1988. Differential response to right and left ansae subcalviae stimulation of early afterdepolarizations and ventricular tachycardia induced by cesium in dogs. Circulation 5: 1241–1250.

12. TAGGART, P., P. SUTTON, T. TREASURE, M. LAB, W. O'BRIEN, M. RUNNALS, R. H. SWANTON & R. W. EMANUEL. 1988. Monophasic action potentials at discontinuation of cardiopulmonary bypass: evidence for contraction-excitation feedback in man. Circulation **77**: 1266–1275.

13. OLSSON, S. B. 1971. Monophasic action potentials of right heart. Suction electrode method in clinical investigations. Thesis. Elanders Boktryckeri AB. Göteborg, Sweden.

14. FRANZ, M. R., D. BURKHOFF, H. SPURGEON, M. L. WEISFELDT & E. G. LAKATTA. 1986. In vitro validation of a new cardiac catheter technique for recording monophasic action potentials. Eur. Heart J. **7**: 34–41.

15. INO, T., H. S. KARAGUEUZIAN, K. HONG, M. MEESMANN, W. J. MANDEL & T. PETER. 1988. Relation of monophasic action potential recorded with contact electrode to underlying transmembrane action potential properties in isolated cardiac tissues: a systematic microelectrode validation study. Cardiovasc. Res. **22**: 255–264.

16. HIRSCH, I., N. EDVARDSSON, S. B. OLSSON & H. BROMAN. 1985. Cardiac monophasic action potentials related to intracellular action potentials. A modeling study. *In* On the Generation, Analysis and Clinical Use of Cardiac Monophasic Action Potentials. Vasastadens Bokbinderi. Göteborg, Sweden.

17. ARLOCK, P. 1979. The influence of the surface electrogram on the rising phase of the mammalian cardiac action potential. Pfluegers Arch. **380**: 139–144.

18. OLSSON, S. B., L. BRORSON, N. EDVARDSSON & E. VARNAUSKAS. 1985. Estimation of ventricular repolarization in man by monophasic action potential recording technique. Eur. Heart J. **6**: 71–79.

19. EDVARDSSON, N., I. HIRSCH & S. B. OLSSON. Effects of lidocaine, procainamide, metoprolol, digoxin and atropine on the conduction of premature ventricular beats in man. Eur. Heart J. **6**: 57–66.

20. DUKER, G., O. ALMGREN & J. AXENBORG. 1988. Computerized evaluation of drug-induced changes in guinea-pig epicardial monophasic action potentials. Pharmacol. Toxicol. **65**: 85–90.

21. OLSSON, S. B. 1989. Class III antiarrhythmic action. *In* Antiarrhythmic Drugs. Editor E. M. Vaughan Williams, Ed. Springer-Verlag. Berlin & Heidelberg.

22. DONALDSSON, R. M., P. TAGGART, H. SWANTON, K. FOX, A. F. RICKARDS & D. NOBLE. 1984. Effect of nitroglycerin on the electrical changes of early or subendocardial ischaemia evaluated by monophasic action potential recordings. Cardiovasc. Res. **18**: 7–13.

23. DONALDSSON, R. M., P. TAGGART, H. SWANTON, K. FOX, D. NOBLE & A. F. RICKARDS. 1983. Intracardiac electrode detection of early ischaemia in man. Br. Heart J. **50**: 213–221.

24. FRANZ, M. R., J. T. FLAHERTY, E. V. PLATIA, B. HEALEY BULKLEY & M. L. WEISFELDT. 1984. Localization of regional myocardial ischemia by recording of monophasic action potentials. Circulation **693**: 593–604.

25. GAVRILESCU, S. & C. LUCA. 1978. Right ventricular monophasic action potentials in patients with long QT syndrome. Br. Heart J. **40**: 1014–1018.

26. BONATTI, V., A. ROLLI & G. BOTTI. 1983. Recording of monophasic action potentials of the right ventricle in long QT syndromes complicated by severe ventricular arrhythmias. Eur. Heart J. **4**: 168–179.

27. BAILIE, D. S., B. S. HIROSHI INOUE, S. KASEDA, J. BEN-DAVID & D. P. ZIPES. 1988. Magnesium suppression of early afterdepolarizations and ventricular tachyarrhythmias induced by cesium in dogs. Circulation **77**: 1395–1402.

28. EL-SHERIF, N., R. H. ZEILER, W. CRAELIUS, W. B. GOUGH & R. HENKIN. 1988. QTU prolongation and polymorphic ventricular tachyarrythmias due to bradycardia-dependent early afterdepolarizations. Afterdepolarizations and ventricular arrhythmias. Circ. Res. **63(2)**: 286–305.

Endocardial and Epicardial Recordings[a]

Correlation of Twelve-Lead Electrocardiograms at the Site of Origin of Ventricular Tachycardia

MARK E. JOSEPHSON[b] AND JOHN M. MILLER

Clinical Electrophysiology Laboratory
Hospital of the University of Pennsylvania
Cardiovascular Section
Department of Medicine
University of Pennsylvania School of Medicine
3400 Spruce Street
Philadelphia, Pennsylvania 19104

The QRS configuration is a representation of the pattern of overall ventricular activation. For many years, it was assumed that the configuration of the QRS could identify the site of ventricular impulse formation. This assumption was based on the hypothesis that impulse formation from specific sites in the ventricle would result in characteristic patterns of ventricular activation and, as a consequence, specific QRS morphologies. However, the QRS morphology of spontaneous ventricular tachycardia (VT) or pacing from multiple ventricular sites is markedly influenced by factors that affect the pattern of ventricular activation, such as the speed and direction of muscle to muscle conduction, participation of the His-Purkinje system in transmitting electrical activity to other areas of the heart, and sites of inexcitable scar tissue. It is, therefore, not surprising that the accuracy of the electrocardiogram in specifically diagnosing the site of origin is limited since most patients with these arrhythmias have cardiac disease which alters these factors.

Over the past 15 years, we have developed endocardial catheter mapping and intraoperative epicardial and endocardial mapping of VT to identify sites of origin in order to develop surgical techniques to ablate these arrhythmias.[1-5] The ability to identify "sites of origin" has allowed us to compare the results of mapping to the 12-lead electrocardiogram (ECG) of these tachycardias in order to develop algorithms to identify the site of origin of the tachycardia. Preliminary studies performed nearly a decade ago in our laboratory demonstrated that for certain VT morphologies, a reasonable approximation of the site of origin of VTs could be made based on the analysis of the 12-lead ECG.[6-8] We have subsequently extended these observations and have provided electrocardiographic algorithms by which one can identify the site of origin of VT to within 10 cm^2 of the earliest site of ventricular activity recorded during catheter and/or intraoperative mapping.[9] The purpose of the present report is to shed light on the use and limitation of the 12-lead ECG in identifying the site of origin by analysis of epicardial and endocardial mapping data.

[a]Supported in part by grants HL28093 and HL07346 from the National Heart, Lung, and Blood Institute, Bethesda, Md., grants from The American Heart Association, Southeastern Pennsylvania Chapter, Philadelphia, Pa., and The Fannie Ripple Trust Fund.

[b]Dr. Josephson is the Robinette Foundation Professor of Medicine (Cardiovascular Diseases).

COMPARISON OF 12-LEAD ECG OF VT AND MAPPING STUDIES

Our data base for relating the 12-lead ECG to the site of origin of VT is based on comparison of the 12-lead ECG of more than 600 VTs the site of origin of which was determined by endocardial catheter and/or intraoperative epicardial and endocardial mapping. The techniques of catheter and intraoperative mapping have been described in detail elsewhere.[1-5] In addition, we have used data obtained from analysis of the 12-lead ECGs resulting from pacing specific sites in the left ventricle in normal and abnormal ventricles.[7,10,11] These results, by and large, confirmed those studies directly

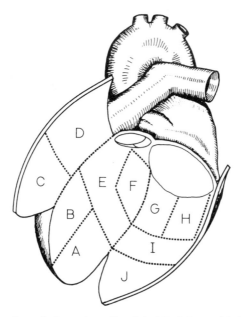

FIGURE 1. Regions of ventricular tachycardia origin. The left ventricle is depicted as having been opened along the lateral wall with anterior wall reflected to the left. Regions are as follows: A, inferoapical septum; B, anteroapical septum; C, anteroapical free wall; D, anterobasal free wall; E, anterobasal and midseptum; F, inferobasal septum; G, inferomedial free wall; H, inferolateral free wall; I midinferior wall; J inferoapical free wall. Areas G and H together constitute the inferobasal free wall. (From Miller *et al.*, with permission.)[9]

comparing mapped sites of origin of VTs with their ECG. Our initial studies demonstrated patterns suggestive of tachycardia originating from the inferobasal parts of the heart (inferior infarction) and those arising in the apical aspects of the heart (i.e., associated with anterior infarction).[6-11] Basal sites of origin were characterized by R waves in leads 1, V_1, V_2, and V_6 while those arising from the apex frequently exhibited Q waves in 1, V_1 or V_2, and V_6. Our results have recently been confirmed by Kuchar *et al.*,[12] who used pace mapping to correlate sites of impulse formation with the 12-lead ECG.

To extend these observations, we retrospectively studied ≈200 VTs, using a more detailed analysis of precordial R wave progression, in order to develop more accurate algorithms for identifying sites of origin.[9] The left ventricle (the sites from which all tachycardias rose) was divided into regions of approximately 10 to 15 cm^2 (FIGURE 1) and tachycardias were divided by both bundle branch block morphology and site of infarction. Eight kinds of R wave progression were defined (FIGURE 2). Tachycardia morphologies for which at least five examples were present were those evaluated for specificity of QRS morphology to a site of origin. Four characteristics were evaluated for each VT: (1) site of prior infarction, (2) bundle branch block pattern; (3) axis deviation; and (4) precordial R wave progression. Among the group of VTs having the same characteristic morphology, a determination was made of which characteristic morphologies were associated with a particular region (A through J in FIGURE 1) with a predictive accuracy of >70%. In other words >70% of VTs with a characteristic morphology had to originate from a specific region. At least five examples of a characteristic morphology were required before the analysis was made.

Overall only 50% of VTs had a specific VT morphology (FIGURE 3). Patients with VT associated with anterior infarction were less likely to have specific morphologies associated with the site of origin than those of the inferior origin (37% vs. 74%). Furthermore, left bundle branch block VTs were clustered at specific sites of origin far more frequently than those with right bundle branch block tachycardias (73% vs. 31%). These observations are likely related to (1) anterior infarctions are larger than inferior infarctions; (2) greater abnormalities of conduction are observed in anterior

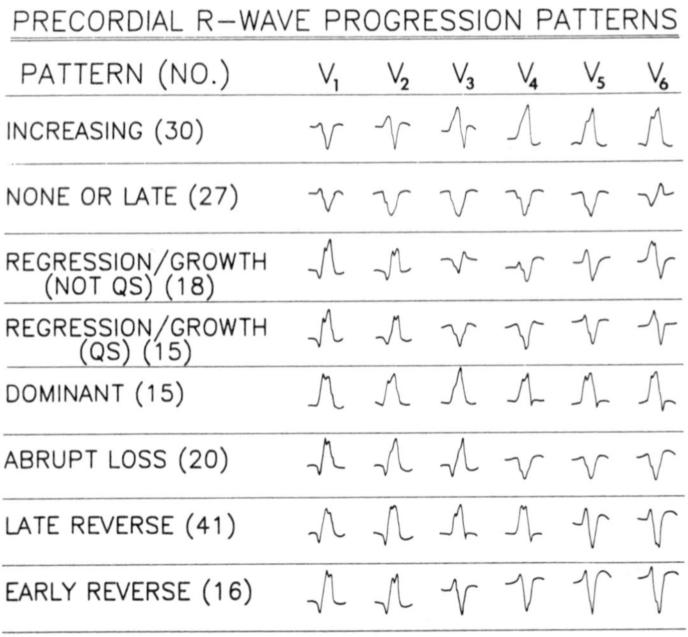

PRECORDIAL R–WAVE PROGRESSION PATTERNS

PATTERN (NO.)	V_1	V_2	V_3	V_4	V_5	V_6
INCREASING (30)						
NONE OR LATE (27)						
REGRESSION/GROWTH (NOT QS) (18)						
REGRESSION/GROWTH (QS) (15)						
DOMINANT (15)						
ABRUPT LOSS (20)						
LATE REVERSE (41)						
EARLY REVERSE (16)						

FIGURE 2. Precordial R-wave patterns (RWP). The eight different patterns seen in this study are listed on the left, with the number of examples in parentheses. Typical R wave patterns for V_1 through V_6 are shown at right. (From Miller *et al.*, with permission.)[9]

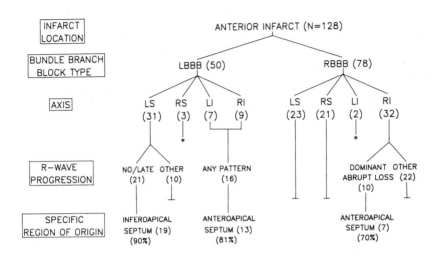

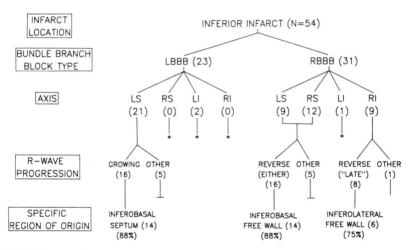

FIGURE 3. Algorithm correlating region of origin to 12-lead ECG of VT. Top, anterior infarct–associated VTs are displayed; bottom, inferior infarct–associated VTs. The first branch point is bundle branch block (BBB) configuration, followed by QRS axis, and RWP. When possible, a "specific region of origin" is indicated. Number of VTs in each group is indicated in parentheses. A vertical line ending in an asterisk indicates inadequate numbers of VT for analysis; a vertical line terminating in a horizontal bar indicates adequate numbers for analysis, but no specific patterns. L = left; S = superior; R = right; I = inferior. (From Miller et al., with permission.)[9]

infarction (as determined by extent of abnormal, fragmented electrograms); and (3) VTs with left bundle branch block all arise from septal or paraseptal regions. However, even within relatively narrow clusters of ECG morphologies, discrepancies could exist between the axes of the tachycardias and the sites of origin. An example of this can be seen in the group of tachycardias with left bundle, left superior axis with anterior infarction (FIGURE 4). Twenty percent of such tachycardias originate from the superior aspects of the apical septum (segment B on superior C in FIGURE 1), a finding that should have produced an inferior axis and not a superior axis. Additionally, virtually identical tachycardia morphologies (right bundle branch block, right superior axis) could come from the septal or free wall of apical infarctions (FIGURE 4).

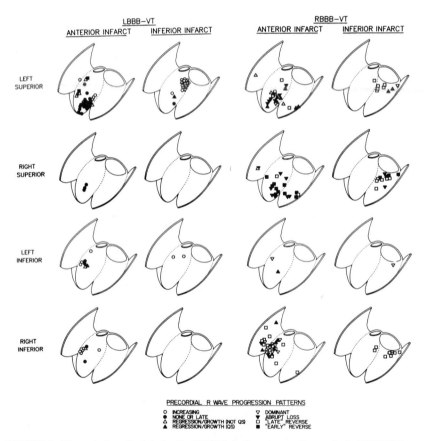

FIGURE 4. Mapped sites of origin for the 182 VTs in the retrospective analysis. LBBB VTs are shown on the left and RBBB VTs on the right; among each bundle branch block type, anterior infarcts are shown on the left and inferior on the right. QRS axis is segregated by horizontal rows, as shown in the far left column. The left ventricular endocardium is displayed as in FIGURE 2, and each individual characteristic morphology is plotted according to the key at bottom. (From Miller *et al.*, with permission.)[9]

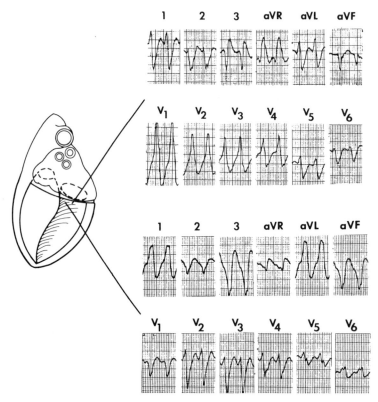

FIGURE 5. Ventricular tachycardia with right and left bundle branch block morphologies originating at the same sites posterobasally (patient 4, Table 3). (From Josephson *et al.,* with permission.)[6]

FACTORS INFLUENCING QRS AND SITE OF ORIGIN

We then sought to establish what factors influenced the QRS morphology of VT associated with myocardial infarction. Size of the infarction, location of the tachycardia within the infarction, the ability to propagate out of the infarct, and the availability of the His-Purkinje system for propagation each contribute to the overall pattern of ventricular activation and resultant QRS morphology.

Prior data from our laboratory suggested that the overall pattern of ventricular activation, particularly that observed during the epicardial mapping, was closely related to the QRS pattern.[3] Thus, the bundle branch block type of tachycardia depended upon the relative activation of the right and left ventricle, and the axis of the tachycardia depended upon the superior/inferior activation of the ventricles. In fact, the epicardial activation sequence bore a closer relation to the QRS morphology than to the site of origin. We found three factors that could affect the discrepancy between epicardial activation patterns and site of origin of VT in coronary disease. The first factor that was apparent was that endocardial activation preceded epicardial activa-

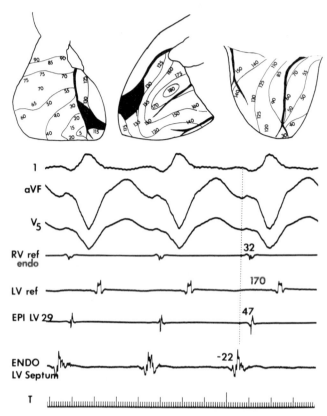

FIGURE 6. Epicardial and endocardial activation in LBBB tachycardia. The epicardial surface of the heart is shown on top (left to right) in the anterior, left lateral, and inferior views. On the bottom, surface leads 1, aVF, and V_5 are shown with electrograms from a right ventricular (RV) endocardial reference electrogram, a left ventricular (LV) reference electrogram, an epicardial electrogram from the left ventricular site 29 (anterolateral LV) and site from the earliest site on the endocardium of the left ventricular septum. The earliest activation in this LBBB tachycardia is on the left ventricular septum, 22 mseconds prior to the onset of the QRS. As can be seen on the epicardial map, typical for VT with LBBB, epicardial breakthrough begins in the right ventricle and activation of the right ventricle is completed prior to that of the left ventricle.

tion in 99% of all tachycardias associated with coronary artery disease, and that the endocardial or subendocardial site of origin was in the left ventricle regardless of QRS morphology.[1-4] Second, was that 64% of the tachycardias had a septal site of origin and, consequently, the site of origin would not be expected to correlate with epicardial activation. Finally, the pattern and rate of propagation from the endocardial site of origin to the muscle producing the QRS was variable. Marked abnormalities of conduction from the site of origin to the muscle mass responsible for generating the QRS occurs in an unpredictable manner. This could lead to VTs with either right or left bundle branch block patterns or different axes based solely on the pattern of propagation from the site of origin within the infarction to tissue outside the infarct. It is well known, and clearly documented, that tachycardias with right bundle branch block morphology and left bundle branch block morphology can arise from the same site (FIGURE 5).[1–4,6,7] We have previously demonstrated that the relative activation of the left and right ventricles is what determines the bundle branch block morphology and not the site of origin.[3] Thus, as shown in FIGURE 6, a tachycardia arising from the left ventricle can have a left bundle branch block morphology as long as the right ventricle is activated relatively early with respect to the left ventricle during the tachycardia. This observation led to the important conclusion that VTs with left bundle branch block patterns should not be classified as *right ventricular tachycardias* unless they are mapped to the right ventricle. VT with a right bundle branch block morphology always arises in the left ventricle in patients with coronary disease. They can originate at the same or different site as VTs with a left bundle branch block pattern. Right bundle branch block pattern occurs when left ventricular activation precedes right ventricular activation (FIGURE 7).

The different patterns of activation from the site of origin to the remainder of the heart occur as a consequence of both the initiation of the tachycardia, which establishes the functional barriers in the reentrant circuit and pathway of impulse propagation in the circuit, and the nonuniform anisotropic properties of the heart following infarction. Because of the dynamic and functional nature of these factors, it is possible

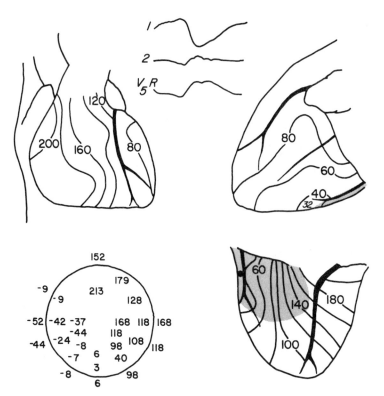

FIGURE 7. Intraoperative mapping during ventricular tachycardia. The epicardial map is displayed with ECG leads 1, 2, and V₅R. The stippled area represents an aneurysm. Early epicardial breakthrough occurs 32 mseconds after the onset of the QRS. Earliest endocardial activation is located 2–3 cm away. (From Josephson et al., with permission.)[2]

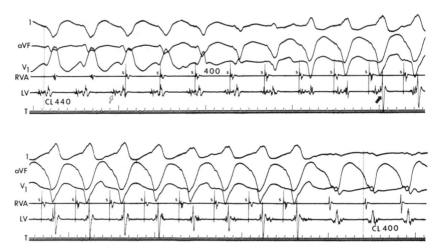

FIGURE 8. Reversal of reentrant loop by ventricular pacing. Surface leads I, aVF, and V₁ are shown with a right ventricular electrogram (RVA) and left ventricular electrogram (LV) at the site of origin of a tachycardia with an RBBB, right superior axis. This electrogram occurred 110 mseconds prior to the onset of the QRS (open arrow). Right ventricular pacing is begun in the top panel and continued through the bottom panel. Note the reversal of the electrogram configuration at the site of origin which develops and then remains fixed during right ventricular pacing. Upon cessation of pacing, the tachycardia loop appears reversed and the QRS morphology now has an LBBB, left axis deviation configuration.

to change the pattern of activation in a reentrant circuit (i.e., clockwise vs. counterclockwise) or exit site from that reentrant circuit by rapid ventricular pacing or ventricular extrastimuli. Such perturbations can reverse the bundle branch block morphology by changing the relative timing of activation of both ventricles (FIGURE 8).

RELATIONSHIP OF EPICARDIAL AND ENDOCARDIAL ACTIVATION TO QRS PATTERN

In patients in whom the earliest epicardial breakthrough occurs in the same region as the earliest endocardial site of activation, there is a reasonable correlation with the surface QRS morphology and that site of origin. An example of such a tachycardia is shown in FIGURE 9 in which the endocardial site of origin and epicardial breakthrough site are located in the same general area. Despite a difference in timing of 55 mseconds, (endocardial earlier than epicardial) there is a reasonable correlation of earliest endocardial activation and epicardial breakthrough. Note the right bundle branch block, right superior axis tachycardia results because, following epicardial breakthrough, ventricular activation proceeds from the inferior, anterolateral left ventricle to superior-basal right ventricle.

Unfortunately, epicardial breakthrough and endocardial activation are more frequently unassociated. This is always true when tachycardias arise on the left ventricular septum, which is the case in 64% of all tachycardias. In which case, the endocardial site of origin is not correlated to epicardial breakthrough. Thus, left bundle branch block tachycardias, which virtually always arise from the septum, or paraseptal areas, typically have right ventricular epicardial breakthrough and/or early right ventricular activation followed by left ventricular activation, yet the earliest site is on the left ventricular septum (see FIGURE 6). This can also lead to a totally disparate axis deviation, with breakthrough superiorly or inferiorly regardless of the site of origin as shown in FIGURE 10. Therefore, tachycardias arising on the septum can have either a right or a left bundle branch block or inferior or superior axis and have the same site of origin. In FIGURE 11, VTs with the same site of origin on the septum demonstrated a right bundle branch pattern but totally different axes because epicardial breakthrough was anterior for one and inferior for the other.

Discrepancies also occur frequently in patients with tachycardia arising in the free wall. As shown in FIGURE 12, the earliest epicardial breakthrough of the right bundle

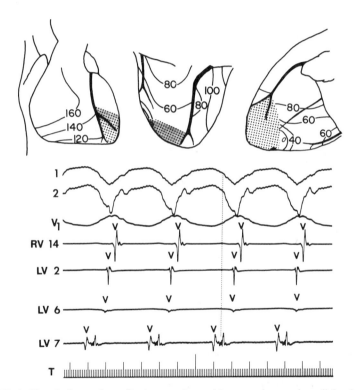

FIGURE 9. Ventricular tachycardia in a patient with concordant endocardial origin and epicardial breakthrough. On top, an epicardial map with 20 msecond isochrones is shown in the anterior, inferior and left lateral views (left to right). The stippled area represents an apical infarction. Epicardial breakthrough and earliest endocardial site (filled circle at lateral edge of the aneurysm) occur within the same area. An endocardial catheter map is shown on the bottom. Leads 1, 2, and V_1 are shown with a reference electrogram from RV site 14 (the anterior RV wall) and three LV sites on the septum (LV-2), the inferobasal part of the left ventricle (LV-6), and the anterolateral left ventricle (LV-7) which was the site of origin. (From Josephson et al., with permission.)[2]

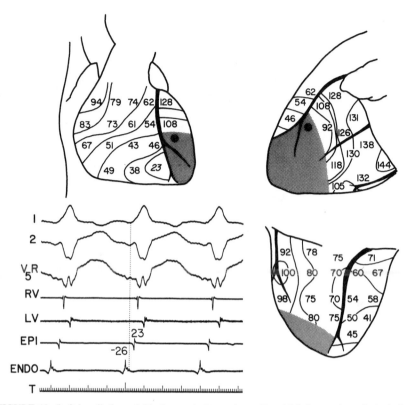

FIGURE 10. Left bundle branch block ventricular tachycardia with left superior axis deviation originating from the high anterior septum. Epicardial isochronic maps are shown in the anterior, left lateral and inferior views (clockwise from top left), and an endocardial map in the left lower corner. The stippled area represents an anterior apical aneurysm. The filled circle represents the site of earliest endocardial activity in the high septum. Earliest epicardial breakthrough is in the right ventricle, 23 mseconds after the onset of the QRS with rapid spread superiorly to the right and eventually left ventricles, giving rise to a superior left axis deviation. Earliest endocardial activation shown in the lower left occurs 26 mseconds prior to the onset of the QRS at the superior aspect of the left ventricular septum.

branch block VT is at the inferoapical portion of the left ventricular aneurysm. The earliest endocardial site of origin is 5 cm away and 70 mseconds earlier in time. The endocardial site of origin is at a superiorly located site on the anterior wall and therefore would be expected to give rise to ventricular tachycardia with an inferior axis. However, since epicardial breakthrough, and the subsequent spread of activation, was initiated at the inferoapical portion of the heart, a superior axis resulted. An even more unusual situation is shown in FIGURE 13 in which VT originates at the endocardium near the border of an inferior wall infarction. The two VTs observed in this patient had earliest epicardial breakthrough on opposite sides of his inferior aneurysm. Thus, abnormalities of conduction within the reentrant circuit and/or infarction can lead to epicardial breakthrough at widely disparate sites leading to totally different overall ventricular activation sequences and QRS morphologies, despite the same site of origin. The abnormalities of impulse propagation responsible for these discrepancies are most likely related to the nonuniform anisotropy produced by the infarction. The effect of anisotropy on propagation from the site of origin of VT arising from the superior septum is shown in FIGURE 14. Presystolic electrograms are seen at many sites but since propagation spreads most rapidly inferiorly, the earliest epicardial activation will be on the inferior surface of the heart, giving rise to a superior axis. A more detailed analysis of how nonuniform anisotropy plays a role in conduction is shown in FIGURE 15 in which detailed activation during two different tachycardias propagating through the same site are shown. These activation patterns, which were recorded from multiple electrodes on a small plaque, differ greatly during the two tachycardias and during sinus rhythm. These different patterns and rates of propagation are due to functional differences in conduction produced by the varying relationship of the direction of the wavefront to the fiber orientation.[13-15] We have observed intermittent failure of conduction in very small areas within the region of tachycardia origin.[16] Such small changes (FIGURE 16) may lead to a change in overall ventricular activation. This, in

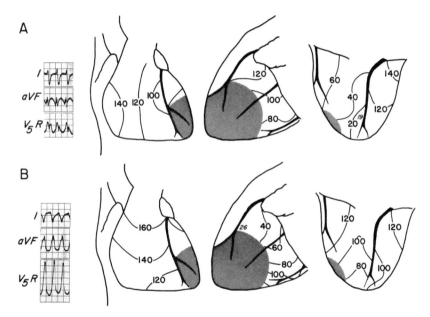

FIGURE 11. Epicardial maps during ventricular tachycardia with right bundle branch block and different frontal plane axes. In both panels the epicardial surface of the ventricles is shown in the anterior (left), lateral (middle), and inferior (right) projections, with ECG leads I, aVF, and V₅R recorded during two VT morphologies in the same patient. Twenty millisecond isochrones are shown. An apical aneurysm is indicated by the stippling. In Panel A, an inferior epicardial breakthrough occurred 19 mseconds after the onset of the QRS along the posterior interventricular groove, 4 cm from the epicardial border of the aneurysm. In panel B, VT with a right bundle branch block morphology and differential frontal plane axis was associated with an anterior epicardial breakthrough 26 mseconds after the QRS. The site of origin of both VTs was located on the midapical septum. (From Horowitz et al., with permission.)[3]

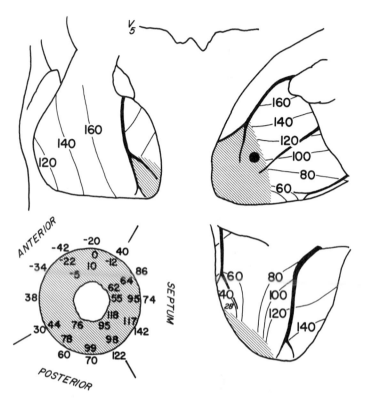

FIGURE 12. Ventricular tachycardia with a right bundle branch block pattern in a patient with an anteroseptal aneurysm. The epicardial map with the site of epicardial breakthrough indicated by the italicized numeral and 20 msecond isochrones are shown with ECG lead V_5 and endocardial activation data (lower left). During VT-RBBB, epicardial breakthrough occurred 28 mseconds after the onset of the QRS complex on the inferolateral left ventricle and the site of origin was located on the anterior epicardial border of the aneurysm (-42 on the endocardial map). This resulted in a disparate axis (superior) for this site of origin.

turn, may lead to a sudden change in morphology which may be slight or great (FIGURE 17). In some instances, it may even cause a change in bundle branch block morphology.

ROLE OF THE HIS-PURKINJE SYSTEM IN VENTRICULAR ACTIVATION

Several factors affect the QRS width. Although muscle mass, and nonuniform anisotropy (see above), play a role in overall duration of activation, we believe that the His-Purkinje system also plays an important role in impulse propagation. Using closely spaced electrodes (e.g., 5 mm), we have been able to discern His bundle activation in nearly 85% of VTs. In occasional patients, we have been able to document morphologically similar tachycardias with different QRS widths. In such cases, the QRS width appears related to His-Purkinje activation and participation in global left ventricular activation.[17] This does not, however, implicate the His-Purkinje system as a component

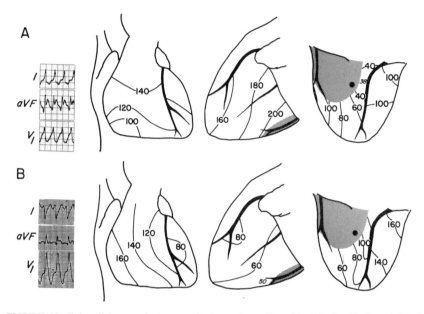

FIGURE 13. Epicardial maps during ventricular tachycardias with right bundle branch block morphology and different frontal axes associated with a posterior aneurysm. In both panels the epicardial surface of the ventricles is shown with ECG leads I, aVF, and V_1 recorded during VT. Isochrones are shown as 20 msecond intervals. The aneurysm is indicated by the stippled area and the endocardial origin is indicated by the solid circle. In panel A, VT-RBBB with a normal axis was associated with epicardial breakthrough 38 mseconds after the onset of the QRS on the medial aspect of the aneurysm. In panel B, VT-RBBB with right axis deviation was associated with epicardial breakthrough 50 mseconds after the onset of the QRS at one lateral border of the aneurysm. The origin of both VTs was at the base of the posterior papillary muscle, which was abnormally positioned. (From Horowitz *et al.,* with permission.)[3]

of the underlying reentrant circuit. For example, in FIGURE 18, two tachycardias of the same morphology are shown, one with a narrow QRS (128 mseconds) and one with a wider QRS (153 mseconds). The tachycardia cycle lengths are similar, but the wider QRS has a much longer VH interval, suggesting that the QRS width but not the tachycardia cycle length is affected by participation of the His-Purkinje system. Occasionally one can see a marked spontaneous increase in tachycardia cycle length, suggesting either slowing of conduction in the reentrant circuit or a change to a larger reentrant circuit, but the VH interval and QRS width remain constant. These situations suggest that the His-Purkinje system is primarily related to overall activation of the heart but has no role in the tachycardia mechanism. Linear regression analysis of five tachycardias from an individual patient showing a direct relationship between VH intervals and QRS widths further supports this concept (FIGURE 19).

Q WAVES DURING VT: RELATION TO DISEASE PROCESS

It has been suggested that Q waves (particularly QR complexes) during VT are diagnostic of tachycardias due to coronary artery disease.[18,19] We disagree with this

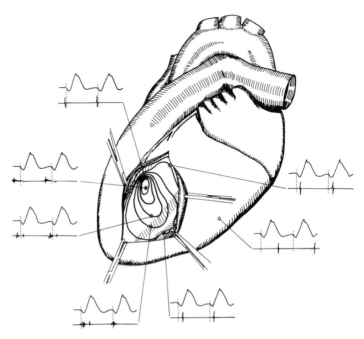

FIGURE 14. Asymmetric endocardial activation during ventricular tachycardia. A schema of the opened LV is shown during VT. The site of origin is at the superior apical septum (second electrogram on left). Isochrones demonstrate rapid activation inferiorly and slow propagation superiorly. This led to a discrepancy in site of origin and epicardial breakthrough and axis. See text for discussion.

suggestion. We have seen Q waves (qs or qR) in patients with cardiomyopathy with both right and left bundle branch block tachycardias (FIGURE 20 and 21). Thus, Q waves are not specific for a disease process and cannot be used to diagnose infarction. We believe the presence of Q waves only suggests propagation of the impulse away from the recording electrode. Thus, Q waves are produced by either fixed scar or functional conduction disturbances secondary to fibrosis of whatever etiology. We agree with Coumel[18] that QRS amplitude is greatest in VT associated with normal hearts. The more diseased the heart, the more "splintered" the QRS.

CONCLUSIONS

The QRS morphology has been useful in regionalizing the origin of VTs but suffers from many limitations. These limitations are related by the presence of myocardial infarction, fibrosis, hypertrophy, ventricular geometry (i.e., aneurysm or postoperative changes), position of the heart in the chest cavity, and, perhaps, metabolic or pharmacologic factors. Epicardial and endocardial mapping has led to a greater understanding of the mechanisms of these limitations. Several conclusions can be reached based on our data: (1) the QRS pattern of VT correlates better with the pattern of global epicardial activation than the endocardial site of origin as a result of very slow, and variable conduction from the origin to the muscle mass generating the QRS complex; (2) the more normal the heart, and the greater the correlation of epicardial and endocardial activation, the higher predictive accuracy of the electrocardiographic pattern for the site of origin; (3) the larger the infarct (i.e., anterior infarction), and the more abnormal the pattern of ventricular activation, the greater the disparity of epicardial and endocardial activation and the lower the predictive accuracy of the electrocardiographic patterns. Despite these limitations, the 12-lead electrocardiogram can provide information that will direct mapping to specific regions. This will facilitate the determination of the site of origin and allow for surgical or nonsurgical ablation of that site in less time.

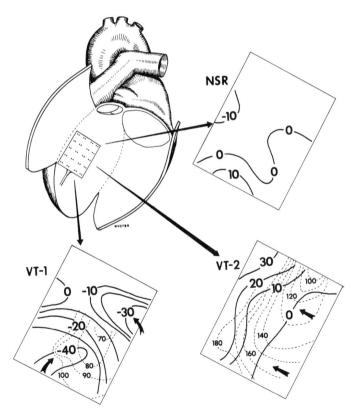

FIGURE 15. Role of nonuniform anisotropy and conduction patterns during ventricular tachycardia. The left ventricle is opened up and a plaque consisting of 20 bipolar electrode pairs (≈ 3 cm^2) is shown. During VT-1 and VT-2, endocardial activation is totally different, being rapid or slow depending upon the wave of activation. In both cases it is much slower than that seen during sinus rhythm (NSR). The rapidity of activation is thus a functional property of the direction of impulse propagation.

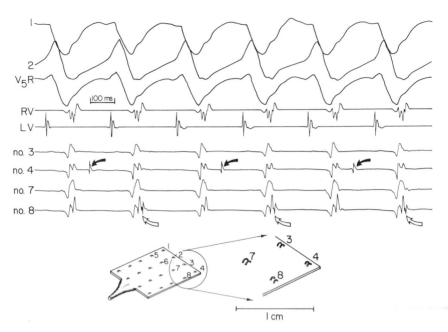

FIGURE 16. Localized nature of conduction failure during ventricular tachycardia. Leads 1, 2, and V_5 are shown with reference electrograms from the right and left ventricles (RV and LV). Recordings from poles 3, 4, 7, and 8 on a multipolar plaque are shown. Bipolar pairs are 4 mm apart. In the recordings from these bipolar electrodes, local conduction failure is observed in numbers 4 and 8 (arrows) but not in numbers 3 and 7 (only 4 mm away). Additionally, local conduction failure occurs on opposite beats in bipolar numbers 4 and 8 (open arrows). (From Miller *et al.*, with permission.)[16]

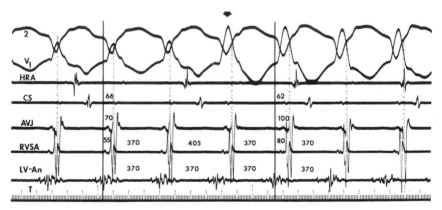

FIGURE 17. Abrupt change in QRS morphology and endocardial activation sequence of ventricular tachycardia. Leads 2 and V_1 are shown with electrograms from the high right atrium (HRA), coronary sinus (CS), AV junction (AVJ), right ventricular septum near the apex (RVSA), and from within the left ventricular aneurysm (LV-AN) at the site of origin of the tachycardia. Following three beats of VT, there is a sudden change in QRS morphology noted by the arrow; however, the electrogram in the LV-AN remains unchanged. The morphological change in the QRS is associated with a one beat delay (370–405 mseconds) in the electrogram recorded at the RVSA, and subsequent change of ventricular activation in the CS, AVJ, and RVSA (vertical lines). A change in ventricular activation which accompanies the change in QRS is abrupt without any change in the tachycardia cycle length. This suggests a change in exit site from the underlying reentrant circuit. (From Josephson *et al.*, with permission.)[1]

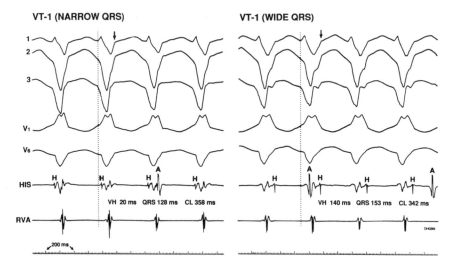

FIGURE 18. Role of His-Purkinje system in determining width of QRS during ventricular tachycardia. Leads 1, 2, 3, V_1, and V_6 are shown with recordings from the His bundle electrogram (HIS) and the right ventricular apex (RVA). VT-1 has a relatively narrow QRS (128 mseconds) and a cycle length of 358 mseconds. The VH interval is short at 20 mseconds. Shortly following the first tracing the QRS of the VT-2 widened without a significant change in the tachycardia cycle length (this actually is slightly shorter at 342 mseconds). The wider QRS of VT-2 is associated with a longer VH interval (VH = 140 mseconds). See text for discussion.

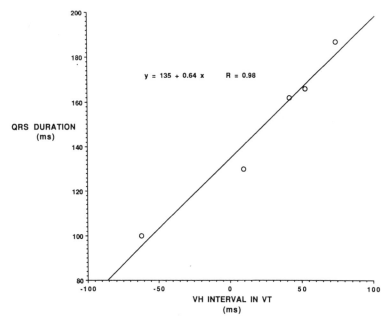

$$y = 135 + 0.64\ x \qquad R = 0.98$$

FIGURE 19. Relationship between VH interval and QRS duration during ventricular tachycardia. VH interval is plotted on the abscissa and QRS duration on the ordinate. Five tachycardias in the same individual are shown in circles. Note the linear correlation between the VH interval and the QRS duration.

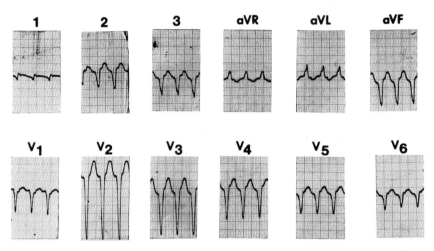

FIGURE 20. Ventricular tachycardia with an LBBB pattern in a patient with idiopathic dilated cardiomyopathy. Q waves are present in leads 1, 2, 3, aVF, and V_3–V_6.

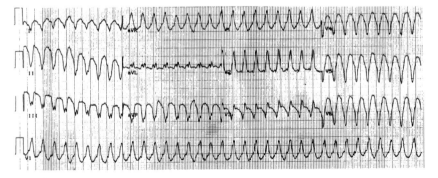

FIGURE 21. Ventricular tachycardia with an RBBB pattern in a patient with idiopathic dilated cardiomyopathy. VT with an RBBB pattern is demonstrated. Q waves are seen in leads 1, 2, 3, aVF, and V_3–V_6. Note the qR pattern in V_3.

REFERENCES

1. JOSEPHSON, M. E., L. N. HOROWITZ, A. FARSHIDI, J. F. SPEAR, J. A. KASTOR & E. N. MOORE. 1978. Recurrent sustained ventricular tachycardia 2. Endocardial mapping. Circulation **57:** 440–447.
2. JOSEPHSON, M. E., L. N. HOROWITZ, S. R. SPIELMAN, A. M. GREENSPAN, C. VANDEPOL & A. H. HARKEN. 1980. Comparison of endocardial catheter mapping with intraoperative mapping of ventricular tachycardia. Circulation **61:** 1227–1238.
3. HOROWITZ, L. N., M. E. JOSEPHSON & A. H. HARKEN. 1980. Epicardial and endocardial activation during sustained ventricular tachycardia in man. Circulation **61:** 1227–1238.
4. JOSEPHSON, M. E., L. N. HOROWITZ, S. R. SPIELMAN, H. L. WAXMAN & A. M. GREENSPAN. 1982. Role of catheter mapping in the preoperative evaluation of ventricular tachycardia. Am. J. Cardiol. **49:** 207–220.
5. MILLER, J. M., A. H. HARKEN, W. C. HARGROVE & M. E. JOSEPHSON. 1985. Pattern of endocardial activation during sustained ventricular tachycardia. J. Am. Coll. Cardiol. **6:** 1280–1287.
6. JOSEPHSON, M. E., L. N. HOROWITZ, H. L. WAXMAN, M. E. CAIN, S. R. SPIELMAN, A. M. GREENSPAN, F. E. MARCHLINSKI & M. D. EZRI. 1981. Sustained ventricular tachycardia: role of the 12-lead electrocardiogram in localizing the site of origin. Circulation **64:** 257–272.
7. JOSEPHSON, M. E., H. L. WAXMAN, F. E. MARCHLINSKI, L. N. HOROWITZ & S. R. SPIELMAN. 1981. Relation between site of origin and QRS configuration in ventricular rhythms. *In* What's New in Electrocardiography. H. J. J. Wellens & H. E. Kulbertus, Eds. Martinus Nijhoff Publishers. The Hague, The Netherlands.
8. JOSEPHSON, M. E. 1982. The origin of premature ventricular complexes—role and limitations of the 12-lead electrocardiogram. Int. J. Cardiol. **2:** 87–90.
9. MILLER, J. M., F. E. MARCHLINSKI, A. E. BUXTON & M. E. JOSEPHSON. 1988. Relationship between the 12-lead electrocardiogram during ventricular tachycardia and endocardial site of origin in patients with coronary artery disease. Circulation **77:** 759–766.
10. JOSEPHSON, M. E., H. L. WAXMAN, M. E. CAIN, M. J. GARDNER & A. E. BUXTON. 1982. Ventricular activation during ventricular endocardial pacing. II. Role of pace-mapping to localize origin of ventricular tachycardia. Am. J. Cardiol. **50:** 11–22.
11. WAXMAN, H. L. & M. E. JOSEPHSON. 1982. Ventricular activation during ventricular endocardial pacing. 1. Electrocardiographic patterns related to site of pacing. Am. J. Cardiol. **50:** 1.
12. KUCHAR, D. L., J. N. RUSKIN & H. GARAN. 1989. Electrocardiographic localization of the site of origin of ventricular tachycardia in patients with prior myocardial infarction. J. Am. Coll. Cardiol. **13:** 893–900.
13. SPACH, M. S., W. T. MILLER, D. B. GESELOWITZ, R. C. BARR, J. M. KOOTSEY & E. A. JOHNSON. 1981. The discontinuous nature of propagation in normal canine cardiac muscle. Evidence for recurrent discontinuities of intracellular resistance that affect membrane currents. Circ. Res. **48:** 39–54.
14. SPACH, M. S., W. T. MILLER, P. C. DOLBER, J. M. KOOTSEY, J. R. SOMMER & C. E. MOSHER, JR. 1982. The functional role of structural complexities in the propagation of depolarization in the atrium of the dog. Cardiac conduction disturbances due to discontinuities of effective axial resistivity. Circ. Res. **50:** 175–191.
15. JOYNER, R. W. 1982. Effects of the discrete pattern of electrical coupling on propagation through an electrical syncytium. Circ. Res. **50:** 192–100.
16. MILLER, J. M., J. A. VASSALLO, W. C. HARGROVE & M. E. JOSEPHSON. 1985. Intermittent failure of local conduction during ventricular tachycardia. Circulation **72:** 1286–1292.
17. MILLER, J. M., C. D. GOTTLIEB, M. D. LESH, F. E. MARCHLINSKI, A. E. BUXTON & M. E. JOSEPHSON. 1989. His-Purkinje activation during ventricular tachycardia: a determinant of QRS duration. J. Am. Coll. Cardiol. **13:** 21A.
18. COUMEL, P. 1987. Diagnostic significance of the QRS wave form in patients with ventricular tachycardia. Cardiol. Clin. **5:** 527–540.
19. COUMEL, P., J. F. LECLERCQ, P. ATTUEL, et al. 1984. The QRS morphology in post-myocardial infarction ventricular tachycardia. A study of 100 tracings compared with 70 cases of idiopathic ventricular tachycardia. Eur. Heart J. **5:** 792.

Body Surface Mapping Including Relationships with Endocardial and Epicardial Mapping

NANCY C. FLOWERS[a] AND LEO G. HORAN[a,b]

[a]Section of Cardiology
Medical College of Georgia
Augusta, Georgia 30912-3105

[b]Cardiology
Veterans Administration Medical Center
Augusta, Georgia 30910

INTRODUCTION

Recording and display of the temporal and spatial distribution of surface potentials recorded from multiple sites on the torso is termed body surface mapping (BSM). The concept of mapping was probably first articulated by Waller at St. Mary's Hospital in an inaugural address, who in 1888 published a torso map of the voltage field about the heart. He based his description upon the concept that the cardiac generator could be represented by a bipole, resulting in positive and negative isopotential lines projected onto the thoracic surface (FIGURE 1).[1] The first recording we are aware of in isopotential map form of successive instants of the QRS complex was by Koch and Schneyer.[2] Instant-by-instant mapping of surface voltage change throughout the cardiac cycle was described by Nahum et al. who demonstrated a surface potential field that was more complex than could likely result from a dipolar source.[3] Nelson first clearly portrayed multipolar sources as multiple peaks and valleys in the curves of instantaneous potential distribution recorded from a band of electrodes about the chest,[4] after which Taccardi in Italy,[5,6] Amirov in Russia,[7] and Horan et al. in the United States[8] published comprehensive maps from both dogs and men in which evidence of both dipolar and nondipolar activity was apparent. Maps were originally drawn from manual measurements of scalar electrocardiograms. The acceleration of interest in BSM is directly related to technological advances making computers available to handle tedious and time-consuming data aquisition and reduction, and to increasingly sophisticated instrumentation.

This review will not explore the basic biophysical underpinnings of the science of mapping or details of efforts to solve the "inverse problem." It will, in the main, deal with physiologic correlations and pathophysiologic relationships. TABLE 1 summarizes the rationale for BSM. The reader is also referred to two recent significant works in the area of BSM: an entire book edited by Mirvis on BSM[9] and a chapter by Ambroggi et al. in a three-volume set on electrocardiology edited by MacFarlane and Laurie.[10]

BSMs from our laboratory have been obtained by two methods. At an early stage we utilized a multichannel Ampex FM tape recorder to store analog signals from an array of 1000-gain low-level amplifiers from 142 equally spaced sites about the torso. Potentials were then digitized, signal-averaged seven channels at a time, and then temporally collated (using the eighth channel) into map format by a digital computer. More recently, we have utilized an array of 35 chest electrodes which had been shown

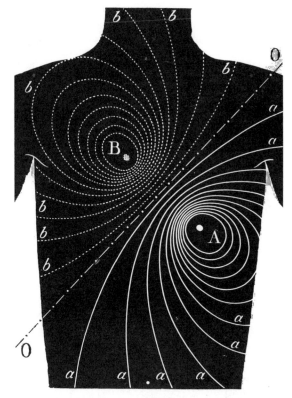

FIGURE 1. Waller's 1888 conception of the electrical field of the heart. The null line is indicated by the dash-dot line. Solid lines (a) represent positive isopotential lines while dotted lines (b) represent negative isopotential lines. Points of maximum and minimum are indicated by A and B respectively. (Reprinted from Reference 1 with permission.)

TABLE 1. Rationale for Recording Body Surface Maps

1. Not all surface electrical information is contained in the electrocardiogram or vector-cardiogram.
2. The heart is not a dipole, and it generates a more complex message than even several simultaneous dipoles can account for. Maps can portray the complexities of tensor potential fields while scalar leads and vectorcardiograms cannot.
3. Instantaneous surface potential maps are also a more physiologically appropriate ana-logue of cardiac depolarization and repolarization than are scalar electrocardiograms or vector loops.
4. Mid and late QRS events which are not easily recognizable in scalar leads can be iso-lated in space and time by the map for analysis.

to permit an excellent reconstruction of the 142-point body surface map when a modification of the estimate of covariance described by Lux *et al.* was utilized.[11,12] These signals acquired at a gain of 1000 are digitized at a sampling frequency of 1000 Hz and recorded through a portable laboratory computer onto floppy discs for subsequent transfer to a DEC PDP 11–34 processor for analysis and display. Maps in this report are displayed as isopotential maps, isointegral maps, or isometric projection maps.

NORMAL MAPS

In FIGURE 2A normal isopotential maps are illustrated. Atrial activation is displayed at 20 msecond intervals beginning at 10 mseconds after onset of atrial

A

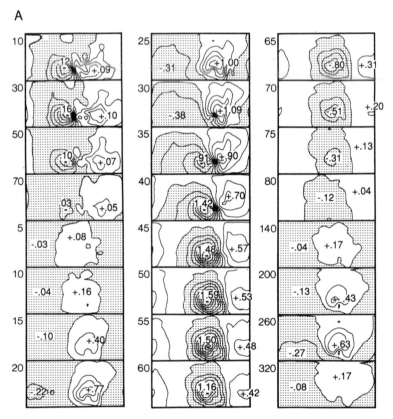

FIGURE 2. Body surface maps of normal subjects. **FIGURE 2A** (above). Isopotential maps of atrial excitation (10–70 mseconds), ventricular excitation (5–80 mseconds) and ventricular recovery (140–320 mseconds). Negative fields are dashed; positive fields are clear. Maxima are indicated with pluses (+); minima are indicated with minuses (−). The middle of each map coincides with the midsternal line while the edges coincide with the vertebral lines. The lower edge is just above the umbilicus while the upper edge is just below the clavicle. See text for discussion.

activity. Ventricular activation maps are illustrated from 5 mseconds through 80 mseconds after onset of ventricular excitation, while ventricular recovery maps are shown at 40 msecond intervals from 140 mseconds through 320 mseconds after onset of ventricular excitation. The middle of each map corresponds to the midsternal line; the map is unrolled so that the edges represent the vertebral line. The top of the map is just below the clavicle, while the bottom is just below the edge of the thorax. By 10 mseconds the potential maximum has moved to the left chest and the V1 electrode site, initially positive, by 10–20 mseconds becomes enveloped by the trailing negative voltage field as excitation precedes leftward. As activation continues the maximum moves to involve the left anterior, lateral, then posterior walls while the minimum moves slightly inferiorly. Complexity of atrial excitation is reflected by pseudopods and secondary maxima noted in the region of the left lateral chest. This activation pattern appears to correlate well with excitation of the right atrium relatively rapidly followed by activation of left atrium. Although not depicted here we have noted that maps of atrial repolarization are similar to maps recorded during the first part of atrial depolarization, but with positive and negative fields reversed. This finding has also been described by others.[9] Early activation of the ventricle is marked by a central sternal maximum representing dominant left to right septal activation. The positivity increases in magnitude and moves to the left while the zone of negativity is located to the right and posteriorly. The early negativity encompasses most of the back area. In some subjects as the anterior minimum increases, a second field of negativity emerges which may remain as a pseudopod or may become separated by a band of relatively higher potential; Taccardi et al. termed this configuration the saddle pattern.[13] Often the anterior voltage field may become separated into two maxima by an invagination of lower voltage or negativity resulting in a breakup into at least two zones of peak positivity. These findings have been associated with right ventricular epicardial breakthrough of the wave of activation. While the map displayed does not show complete breakup into classic multiple extrema, the pseudopods and invaginations, e.g., at 15–35 mseconds, are apparent. In the present illustration, at 40 mseconds a large anterior and right field of negativity which earlier occupied most of both the anterior and posterior chest moves somewhat to the left and inferiorly. By 50 mseconds the minimum and a very large anterior zone of negativity dominate. This is occurring as a result of both left and right ventricular epicardial breakthrough and the movement of the activation wave from apex toward the base, and from a relatively anterior to a relatively posterior direction. The positive zone continues to move further leftward and posteriorly while, in the latter part of activation, the maximum positivity remains at the far left lateral extreme and posteriorly. Sometimes a second anterior maximum appears at the end of excitation reflecting late excitation of the base near the valve rings, or possibly of the region of the right ventricular outflow tract. Repolarization is marked by a maximum on the sternal or precordial area with low level negativity surrounding. In contrast with the excitation, the spatial pattern of repolarization shifts only slightly as voltage increases. FIGURE 2B illustrates the normal electrocardiogram and isoarea maps of QRS, ST-T, and QRST of the subject whose isopotential maps of ventricular excitation and recovery are illustrated in FIGURE 2A. Isoarea maps represent the algebraic sum of voltages occurring throughout a specified portion of the cardiac cycle integrated from each individual electrode site. Thus, at a glance, one may see the reduced data depicting the dominant spatial information in the isopotential maps and gain a general sense of the mean direction and magnitude of the portion of the cycle examined. This is largely of dipolar content in the normal QRS. The QRST isoarea map is an expression of the ventricular gradient, an estimate of the differences in the electrical properties of ventricular repolarization.[14]

Another method of display is an isometric projection in which the map can be considered as unrolled from the chest, and tilted in order to produce a pseudo-three-dimensional effect. Peaks indicate positive potentials, and valleys indicate negative potentials. Each side of the map is the vertebral line, while the midline is the midsternal line; the upper border is subclavicular, and the lower border is just above the umbilicus. The plane above the map is set at 1 mV. FIGURE 2C is an example of this format from a normal subject. Note how the mound of voltage representing septal activation rises along the midsternal line (S) and slightly leftward. This activation mound increases, develops a sink at the time of right ventricular epicardial breakthrough, and grows as breakthrough at the left ventricular apex also expands (30–40 mseconds). The positive peaks move leftward and posteriorly (50 mseconds and beyond) as the negative valleys

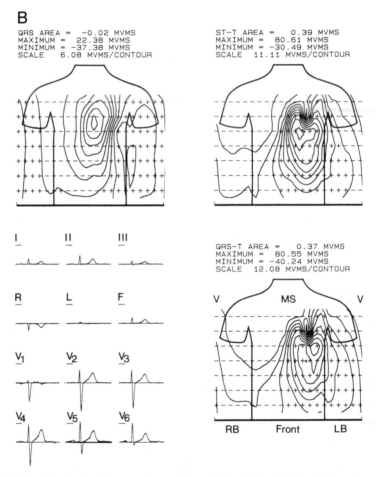

FIGURE 2B. The standard electrocardiogram (lower left) with the isointegral (isoarea) map for the QRS (upper left), the STT (upper right), and the QRST (lower right). Midsternal line (MS); right back (RB); left back (LB); vertebral line (V). The maps are viewed as if unrolled so that each edge represents the vertebral line. See text for discussion.

C

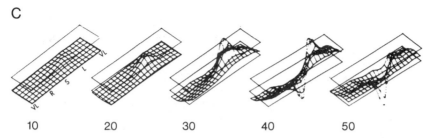

10   20   30   40   50

FIGURE 2C. Isometric projection maps in which each line intersection is a recording site; the plane above the grid represents 1 mV. Positive potentials distort the map upward and negative potentials downward. Midsternal line (S); right midaxillary line (R); left midaxillary line (L); vertebral line (VL). Maps at 10 msecond intervals through 50 mseconds are depicted from a normal male subject. At 10 and 20 mseconds buildup of voltage occurs in the septum and is reflected on the map as a central bulge; as the anterior left ventricular wall is activated the peaks move leftward. By 30 mseconds, right ventricular breakthrough has occurred. Excitation proceeds leftward and posteriorly with the maximum just above 1 mV and the minimum just under 1 mV. By 40 and 50 mseconds, the minimum increases significantly reflecting completion of ventricular activation with the negative face of the excitation wavefront prominent anteriorly while terminal positivity is seen mainly in the left back. See text for further discussion.

increase in magnitude and area, as more and more of both ventricles become depolarized.

MYOCARDIAL INFARCTION

The first group of patients with distinct lesions to be studied were patients with myocardial infarction (MI). FIGURE 3 contains data recorded from a patient with a large anteroseptal MI. He also had significant left atrial enlargement which is highlighted in the isopotential P wave maps illustrated at 10–70 mseconds (FIGURE 3A). The large relatively diphasic aspect of atrial excitation with a relatively large minimum is located anteriorly with the negative field extending during the last half of atrial activation to encompass the right anterior and lateral thorax. During ventricular excitation the minimum during the first 5–10 mseconds is located inferiorly, near and slightly left of the midsternal line. FIGURE 3A is illustrative of the pattern that obtains in many individuals with significantly large anterior infarctions, with the minimum remaining centrally and anteriorly during most of the QRS time zone. This is contrasted with the normal situation in which the minimum initially is at a very low level in the back and laterally, and builds predominantly in the right back and moves to the right anterior thorax, eventually occupying much of the anterior portion of the midsternal area and slightly to the left, where it remains during most of the rest of activation (FIGURE 2A). Mirvis has commented on the abnormal ST segment patterns that can be tracked back into the QRS complex in patients with an acute anterior MI,[9] demonstrating a temporal overlap with late QRS with its ST maximum anteriorly and leftward (FIGURE 3A). The continuity of the emerging repolarization-and-injury pattern is best seen in the last part of the QRS and early ST segment, extending varying durations into the ST. This is the time period of the marked elevation of the ST segment and prior to the T wave which may later become negative over much of the precordium. Mirvis has noted the increased amount of dipolarity during a period of

myocardial injury in contrast to that found in a normal heart.[9] FIGURE 3A supports this
concept with positive and negative voltages developing relatively early on opposite sides
of the chest. FIGURE 3B demonstrates the QRS isoarea map of the same patient with
anteroseptal MI, again pointing to the dominant integrated negativity occupying the
entire anterior chest with the back reflecting the oppositely directed positivity. The
elevated ST segments on the anterior chest are seen in interval map form with the
domination of the anterior chest by positive field and the QRST area map is more
complex with multiple maxima representing the altered properties of repolarization.

It became apparent, however, that some means of isolating the infarct zone for
analysis was desirable. Therefore, our group developed in dogs the concept of the
difference map.[15] FIGURE 4 demonstrates this approach in which the voltages from the
post-MI map may be subtracted from the normal or pre-MI map at each instant to
yield a difference map. In a dog in which a posterior MI (PMI) was produced, the
difference map, with the shallow sink of anterior negativity, reflects the net size and

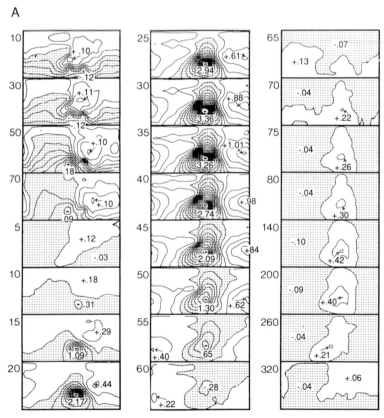

FIGURE 3. Body surface maps of a subject with an acute anteroseptal myocardial infarction.
FIGURE 3A (above). Isopotential maps of atrial activation, ventricular activation, and ventricular
recovery. The format is the same as for FIGURE 2A. Contrast these maps with the normal
illustrated in FIGURE 2A. See text for discussion.

B

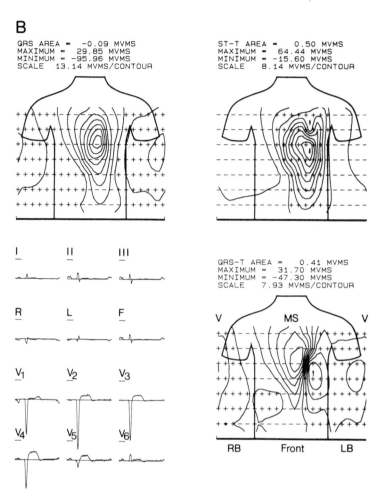

FIGURE 3B. A standard 12-lead electrocardiogram and isointegral maps of the QRS, ST-T, and QRST. The format is the same as for FIGURE 2B. See text for discussion.

orientation of the activation wavefront at this instant which had been removed by the PMI. The negative wake of the activation front which was directed posteriorly is reflected on the anterior chest as a sink. Conversely, in anteroseptal MI, the post-MI map shows an anterior sink, secondary to the loss of septal and anterior forces, while the difference map highlights the isolated dimension of this zone of loss. In dogs, we compared the effectiveness of infarct sizing using 142 lead BSM difference maps, vectorcardiogram (VCG) difference magnitudes, and 35 lead simple precordial grid difference maps with anatomically measured infarct mass. Worst and best correlations using instantaneous and integral analyses were grid, $r = 0.5$–0.7; VCG, $r = 0.7$–0.8; BSM, $r = 0.85$–0.88.[16]

Because it would be unusual if large numbers of patients had a pre-MI BSM from which to subtract their post-MI map, we developed the technique of departure mapping.[17] A large normal population was characterized as to surface potential mean voltage plus or minus two standard deviations (SD) at each electrode site, at one msecond intervals. FIGURE 5 is a diagrammatic representation of this approach. The acceptable normal range is characterized by the shaded region between curves; a hypothetical patient's infarct instantaneous voltage, along a single line of latitude around the chest, is characterized by the bold curve and is subtracted from the normal zone. The dashed line depicts the departure potentials at this level at a single instant outside the normal zone emphasizing the loss produced by infarction. In FIGURE 6, from a patient with an ECG showing a Q wave anteroseptal MI (Q > 30 mseconds, avL, V_1–V_3), the departure maps demonstrate that the patient's surface voltage pattern departed from the limits of normal during the Q time zone for 25 mseconds centered over the anterior left parasternal area and precordium. Most valuable, however, are instances in which the departure maps demonstrate abnormalities in which the standard ECG is either ambiguous or does not confirm infarction with changes in the Q time zone.[18] FIGURE 7 is an example of this phenomenon. This patient was known by cardiac enzyme assay and serial ECGs to have had an inferior MI (IMI). As frequently happens, the diagnostic Q waves of infarction had narrowed to within the limits of normal. The departure map indicated no potential distribution outside the normal range in the early Q time zone. Yet at 25 mseconds a mound of positivity arose

Posterior MI

8 MS

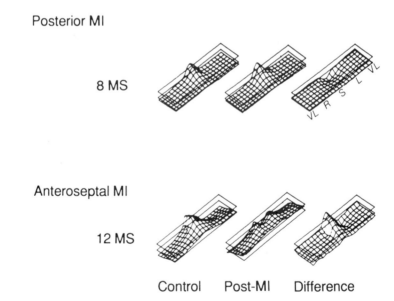

Anteroseptal MI

12 MS

Control   Post-MI   Difference

FIGURE 4. Body surface isometric projection maps from dogs with experimentally produced closed-chest posterior and anteroseptal myocardial infarctions (MI). Maps are obtained before (control) and after infarction (post-MI); difference maps are produced by subtracting the post-MI map from the control map. In posterior MI, the difference map shows the retreating lost potential from the posterior free wall as seen from the midanterior chest appearing as a central bowl-shaped sink. In anteroseptal MI, note the midsternal and anterior sink reflecting the loss of anteroseptal forces while the difference map reports the lost potentials of MI, their location, and magnitude. Vertebral line (VL); right lateral (RL); midsternal (S); left lateral (L).

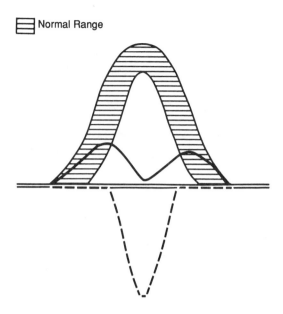

Abnormal - Normal Range = Departure

FIGURE 5. The departure principle. A modification of difference mapping applicable to human subjects in which an envelope bounded by ±2 standard deviations (SD) from the normal population mean is depicted. The shaded area represents the normal range for a hypothetical line of latitude on the body surface map. The bold curve represents the actually recorded voltages along that line from an infarct patient. "Departure" is the voltage value outside the envelope and is determined by subtracting the expected nearest boundary of the normal range from the recorded value for that electrode site at the precise instant in time.

exceeding +2 SD of normal, best demonstrated in the 30 msecond map and indicating abnormal departure. In 6 of 22 patients with IMI, this finding occurred, often arising as early as 15 mseconds after the onset of QRS and usually ending between 30 and 35 mseconds. This is an example of a mid-QRS abnormality in a patient with a definite MI that was not in evidence by the standard ECG method of noting Q waves in excess of 30 mseconds in the inferior leads. This technique is also valuable in non-Q MI.

The abnormalities in the mid and the late portions of ventricular excitation may sometimes reflect the loss of infarcted tissue which normally would be excited outside the Q time zone, and can be appreciated only as instantaneous voltage patterns departed from the normal expectation. This is especially valuable in non-Q MIs, or in instances of smaller lateral or posterior lesions. A second mechanism of mid and late abnormalities likely relates to local delayed conduction velocity, which permits the wave of excitation to arrive relatively late at a site distal to the infarct zone, and to have avoided the time in which it would have been canceled by opposing forces during normal excitation. These abnormalities are frequently seen toward the end of QRS complex. Many departures from normal may occur simply from the absolute loss of the infarcted myocardium and its immediate contribution to the simultaneous activation process involving other parts of the myocardium; the consequent *lack* of cancellation results in "departure" from normal. Nonuniform anisotropy may result in directional

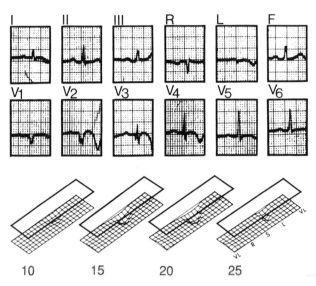

FIGURE 6. Scalar electrocardiogram and departure maps recorded from a patient with an overt anteroseptal Q wave myocardial infarction. Note pathologic Q waves in leads V1–V3, elevated ST segments, and inverted T waves. Enzymes were appropriately elevated for definitive diagnosis. Departure maps would be flat if, when the normal range is subtracted from a patient's map, no departure from the normal ±2 standard deviations exists at any millisecond, at any electrode site. Instants and locations of departure highlight the abnormalities introduced by infarction. Note surface voltage becomes abnormally negative only during the Q time zone. Compared to the electrocardiogram, departure map yielded no additional information other than locational information. Vertebral line (VL); right lateral (RL); midsternal (S); left lateral (L).

changes and slowed conduction velocity during excitation, or, more grossly, detours may be taken around intramural scarred areas that are interspersed with normal tissue. Such directional changes may result in departures in surface potential from the normal range. Although it is impossible to cite all, many contributors to the field of BSM in MI have expanded our knowledge in this area.[17–45] The departure concept has been extended to form index maps indicating how the primary map potentials may be ranked in terms of the isocontours of standard deviations from the mean normal expectation.[44] The predictive value of methods of detecting MI from several laboratories have been summarized by Mirvis.[46] Of all the studies reported, those in the group listed in TABLE 2 allow statistical conclusions to be drawn. There were 95 patients who had definite MI but who did not have a diagnostic standard ECG. In 82.1% there were characteristic map abnormalities. It is clear that mapping offers a distinct advantage in the diagnosis of electrocardiographically subtle or silent MI, and unlike alternative noninvasive methods, it appears equally valuable in inferoposterior as in anterior lesions.

VENTRICULAR HYPERTROPHY

Blumenschein *et al.* recorded BSM in children with right ventricular hypertrophy (RVH).[47] The groups included RVH of the crista supraventricularis secondary to secundum atrial septal defect, RVH of the outflow tract secondary to pulmonic stenosis, and RVH between the tricuspid valve and the infundibulum resulting in infundibular stenosis. As might be expected, the positive voltage peaks in RVH migrate toward the right chest rather than moving from the precordial area toward the left and then the back. The movement of positivity on the right thorax, however, differs according to the pathological condition involved. In this study, because a number of patients went to surgery, it was possible to relate the surface potential patterns to the spread of excitation through the right ventricular wall. In atrial septal defect, the latest epicardial events were recorded along the atrioventricular groove and appeared to give rise to the peak positivity in the right chest. Yet, after completion of epicardial excitation on the ventricular surface, the peak positivity persisted in the upper sternal region. This very likely corresponded to the R' in V1 or V2 seen in association with the atrial septal defect and represented terminal excitation which is associated with volume overload pattern. In pulmonic stenosis, the wavefront moved laterally across the epicardial surface of the right ventricular free wall and produced peak positivity over the right chest with peak negativity over the left precordium. Terminal excitation spread superiorly through the outflow tract of the right ventricle and gave rise to the upper sternal maximum positivity. Sohi et al. recorded surface maps in adult patients with mild to moderate valvular pulmonic stenosis and, using the departure map technique, observed a delayed appearance of the sternal negativity that has been attributed to right ventricular breakthrough.[48] Abnormal positivity was located in the upper anterior chest, similar to the upper sternal maximum in children, attributed to spread through the outflow tract of the right ventricle.

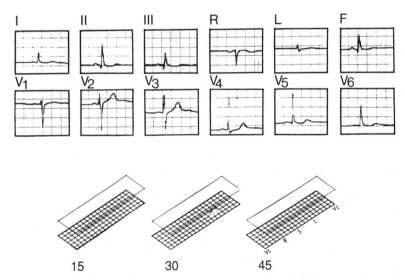

FIGURE 7. Scalar electrocardiogram and departure maps recorded from a patient with a documented inferior infarction. This patient's diagnostic Q waves narrowed to within normal limits during a period of convalescence. From 1–15 mseconds and from 45 mseconds to the end of activation, the departure maps indicate very little potential distribution outside the normal range. However, beginning at about 25 mseconds and ending shortly after 35 mseconds, in the zone of the left anterior chest, a mound of positivity (illustrated at 30 mseconds) appears exceeding 2 standard deviations. Vertebral line (VL); right lateral (RL); midsternal (S); left lateral (L).

TABLE 2. Prevalence of Abnormal Body Surface Maps and Standard
Electrocardiogram (ECG) in Patients with Prior Myocardial Infarction (MI)

Author (Year)	MI Site	Number of Patients	Abnormal Map	Abnormal ECG	Normal ECG/ Abnormal Map
Flowers et al.[16] (1976)	AMI	26	26 (100%)	24 (92%)	2 (100%)
Flowers et al.[17] (1976)	IMI	22	19 (86%)	8 (35%)	11 (79%)
Vincent et al.[30] (1977)	IMI	28	28 (100%)	20 (71%)	8 (100%)
Hirai et al.[25] (1984)	AMI	32	26 (81%)	0[a] —	26 (81%)
Osugi et al.[32] (1984)	IMI	24	20 (83%)	0[a] —	20 (83%)
De Ambroggi et al.[43] (1986)	IMI	15	15 (100%)	15 (100%)	0 —
	IMI	15	11 (73%)	0[a] —	11 (73%)
Kornreich et al.[38] (1986)	AMI	114	110 (97%)	101 (89%)	—
	IMI	144	135 (94%)	122 (85%)	—

[a]Studies include only patients with nondiagnostic ECG. Anterior myocardial infarction (AMI); inferior myocardial infarction (IMI). Percentages connote recognition of infarction. (Modified and reprinted from Reference 9 with permission of Kluwer Academic Publishers.)

Patients with left ventricular hypertrophy from aortic valvular stenosis were also studied, noting that departure maps demonstrated abnormal positivity in the upper chest anteriorly, appeared later, and lasted longer than in the depolarization sequence of maps from pulmonic stenosis patients.[48] In aortic stenosis, peak positivity occurred later and was more discrete and consistent in timing than in pulmonic stenosis. Delayed and longer lasting positivity in left ventricular hypertrophy is to be expected as this dominant chamber gains even more mass and cardiac electrical events become predictably delayed. In small part, this may be because the advancing wavefront has farther to travel; more importantly, the wavefront likely encounters areas of slowed conduction velocity or altered pathway, as minor degrees of conduction defect develop. The abnormality of upper left positivity in the pulmonic stenosis patient began earlier (about 20 mseconds) after onset of activation whereas in aortic stenosis it developed at 35 mseconds or later. In RVH this abnormality was diffuse in location and scattered in time. Evidence of right ventricular and left ventricular breakthrough was delayed in the aortic stenosis patients even more than in pulmonic stenosis. In the Blumeschein study[47] and in a study by Wallace et al.,[49] right ventricular electrical events were delayed and in patients who had moderate-to-severe RVH the depolarization process sometimes continued in the right ventricle later than in the left. In the Sohi study of patients with mild-to-moderate right ventricular outflow obstruction, abnormalities were detected earlier in the depolarization sequence than in the more severe group and did not last as long.[48]

A study of left ventricular mass as related to surface map patterns was undertaken by Holt et al., who demonstrated the correlation coefficient between left ventricular mass determined at angiography and that determined by BSM was high ($r = 0.85$).[50,51] This correlation was much higher than the correlation resulting from using the standard ECG or VCG for data acquisition and analysis.

CARDIOMYOPATHIES

We studied 19 patients with hypertrophic obstructive and dilated cardiomyopathy.[52] In the dilated group, the findings were more similar to normal QRS maps, but demonstrated a more prominent apical breakthrough pattern. In the obstructive group, high positive potentials and delayed breakthrough negativities were observed, resulting from the marked thickness of the ventricular walls, coupled with some conduction delay.

CONDUCTION DEFECTS

Right bundle branch block (RBBB) has been studied in several laboratories.[52–56] In early activation (FIGURE 8), the surface potential distribution was similar to that recorded from normal subjects; the maximum was located midsternally, or left, parasternally. Positivity manifest on the anterior left chest moved toward the back (FIGURE 8, 15 and 30 mseconds). The absence of normal right ventricular break-through was manifest by a failure of the relatively early negativity to appear centrally between 15 and 40 mseconds after QRS onset. This negativity occurred later in RBBB and appeared in each of the studies in the left anterior chest. A second minimum often occurred slightly to the right of the peak positive potential (maximum) located on the left precordium. The maximum was attributed to the activation of the left ventricular wall while the minimum was thought to represent left ventricular breakthrough. In our studies, epicardial breakthrough was abnormally located on the left and varied in its appearance from 30–60 mseconds with an average of 45. During late QRS, evidence of delayed right ventricular excitation persisted well beyond 80 mseconds and into the early phases of repolarization. Taccardi *et al.* point out that, as the activation maximum and minimum move to the right, the recovery maximum appears in the left mammary region sometimes giving as many as three repolarization maxima.[53] The recovery minimum in the sternal or right mammary region persisted as did a recovery maximum in the left mammary area suggesting a mirror image of potential distribu-tion during the last phase of ventricular activation. This reflects the effect of the altered activation sequence on repolarization order. We found five different patterns of abnormal repolarization in RBBB.[56] The most common was the onset of repolarization manifesting as negativity that was anterior and to the right of the midline. As this process progressed, a second front appeared anteriorly in the form of positivity over the left chest. These coexisted until the end of repolarization. The second most common pattern consisted of a negative front on the right of the midline without the associated positive potentials described previously. The positive potentials manifested only in the anterior left upper chest in some patients while in others the abnormal repolarization was noted in the precordium to the left of the midline in the form of negative potentials. A subject who had undergone a tetralogy of Fallot repair demonstrated the onset of repolarization to the right of the sternum which later moved to the left of the midline. Many valleys and peaks were noted in the right upper chest positivity and both positive and negative potentials were present in the late 105 msecond map indicating that the repolarization process had begun while depolarization was still proceeding. Leibman *et al.* studied children with varying degrees of RBBB.[57] Many of their findings are similar to those in adults, while there are interesting nuances in certain individual pediatric patients that are unique.

Our group studied 25 subjects with left bundle branch block (LBBB) with (10) and without (15) left axis deviation.[58] In 19 of the 25 subjects, the early upper sternal

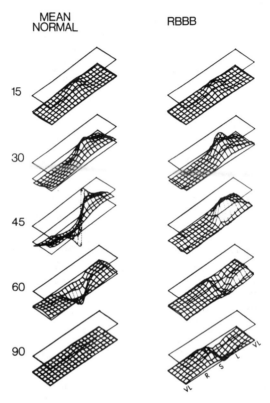

FIGURE 8. Mean body surface maps of the progression of depolarization in a group of normal patients compared to a patient with right bundle branch block (RBBB). Upper anterior positivity (15 mseconds) is present in both conditions. The right anterior sink of negativity in normals at about 30 mseconds (representing epicardial breakthrough) is absent in RBBB. This negativity progresses in the normal, engulfing a large area of the map on the right of the midline; in RBBB, this negativity never appears on the right of the midline. Conversely, in RBBB, negative potentials (45 mseconds) appear on the left of the midline and increase in strength involving most of the precordium; thus epicardial breakthrough is abnormally located and delayed. Note also in RBBB the right anterior upper positivity at 60 mseconds and continuing to the end. Vertebral line (VL); right lateral (RL); midsternal (S); left lateral.

positivity was similar to that reported in normal subjects indicative of timely, although by necessity oppositely directed, septal activation. It may be that some of the early upper sternal positivity was right ventricular free wall activation in these patients. In LBBB, right ventricular breakthrough, which in the normal subject occurs between 15–40 mseconds after QRS onset, was similarly located centrally but occurred *earlier* due to the delay of QRS onset implicit in LBBB. Positivity produced by left ventricular activation located in the upper anterior left chest was similar in the patients with and without left axis deviation, but the onset was delayed in both compared with normal subjects. Presumably as a result of the time required for right-to-left septal activation, followed by excitation of the left ventricle, some of which is not via the Purkinje network, the total duration of the positivity was longer than in the normal and extended considerably beyond 90 mseconds indicating prolonged activation of the anterior wall of the left ventricle. In the patients with a normal axis, this upper anterior positivity remained anterior throughout the depolarization process; in subjects with left axis deviation it moved toward the left shoulder and into the left superior and lateral aspect reflecting the dominance of excitation via the inferoposterior fascicle. The maximum during the last half of excitation, then, in patients with left axis deviation, was thought to be due to the late activation of the anterobasal portion of the left ventricle caused by relatively greater involvement of the left anterior fasicle.

Musso et al. found in uncomplicated LBBB that 10–20 mseconds before the end of QRS a new maximum appeared in the upper sternal region.[59] This maximum increased in voltage, lasted throughout the ST-T, and was assumed to be an early manifestation of repolarization. These authors interpreted the findings to suggest that repolarization originating in the right ventricle begins before left ventricular depolarization is completed. Further they reasoned that the left ventricle behaves as a sink during much of the recovery process because of its delayed repolarization resulting from the delayed activation. Preda et al.[60] and Musso et al.[61] have some experience with LBBB associated with MI. Preda et al. state that, with anterior MI, the middle third of the anterior chest remains negative during the final phases of the QRS. This finding was attributed to the lack of excitation of the anterobasal portion of the left ventricle due to the presence of necrosis. In inferoposterior MI a persistent negativity was noted during the mid QRS in the lower back, chest, or in the left lateral or posterior areas. This negativity moved to the right side of the back.[60] Musso et al. did not confirm these findings,[59,61] rather, they were unable to identify any potential pattern uniquely found in a given group with LBBB. They stated that generally high voltages were present in patients with hypertrophy, and lower voltages in patients with MI.

In a study of 25 subjects with left anterior fascicular block (LAFB), we noted three characteristic abnormalities.[62] In the early and mid portion of QRS, 20 of the 25 demonstrated abnormal anterosuperior positivity beginning in the precordial area and proceeding toward the subclavicular area. The explanation was believed to be the relatively delayed, dysynchronous, and superiorly directed altered sequence of depolarization of the anterior left ventricle. All 25 subjects demonstrated left lower abnormal negativity. This was thought to represent the unopposed receding activation front after left ventricular breakthrough posteroinferiorly as well as the negative aspect of the abnormally directed superior positivity (activation via the left posterior fasicle). Finally, 11 subjects showed abnormal negative potentials in the right lower chest. This was thought to represent the partially unopposed activation front of the right ventricular free wall seen after right ventricular epicardial breakthrough because of the absence of the usual canceling normal forces from the anterior portion of the left ventricle. The surface manifestations of the septal depolarization were found to be indistinguishable from normal.

DIFFERENTIATION OF LAFB AND INFERIOR MI BY BSM

In 38 patients (LAFB, 19; IMI, 19) three distinguishing features were detected[63] (FIGURE 9). Abnormal high anterior positivity was noted in both LAFB and IMI; this

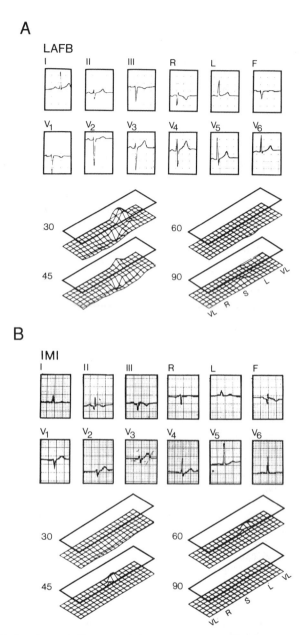

FIGURE 9. Scalar electrocardiogram and departure maps recorded from a patient with left anterior fascicular block (LAFB) in A and a patient with an inferior myocardial infarction (IMI) in B. The LAFB patient demonstrates left axis deviation ($-45°$) and the presence of R waves in leads II, III, and F. The IMI patient demonstrates diagnostic Q waves in leads II, III and F, and a lower right and central band of shallow negativity (30 msecond map). Abnormal upper positivity is present in both conditions but occurs earlier in LAFB. There is abnormal central and right lower negativity in both but in LAFB this negativity lasts longer and is more impressive. The abnormal left lower negativity prominent in LAFB is not seen in IMI. These distinguishing features are particularly valuable when the ECG distinction is uncertain (See text). Vertebral line (VL); right lateral (RL); midsternal (S); left lateral (L).

occurred earlier in LAFB, before 30 mseconds (FIGURE 9A), while beginning at 45 mseconds or later in IMI (FIGURE 9B). The rim of abnormal lower negativity centering sternally and slightly to the right was noted in both groups but in IMI it occurred within the first 40 mseconds while in LAFB it was found in the mid and latter parts of depolarization. Abnormal left lower negativity was noted in all the patients with LAFB, but was absent in all with IMI. The earlier left infraclavicular positivity encountered in LAFB is in a slightly more lateral location than in IMI and is explained by the fact that departure from normal does not manifest itself until well within or after the normal Q time zone in IMI. Perhaps because the early transeptal forces may be maintained intact, the abnormal, superiorly directed forces in LAFB arise from the slight initial delay, the sustained dysynchrony and the abnormality of direction of activation of the geographic zone supplied by the left anterior division. The left lower negativity in hemiblock may be due to abnormalities of timing of epicardial breakthrough and the superior orientation of the excitation front as a result of the altered sequence of depolarization. The same is suggested as the likely explanation of a right lower abnormal negativity in this group. The earlier right lower and central negativity in the IMI however appears to be due to the direct loss of inferior forces in IMI manifested in the early Q time zone. The combined group that showed indistinguishable standard ECG changes had BSM instantaneous changes more similar to LAFB than to IMI, in that the abnormal left high lateral anterior positivity was displayed and all had left lower negativity in contrast with uncomplicated IMI, in which lower negativity is most obvious centrally and slightly to the right. Therefore, this group (all without MI history) probably consisted of patients with hemiblock rather than MI. The analysis of BSM in IMI and those with hemiblock known not to have MI showed some similarities, but distinctive patterns can be seen when instantaneous maps are analyzed, both from a temporal and a topographical standpoint. Thus, the BSM not only amplifies electrophysiologic understanding but also may pragmatically aid in differentiation in instances of confusion.

ARRHYTHMIC POTENTIAL SUGGESTED BY MAPS

It has been determined that the normal QRST isoarea map has a relatively dipolar character as referred to earlier with two simple extrema. In contrast, Burgess[64] and Abildskov and coworkers[65] noted that many of the QRST isoarea maps of patients with ventricular tachycardia (VT) or ventricular fibrillation (VF) have multiple peaks and valleys as well as pseudopods. Horacek *et al.* also noted that the span of amplitudes between the principal maximum and the principal minimum of the QRST interval distribution was larger in the normal subjects than in their patients with VT or VF (FIGURE 10).[66] It appears then that the patients with VF or recurrent sustained VT have much more multipolarity in their QRST integral maps, manifested by more than a single maximum and minimum. (Note multiple pluses and minuses.) This appears to be a reflection of heterogeneous recovery of sufficient degree to render the myocardium vulnerable to these arrhythmias. De Ambroggi *et al.* studied BSM in the long QT syndrome noting an abnormally high nondipolar component suggesting regions of disparity in repolarization,[67] thus a potential substrate for VT or VF.

Several groups have studied BSM in preexcitation.[66-74] Horacek *et al.* demonstrated that the ventricular preexcitation site may be approximated by noting the vectorial characteristics of the delta wave (FIGURE 11).[66] Kamakara *et al.* selected surface leads for correlation based on surface potential maps.[70] Cobb *et al.* performed surface mapping preoperatively followed by intraoperative epicardial mapping in order to localize precisely the site of anomalous activation.[71] Yamada *et al.* studied 22 patients with the Wolff-Parkinson-White syndrome by surface mapping to determine how closely the spatial patterns correlated with the conventional diagnostic classification.[72] They were able to classify their patients into three distinct groups but had no further electrophysiological confirmation. De Ambroggi *et al.* concluded after studying 42 patients with both surface and intracardiac mapping that, in general, the results were encouraging and demonstrated that the surface potential pattern provided more information on the probable location of the preexcited area than did the conventional ECG.[68] More importantly, they gained the insight that during the delta wave an opportunity arose to expand our ability to solve the inverse problem in

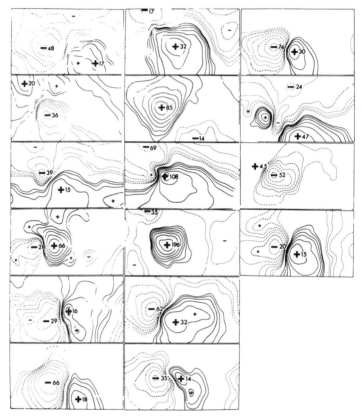

FIGURE 10. QRST isoarea maps of 16 individual subjects with a history of ventricular tachycardia or ventricular fibrillation. The right and left edges of each rectangle correspond to the right midaxillary line. The upper border of the map is at the neck and the lower border at the waist. Solid contour lines indicate positive values; interrupted contour lines indicate negative values. The contours are plotted to progress logarithmically (10, 15, 22). The positive and negative extrema are identified with a numerical value of the amplitude in microvolt seconds. Additionally, the local extrema and the pseudopods indicating breakup into a multipolar pattern are marked with an asterisk. These were counted in the multipolarity index for each map. Note the multiple extrema in these maps in contrast to the marked dipolarity in the normal maps of FIGURE 2B. (Reprinted from Reference 64 with permission of Kluwer Academic Publishers.)

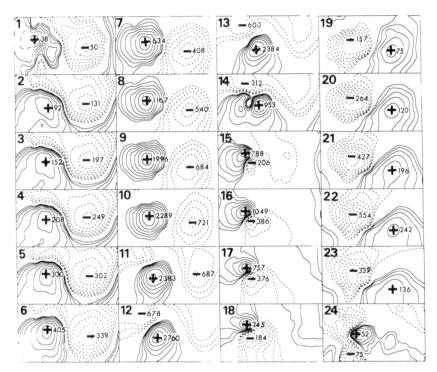

FIGURE 11. Isopotential map of a patient with Wolff-Parkinson-White syndrome with a left lateral accessory pathway. Maps 1–18 are 8 mseconds apart; maps 18–24 (during ventricular repolarization) are 40 mseconds apart. The first 10 maps correspond to the delta wave in the electrocardiogram, while the next 3 maps correspond to activation that has now engaged the His-Purkinje system. Note the vectorial characteristics of this portion of activation. The repolarization sequence starts at map 19; note that it is the reverse of the delta wave distribution seen in the earlier maps. Map 24 likely reflects repolarization of the right ventricle whose depolarization is seen in maps 15–18. (Reprinted from Reference 64 with permission of Kluwer Academic Publishers.)

electrocardiography because there is only one wavefront occurring during the delta wave. The localization of this front by solving the inverse problem may be expected to be easier than during normal, complex, multipolar excitation. Spach et al., from experiments in which preexcitation was produced by stimulating seven different ectopic sites,[73] were the first to note that the delta wave produced a body surface maximum within a relatively small area on the anterior chest, while the position of the more distant low level minimum was spatially related to the stimulation site. Stimulation sites as close as 2–3 cm produced differences in the distant low-level surface potential areas not only during excitation, but during repolarization. In fact, ST-T patterns were also as useful in these authors' opinion as was the QRS in determining the preexcitation site. More recent studies have used numerous electrocardiographic techniques to improve the ability to confirm the preexcitation site.[74,75] No method is perfect, and there is controversy as to the best approach. At present, confirmation by intraoperative epicardial mapping is recommended.

FUTURE NOTES

BSM (FIGURE 12) has been utilized to track the dynamic pathway of His-Purkinje activation.[76,77] Above are maps of atrial repolarization and His-Purkinje activity superimposed in time as they frequently are. Below are maps from which the contribution of atrial activation to the pattern has been subtracted leaving predominantly the dipolar pattern of His activity seen at 45, 40, and ceasing at 30 mseconds before QRS. As the technology improves undoubtedly refinements of the originally described technique will occur and it is only a matter of time until discrete portrayal of this portion of the conduction system will be practical.

Recently, Horan *et al.* have described the quantitative relationship between the ventriculographic silhouette and the topography of body surface potential in a series of

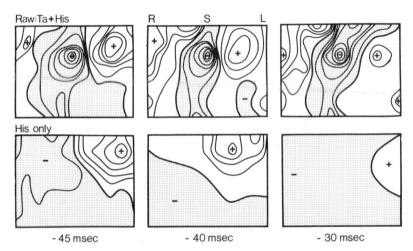

FIGURE 12. Characterization of His-Purkinje by eliminating unwanted atrial repolarization signals (Ta). From a span of PR segment well away from the expected time of major His-Purkinje activity and well before QRS, a total chest pattern of Ta was recorded. Having identified this pattern, the amount found in each millisecond throughout the PR segment was subtracted from the period in which Ta and His are likely to overlap in time (upper panel), leaving a residual which is predominantly His-Purkinje (lower panel). Right lateral (R); midsternal (S); left lateral (L). (Modified and reprinted from Reference 75 by permission of the American Heart Association, Inc.)

180 subjects without conduction defect who had coronary arteriograms, left ventriculograms, and BSM.[78] A method for quantitating left ventricular segmental wall motion as described by Ingels *et al.* was used.[79] The differences in ray lengths in systole and diastole were taken as estimates of wall motion at local sites (FIGURE 13). Paralactic distortion in measurements was corrected by a factor derived from the reference disc projection recorded before each ventriculogram. BSM were obtained from these patients as well as from 63 normal subjects. With any fraction of the heart cycle, the potential at a body surface site may be expected to be a function of the heart muscle elements electrically active during that interval. If we hypothesize that the position of each ventriculographic boundary element is also dependent upon certain properties defining the integrity of heart muscle in common with those that produce the electrical

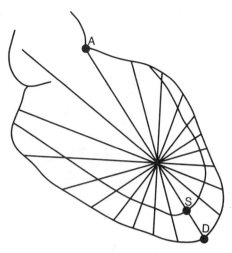

FIGURE 13. Ventriculographic outline (traced from cineangiographic projections) of the end systolic (S) and end diastolic (D) image from a patient's right ventricular oblique projection of the left ventriculogram. The centroid, or polar origin for reference, is defined as 69% of the distance along a line from the anterolateral aortic edge (A) to the apex at end systole. From the centroid, then, rays are projected outward at 18° separations to intersect the superimposed perimeters drawn from angiographic projections at end systole and end diastole. The difference in the ray lengths in systole and diastole are taken as estimates of wall motion at that time. Regional and global wall motion can be thus described.

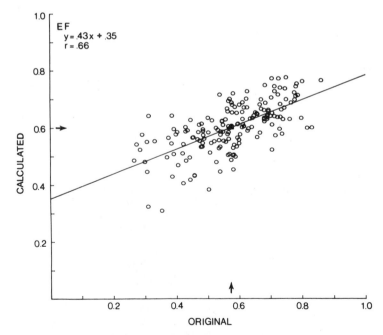

FIGURE 14. Ejection fractions (EF) predicted from body surface maps versus those obtained from cineangiograms. On the abscissa are ejection fractions directly obtained from cineangiographic catheterization data. On the ordinate are ejection fractions calculated from body surface maps. Correlation was $r = 0.66$. (Reprinted from Reference 75 with permission.)

A

MI without VT

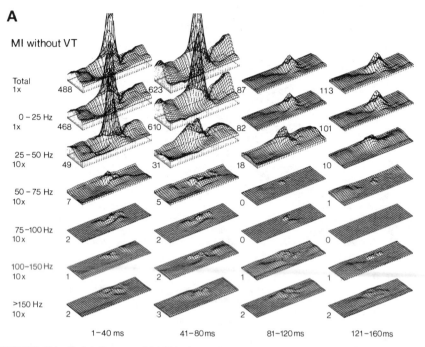

FIGURE 15A. Serial 40 msecond RMS isointegral voltage maps from onset of QRS through 160 mseconds after onset are displayed with the time periods indicated along the bottom line. Each isointegral map (top row) is depicted in isometric projection map form using the format described for FIGURE 2C. Each lower row represents maps reconstructed only from the component frequency bands indicated on the ordinate. Maps for frequency bands above 25 Hz are amplified with a gain of 10. The maps were obtained from a patient with myocardial infarction (MI) without ventricular tachycardia (VT). The mean microvolt level (for mean electrode site) for the time period indicated is listed to the left of each map. Note during the time period beyond 81 mseconds that frequencies above 50 Hz have relatively low voltage expressions in the maps and in the instance of three maps the average voltage per electrode site was effectively zero.

signal, then we may further hypothesize a secondary dependency of electrical potential distribution on wall contour or vice versa. If we then make the assumption that this dependency is linear, then the muscle parameter (the ray length) at each radius of the ventriculogram may be expressed arithmetically. For the wall boundary characteristics, each diastolic and systolic ray length was utilized. A training set was developed in which the surface potential patterns were correlated with the wall motion at each site serially examining a relationship for each ray length and a 70 by 40 transformation matrix which converted 70 voltage values into 40 ray length values. The transformation coefficients thus derived were applied to a test set with preliminary results demonstrating the progressively smaller error for calculating the reconstruction of the diastolic and systolic images obtained at catheterization as the size of the training set increased. Further, ejection fractions obtained at catheterization were correlated with ejection fractions predicted from the BSM with a resulting correlation coefficient of 0.66 (FIGURE 14). This work should be viewed as an early attempt to make quantitative transfers possible, yet the growing expertise in data acquisition as well as imaging technology suggests optimism for what may ultimately be achieved.

Recently, we have tested several approaches of analysis and display of the spatial distribution of various frequency bands of ventricular late potentials in normal subjects and in subjects with MI without and with VT. Though our results are tentative, using BSM techniques we are able to identify the dominant frequency band in normal subjects (0–25 Hz) and to contrast this with the location and expression of various frequency bands in infarct patients without VT and with VT. FIGURES 15A and 15B are two such examples from a patient without VT and one with VT. Note both the greater expression of frequencies above 50 Hz and their more diffuse distribution in the infarct patient with VT beginning at 81 mseconds and extending through 160 mseconds. Note also the greater *relative* contribution of frequencies above 50 Hz compared to those below 50 Hz appearing in the 81–120 msecond time zone in the VT patient compared with the non-VT patient. Using this technique we are able to specify the location, the magnitude, and the timing of the various frequency bands and thus to compare different subgroups of patients with coronary artery disease as to their frequency content. It should be acknowledged that the work of Cain *et al.* has been both complementary and instructive in this area of investigation.[80]

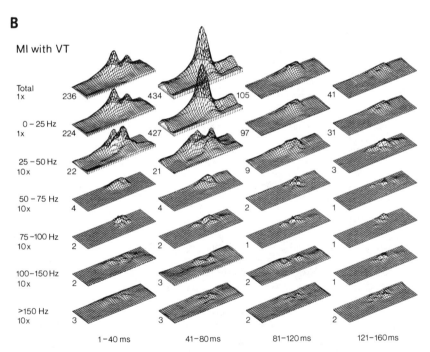

B

MI with VT

Total 1x

0 – 25 Hz 1x

25 – 50 Hz 10x

50 – 75 Hz 10x

75 –100 Hz 10x

100–150 Hz 10x

>150 Hz 10x

1–40 ms   41–80 ms   81–120 ms   121–160 ms

FIGURE 15B. Using the same format of decomposition into maps representing the component frequency bands, an MI patient with VT not only displays relatively less power in the 0–50 Hz range but has slightly more absolute power in the range above 75 Hz. In the zone between 81 and 160 mseconds, the distribution of frequencies on the chest is more diffuse and the absolute voltage slightly greater in the bands beyond 50 Hz than in the case of the patient without VT.

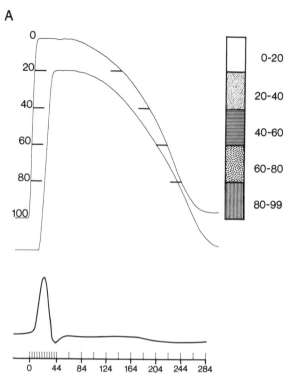

FIGURE 16. Time correlation of left ventricular endocardial, total ventricular epicardial and body surface potential distributions in a dog. **FIGURE 16A** (above). The time courses of monophasic action potential for the left ventricular endocardium (above), the biventricular epicardium (middle), and the simultaneous surface potential in a left axillary chest lead. The two upper curves represent the instant-by-instant spatial root-mean-square of monophasic action potential on the respective ventricular surfaces in which all recordings have been normalized to common amplitude between plateau (0% polarization) and resting level (100% repolarization) with bands of 20% span identified for interpretation of the relative rate of repolarization in panel C.

Recently we have focused on the relationship between the BSM and endocardial and epicardial monophasic action potential mapping (FIGURE 16A). The top curve is an endocardial monophasic action potential, the middle curve the epicardial monophasic action potential, and the lower curve a surface electrocardiographic lead. Approximately 90 sites on the endocardium and epicardium were recorded. In this animal the endocardium completed repolarization first. The maps (FIGURE 16B) demonstrate this feature as well as the following other observations: (1) The beginning of endocardial depolarization is responsible for the first evidence of electrical effect in the BSM while the epicardium remains polarized; therefore, it should be very clear that the early BSM should not be interpreted as reflecting epicardial isochrones of activation (FIGURE 16B; 8 mseconds). (2) The beginning of epicardial depolarization correlates with the saddle on the BSM as has been previously suggested.[6] (3) During the plateau phase of both endocardial and epicardial monophasic action potential recordings, there is little difference in potential and therefore there is little surface effect during early ST-T (FIGURE 16A and 16B). (4) The precordial T surface pattern is an expression of relative rates of repolarization of the endocardial and epicardial surfaces; therefore, it is predominantly positive if the epicardium recovers faster and is negative in instances in which the endocardium recovers faster.

In summary, investigators from many laboratories have pursued insight into the surface expression of cardiac electrophysiologic events portrayed by the BSM. While this pursuit has been ongoing, a rapid multigenerational evolution of computational machinery has occurred. It seems likely that the merger of enhanced clinical understanding from the BSM literature with the compact, portable, advanced imaging microcomputer of today is about to lead to an explosive widespread application in noninvasive cardiologic diagnosis and study.

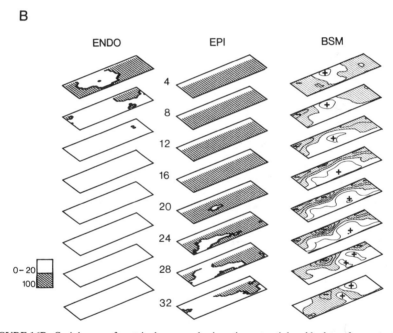

FIGURE 16B. Serial maps of ventricular monophasic action potential and body surface potential during depolarization. Each surface has been unrolled so that its most ventral aspect is central on the map and that the lateral borders represent the dorsal meridian (corresponding to the midvertebral lines which border the body surface maps). In the endocardial series (left column) and epicardial series (middle column), the key indicates that the heavy stippling represents resting level; clear area represents plateau level. The bold line separating resting from fully depolarized is composed of the compression of contours (80, 60, 40, 20) during the rapid local upstroke of phase 0 as the myocardium undergoes activation. The surface electrocardiographic potential (right column) is divided into regions of positivity (clear) and negativity (light stippling) with contour separations of 0.5 mV. Note that the epicardium remains at rest for at least the first 16 mseconds and that early body surface evolution of anterior positivity relates to endocardial and possibly intramural events. Epicardial breakthrough over the right ventricular and then left ventricular apex is accompanied by a pseudopod of negativity dipping down from the upper right chest into the region of anterior positivity on the body surface.

C

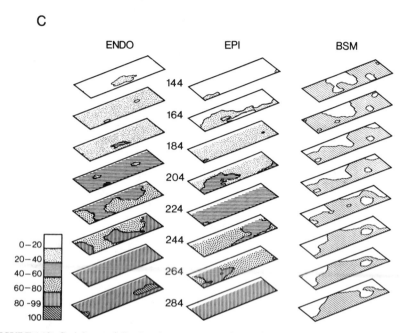

FIGURE 16C. Serial maps following the same conventions as in B but now during repolarization (144 mseconds–284 mseconds after onset). The scale from panel A has been reproduced to indicate by shading the 20% ranges of recovery seen in the left ventricular endocardial and biventricular epicardial monophasic action potential maps. Note that the endocardial maps in this particular animal slightly precede the epicardial maps toward full repolarization and that this is accompanied by dominant anterior T-wave negativity on the body surface.

ACKNOWLEDGMENTS

The technical assistance of Anita Wylds, Sandra Cliff, Sherry Thurmond, Pat Orander and Judith Hubbard is gratefully acknowledged.

REFERENCES

1. WALLER, A. D. 1888. The electromotive properties of the human heart. Br. Med. J. **2:** 751–754.
2. KOCH, E. & K. SCHNEYER. 1934. Weitere untersuchungen uber die topographie der aktionspotentiale des herzens auf der vorderen brustwand. Z. Kreislaufforsch. **26:** 916–922.
3. NAHUM, L. H., A. MAURO, H. M. CHERNOFF & R. S. SIKAND. 1951. Instantaneous equipotential distribution on the surface of the human body for various instants in the cardiac cycle. J. Appl. Physiol. **3:** 454–464.
4. NELSON, C. V. 1957. Human thorax potentials. Ann. N.Y. Acad. Sci. **65:** 1014–1050.
5. TACCARDI, B. 1958. La distribution spatiale des potentiels cardiaques. Acta Cardiol. **13:** 173–189.
6. TACCARDI, B. 1963. Distribution of heart potential on the thoracic surface of normal human subjects. Circ. Res. **12:** 341–352.
7. AMIROV, R. Z. 1961. Cardiotoposcopy. Kardiologia **2:** 55–61.

8. HORAN, L. G., N. C. FLOWERS & D. A. BRODY. 1963. Body surface potential distribution: comparison of naturally and artificially produced signals as analyzed by digital computer. Circ. Res. **13**: 373–387.
9. MIRVIS, D. M., Ed. 1988. Body Surface Electrocardiographic Mapping. Kluwer Academic Publishers. Boston, Mass.
10. DE AMBROGGI, L., E. MUSSO & B. TACCARDI. 1988. Body surface mapping. *In* Comprehensive Electrocardiology, Theory and Practice in Health and Disease. P. W. Macfarlane & T. D. V. Lawrie, Eds. **2**: 1015–1045. Pergamon Press. New York, N.Y.
11. HORAN, L. G., R. C. HAND & N. C. FLOWERS. 1984. Electrode number and body surface potential map reconstruction. *In* Computerized Interpretation of the Electrocardiogram. R. H. Selvester & D. B. Geselowitz, Eds.: 333–341. Engineering Foundation. New York, N.Y.
12. LUX, R. L., C. R. SMITH, R. F. WYATT & J. A. ABILDSKOV. 1978. Limited lead selection for estimation of body surface potential maps in electrocardiography. IEEE Trans. Biomed. Eng. **25**: 270–276.
13. TACCARDI, B., L. DE AMBROGGI & C. VIGANOTTI. 1976. Body-surface mapping of heart potentials. *In* The Theoretical Basis of Electrocardiology. C. V. Nelson & D. B. Geselowitz, Eds.: 436–466. Clarendon Press. Oxford, England.
14. WILSON, F. N., A. F. MACLEOD, P. S. BARKER & F. D. JOHNSTON. 1934. The determination and the significance of the areas of the ventricular deflections of the electrocardiogram. Am. Heart J. **10**: 46–61.
15. MCLAUGHLIN, V. W., N. C. FLOWERS, L. G. HORAN & H. A. KILLAM. 1974. Surface potential contributions from discrete elements of ventricular wall. Am. J. Cardiol. **34**: 302–308.
16. FLOWERS, N. C., R. C. HAND, M. R. SRIDHARAN, L. G. HORAN & G. S. SOHI. 1978. Surface reflections of cardiac excitation and the assessment of infarct volume in dogs: a comparison of methods. Circ. Res. **43**: 406–413.
17. FLOWERS, N. C., L. G. HORAN & J. C. JOHNSON. 1976. Anterior infarctional changes occurring during mid and late ventricular activation detectable by surface mapping techniques. Circulation **54**: 906–913.
18. FLOWERS, N. C., L. G. HORAN, G. S. SOHI, R. C. HAND & J. C. JOHNSON. 1976. New evidence for inferoposterior myocardial infarction on surface potential maps. Am. J. Cardiol. **38**: 576–581.
19. SUGIYAMA, S., M. WADA, J. SUGENOYA, H. TOYOSHIMA, J. TOYAMA & K. YAMADA. 1977. Experimental study of myocardial infarction through the use of body surface isopotential maps: ligation of the anterior descending branch of the left coronary artery. Am. Heart J. **93**: 51–59.
20. YAMADA, K., J. TOYAMA, J. SUGENOYA, M. WADA & S. SUGIYAMA. 1978. Body surface isopotential maps. Clinical application to the diagnosis of myocardial infarction. Jpn. Heart J. **19**: 28–45.
21. HAYASHI, H., Y. WATANABE, T. ISHIKAWA, M. WADA, H. UEMATSU & H. INAGAKI. 1980. Diagnostic value of body surface map in myocardial infarction: assessment of location, size and ejection fraction as compared with coronary cineangiography and 201-Tl myocardial scintigraphy. Jpn. Circ. J. **44**: 197–208.
22. OHTA, T., J. TOYAMA, J. OHSUGI, A. KINOSHITA, S. ISOMURA, F. TAKATSU, H. ISHIKAWA, T. NAGAYA & K. YAMADA. 1981. Correlation between body surface isopotential maps and left ventriculograms in patients with old anterior myocardial infarction. Jpn. Heart J. **22**: 747–761.
23. TOYOMA S., K. SUZUKI, M. KOYAMA, K. YOSHINO & K. FUJIMOTO. 1982. The body surface isopotential mapping of the QRS wave in myocardial infarction. A comparative study of the scintigram with thallium-201. J. Electrocardiol. **15**: 241–248.
24. TONOOKA, I., I. KUBOTA, Y. WATANABE, K. TSUIKI & S. YASUI. 1983. Isointegral analysis of body surface maps for the assessment of location and size of myocardial infarction. Am. J. Cardiol. **52**: 1174–1180.
25. KUBOTA, I., K. IKEDA, M. YAMAKI, Y. WATANABE, K. TSUIKI & S. YASUI. 1984. Determination of the left ventricular asynergic site by QRST isointegral mapping in patients with myocardial infarction. Jpn. Heart J. **25**: 311–324.

26. HIRAI, M., T. OHTA, A. KINOSHITA, J. TOYAMA, J. NAGAYA & K. YAMASHITA. 1984. Body surface isopotential maps in old anterior myocardial infarction undetectable by 12-lead electrocardiograms. Am. Heart J. **108:** 975–982.

27. OHTA, T., J. TOYAMA, S. SUGIYAMA & K. YAMADA. 1985. Sequential changes in the difference maps of potential distributions and the extent of myocardial infarctions. Jpn. Heart J. **24:** 391–398.

28. IKEDA, K., I. KUBOTA, A. IGARASHI, M. YAMAKI, K. TSUIKI & S. YASUI. 1985. Detection of local abnormalities in ventricular activation sequence by body surface isochrone mapping in patients with previous myocardial infarction. Circulation **72:** 801–809.

29. TOYAMA, S., K. SYZYUKI, T. TAKAHASHI & Y. YAMASHITA. 1985. Epicardial isopotential mapping from body surface isopotential mapping in myocardial infarction. J. Electrocardiol. **18:** 277–286.

30. KUBOTA, I., K. IKEDA, T. KANAYA, M. YAMAKI, I. TONOOKA, Y. WATANABE, K. TSUIKI & S. YASUI. 1985. Noninvasive assessment of left ventricular wall motion abnormalities by QRS isointegral maps in previous anterior infarction. Am. Heart J. **109:** 464–471.

31. VINCENT, G. M., J. A. ABILDSKOV, M. J. BURGESS, K. MILLAR, F. L. LUX & R. F. WYATT. 1977. Diagnosis of old inferior myocardial infarction by body surface isopotential mapping. Am. J. Cardiol. **39:** 510–515.

32. OHTA, T., A. KINOSHITA, J. OHSUGI, S. ISOMURA, F. TAKATSU, H. ISHIKAWA, J. TOYAMA, T. NAGAYA & K. YAMADA. 1982. Correlation between body surface isopotential maps and left ventriculograms in patients with old inferoposterior myocardial infarction. Am. Heart J. **104:** 1262–1270.

33. OSUGI, J., T. OHTA, J. TOYAMA, F. TAKATSU, T. NAGAYA & K. YAMADA. 1984. Body surface isopotential maps in old inferior myocardial infarction undetectable by 12 lead electrocardiogram. J. Electrocardiol. **17:** 55–62.

34. SUGIYAMA, S., J. SUGENOYA, M. WADA, N. NIIMI, J. TOYAMA & K. YAMADA. 1977. Diagnosis of high posterior infarction: experimental study through the use of body surface isopotential maps. J. Electrocardiol. **10:** 251–256.

35. SUGIYAMA, S., M. WADA, J. SUGENOYA, H. TOYOSHIMA, J. TOYAMA & K. YAMADA. 1977. Diagnosis of right ventricular infarction: experimental study through the use of body surface isopotential maps. Am. Heart J. **94:** 445–453.

36. MONTAGUE, T. J., D. E. JOHNSTONE, C. A. SPENCER, L. D. LALONDE, M. J. GARDNER, M. G. O'REILLY & B. M. HORACEK. 1986. Non-Q-wave acute myocardial infarction: body surface potential map and ventriculographic patterns. Am. J. Cardiol. **58:** 1173–1180.

37. TOYAMA, S., K. SUZUKI, K. YOSHINO & K. FUJIMOTO. 1984. A comparative study of body surface isopotential mapping and the electrocardiogram in diagnosing myocardial infarction. J. Electrocardiol. **17:** 7–14.

38. PHAM-HUY, H., R. M. GULRAJANI, F. A. ROBERGE, R. A. NADEAU, G. E. MAILLOUX & P. SAVARD. 1981. A comparative evaluation of three different approaches for detecting body surface isopotential map abnormalities in patients with myocardial infarction. J. Electrocardiol. **14:** 43–56.

39. KORNREICH, F., T. J. MONTAGUE, P. M. RAUTAHASJU, P. BLOCK, J. W. WARREN & B. M. HORACEK. 1986. Identification of best electrocardiographic leads for diagnosing anterior and inferior myocardial infarction by statistical analysis of body surface potential maps. Am. J. Cardiol. **58:** 863–871.

40. SUZUKI, K., S. TOYAMA, K. YOSHINO & Y. FUDEMOTO. 1984. Relation between the location of the infarcted area in body surface isopotential mapping and the location of myocardial infarction in vectorcardiography. J. Electrocardiol. **17:** 47–54.

41. IKEDA, K., I. KUBOTA, I. TONOOKA, K. TSUIKI & S. YASUI. 1985. Detection of posterior myocardial infarction by body surface mapping: a comparative study with 12 lead ECG and VCG. J. Electrocardiol. **18:** 361–370.

42. MONTAGUE, T. J., E. R. SMITH, C. A. SPENCER, D. E. JOHNSTONE, L. D. LALONDE, R. M. BESSOUDO, M. J. GARDNER, R. N. ANDERSON & B. M. HORACEK. 1983. Body surface electrocardiographic mapping in inferior myocardial infarction. Circulation **67:** 665–673.

43. MONTAGUE, T. J., E. R. SMITH, D. E. JOHNSTONE, C. A. SPENCER, L. D. LALONDE, R. M.

BESSOUDO, M. J. GARDNER, R. N. ANDERSON & B. M. HORACEK. 1984. Temporal evolution of body surface map patterns following acute inferior myocardial infarction. J. Electrocardiol. **17:** 319–328.

44. DE AMBROGGI, L., T. BERTONI, C. RABBIA & M. LANDOLINA. 1986. Body surface potential maps in old inferior myocardial infarction. Assessment of diagnostic criteria. J. Electrocardiol. **19:** 225–234.

45. BODENHEIMER, M. M., V. S. BANKA, R. G. TROUT, H. PASDAR & R. H. HELFANT. 1976. Correlation of pathologic Q waves on the standard electrocardiogram and the epicardial electrogram of the human heart. Circulation **54:** 213–218.

46. MIRVIS, D. M. 1988. Chronic myocardial infarction. In Body Surface Electrocardiographic Mapping. D. M. Mirvis, Ed.: 137–152. Kluwer Academic Publishers. Boston, Mass.

47. BLUMENSCHEIN, S. D., M. S. SPACH, J. P. BOINEAU, R. C. BARR, T. M. GALLIE, A. G. WALLACE & P. A. EBERT. 1968. Genesis of body surface potentials in varying types of right ventricular hypertrophy. Circulation **38:** 917–932.

48. SOHI, G. S., E. W. GREEN, N. C. FLOWERS, D. F. MCMARTIN & R. R. MASDEN. 1979. Body surface potential maps in patients with pulmonic valvular and aortic valvular stenosis of mild to moderate severity. Circulation **59:** 1277–1283.

49. WALLACE, A. G., M. S. SPACH, E. H. ESTES & J. P. BOINEAU. 1968. Activation of the normal and hypertrophied human right ventricle. Am. Heart J. **75:** 728–735.

50. HOLT, J. H., JR., A. C. L. BARNARD & M. S. LYNN. 1969. A study of the human heart as a multiple dipole electrical source. II. Diagnosis and quantitation of left ventricular hypertrophy. Circulation **40:** 697–710.

51. HOLT, J. H., JR., A. C. L. BARNARD & J. O. KRAMER, JR. 1978. Multiple dipole electrocardiography: a comparison of electrically and angiographically determined left ventricular masses. Circulation **57:** 1129–1133.

52. FLOWERS, N. C. & L. G. HORAN. 1973. Comparative surface potential patterns in obstructive and nonobstructive cardiomyopathy. Am. Heart J. **86:** 196–202.

53. TACCARDI, B., L. DE AMBROGGI & D. RIVA. 1969. Chest maps of heart potentials in right bundle branch block. J. Electrocardiol. **2:** 109–116.

54. SUGENOYA, J., S. SUGIYAMA, M. WADA, N. NIIMI, H. OGURI, J. TOYAMA & K. YAMADA. 1977. Body surface potential distribution following the production of right bundle branch block in dogs: effects of breakthrough and right ventricular excitation on the body surface potentials. Circulation **55:** 49–54.

55. SUGENOYA, J. 1978. Interpretation of the body surface isopotential maps of patients with right bundle branch block. Determination of the region of the delayed activation within the right ventricle. Jpn. Heart J. **19:** 12–27.

56. SOHI, G. S. & N. C. FLOWERS. 1980. Body surface map patterns of altered depolarization and repolarization in right bundle branch block. Circulation **61:** 634–640.

57. LIEBMAN, J., C. W. THOMAS & Y. RUDY. 1988. Conduction abnormalities and ventricular hypertrophy. In Body Surface Electrocardiographic Mapping. D. M. Mirvis, Ed.: 153–166. Kluwer Academic Publishers. Boston, Mass.

58. SOHI, G. S., N. C. FLOWERS, L. G. HORAN, M. R. SRIDHARAN & J. C. JOHNSON. 1983. Comparison of total body surface map depolarization patterns of left bundle branch block and normal axis with left bundle branch block and left axis deviation. Circulation **67:** 660–664.

59. MUSSO, E., D. STILLI, E. MACCHI, G. REGOLIOSI, C. BRAMBILLA, P. FRANCESCON, M. BO, A. ROLLI, G. BOTTI & B. TACCARDI. 1987. Body surface maps in left bundle branch block uncomplicated or complicated by myocardial infarction, left ventricular hypertrophy or myocardial ischemia. J. Electrocardiol. **20:** 1–20.

60. PREDA, I., Z. ANTALOCZY, I. BUKOSZA, G. KOZMANN & A. SZEKELY. 1979. New electrocardiological infarct criteria in the presence of left bundle branch block (surface mapping study). In Progress in Electrocardiology. P. W. Macfarlane, Ed.: 231–235. G. K. Hall Publications. Boston, Mass.

61. MUSSO, E., D. STILLI, C. BRAMBILLA, G. REGOLIOSI, I. PREDA, G. KOZMANN, T. ROCHILITZ, Z. ANTALOCZY & B. TACCARDI. 1986. Validation (test set) of a method for detecting associated heart conditions in LBBB by means of BSM. In Electrocardio-

graphic Body Surface Mapping. R. T. van Dam & A. van Oosterom, Eds.: 91–94. Martinus Nijhoff Publishers. Dordrecht, the Netherlands.

62. SOHI, G. S. & N. C. FLOWERS. 1980. Effects of left anterior fascicular block on the depolarization process as depicted by total body surface mapping. J. Electrocardiol. 13: 143–152.

63. SOHI, G. S. & N. C. FLOWERS. 1979. Distinguishing features of left anterior fascicular block and inferior myocardial infarction as presented by body surface potential mapping. Circulation 60: 1354–1359.

64. BURGESS, M. J. 1982. Ventricular repolarization and electrocardiographic T wave form and arrhythmia vulnerability. In Excitation and Neural Control of the Heart. M. N. Levy & M. Vassalle, Eds.: 181–202. American Physiological Society. Bethesda, Md.

65. ABILDSKOV, J. A., L. S. GREEN & R. L. LUX. 1985. Detection of disparate ventricular repolarization by means of the body surface electrocardiogram. In Cardiac Electrophysiology and Arrhythmias. D. P. Zipes & J. Jalife, Eds.: 495–499. Grune & Stratton. New York, N.Y.

66. HORACEK, B. M., T. J. MONTAGUE, M. J. GARDNER & E. R. SMITH. 1988. Arrhythmogenic conditions. In Body Surface Electrocardiographic Mapping. D. M. Mirvis, Ed.: 167–180. Kluwer Academic Publishers. Boston, Mass.

67. DE AMBROGGI, L., T. BERTONI, E. LOCATI, M. STRAMBA-BADIALE & P. J. SCHWARTZ. 1986. Mapping of body surface potentials in patients with the idiopathic long QT syndrome. Circulation 74: 1334–1345.

68. DE AMBROGGI, L., B. TACCARDI & E. MACCHI. 1976. Body-surface maps of heart potentials: tentative localization of pre-excited areas in forty-two Wolff-Parkinson-White patients. Circulation 54: 251–263.

69. TONKIN, A. M., G. S. WAGNER, J. J. GALLAGHER, G. D. COPE, J. KASELL & A. G. WALLACE. 1975. Initial forces of ventricular depolarization in the Wolff-Parkinson-White syndrome. Circulation 52: 1030–1036.

70. KAMAKURA, S., K. SHIMOMURA, T. OHE, M. MATSUHISA & H. TOYOSHIMA. 1986. The role of initial minimum potentials on body surface maps in predicting the site of accessory pathways in patients with Wolff-Parkinson-White syndrome. Circulation 74: 89–96.

71. COBB, F. R., S. D. BLUMENSCHEIN, W. C. SEALY, J. P. BOINEAU, G. S. WAGNER & A. G. WALLACE. 1968. Successful surgical interruption of the bundle of Kent in a patient with Wolff-Parkinson-White syndrome. Circulation 38: 1018–1029.

72. YAMADA, K., J. TOYAMA, M. WADA, S. SUGIYAMA, J. SUGENOYA, H. TOYOSHIMA, Y. MIZUNO, I. SOTOBATA, T. KOBAYASHI & M. OKAJIMA. 1975. Body surface isopotential mapping in Wolff-Parkinson-White syndrome: noninvasive methods to determine the localization of the accessory atrioventricular pathway. Am. Heart J. 90: 721–734.

73. SPACH, M. S., R. C. BARR & C. F. LANNING. 1978. Experimental basis for QRS and T wave potentials in the WPW syndrome: the relation of epicardial to body surface potential distributions in the intact chimpanzee. Circ. Res. 42: 103–118.

74. IWA, T. & T. MAGARA. 1981. Correlation between localization of accessory conduction pathway and body surface maps in the Wolff-Parkinson-White syndrome. Jpn. Circ. J. 45: 1192–1198.

75. BENSON, D. W., R. STERBA, J. J. GALLAGHER, A. WALSTON & M. S. SPACH. 1982. Localization of the site of ventricular preexcitation with body surface maps in patients with Wolff-Parkinson-White syndrome. Circulation 65: 1259–1268.

76. HORAN, L. G., N. C. FLOWERS & J. C. JOHNSON. 1982. The dynamic pathway of His bundle activation as derived from body surface potential maps. In Advances in Body Surface Potential Mapping. K. Yamada, K. Harum & T. Musha, Eds.: 189–194. The University of Nagoya Press. Nagoya, Japan.

77. FLOWERS, N. C. 1987. Signal averaging as an adjunct in detection of arrhythmias. Circulation 75(Suppl. III):III-74–III-78.

78. HORAN, L. G., H. A. W. KILLAM, N. C. FLOWERS, M. R. SRIDHARAN, R. HARP, P. C. ORANDER & R. C. HAND. 1989. The relationship between the ventriculographic silhouette and the topography of thoracic potential in coronary artery disease. Am. J. Cardiol. 64: 20C–28C.

79. INGELS, N. B., JR., G. T. DAUGHTERS II, E. B. STINSON & E. L. ALDERMAN. 1980. Evaluation of methods for quantitating left ventricular segmental wall motion in man using myocardial markers as a standard. Circulation **61:** 966–972.

80. CAIN, M. E., H. D. AMBOS, J. MARKHAM, A. E. FISCHER & B. E. SOBEL. 1985. Quantification of differences in frequency content of signal-averaged electrocardiograms in patients with compared to those without sustained ventricular tachycardia. Am. J. Cardiol. **55:** 1500–1505.

Signal Averaging

GÜNTER BREITHARDT, MARTIN BORGGREFE, AND
ANTONI MARTINEZ-RUBIO
Hospital of the Westfälische Wilhelms-University
Department of Internal Medicine (Cardiology, Angiology)
Münster, Federal Republic of Germany

The standard level of amplification as used for routine electrocardiographic (ECG) recording does not make use of the full range of information contained in the electrocardiographic signal on the body surface. Under physiologic and pathologic conditions, low-amplitude signals can be recorded directly from the epicardium or endocardium of the heart that may be clinically useful. Due to the progress of the last decade, recording of these low-amplitude signals from the body surface by "high-resolution electrocardiography" has been achieved. The most widely used technique is the signal-averaging technique which was used as early as in 1973 by Stopczyk *et al.* to perform surface recordings of the electrical activity during the P-R segment in man.[1] The usefulness of this approach has subsequently been shown in various studies.[2] However, despite great efforts, noninvasive recording of His-bundle potentials within the P-R segment has not gained great acceptance as a routine clinical technique. Neither have there been any large-scale prospective studies in patients with atrioventricular or intraventricular conduction disease. In contrast, signal averaging has attracted substantial interest since initial reports[3,4] showed that this technique is able to detect delayed ventricular activation on the body surface.[5–14] In the early 1980s, Simson,[9,10] Rozanski *et al.*,[8] Breithardt *et al.*,[5,6] and Hombach *et al.*[7] presented their early experience with the signal-averaging technique in patients with ventricular tachyarrhythmias. The subsequent experimental and clinical studies have improved our understanding of the pathophysiological mechanisms as well as of the clinical significance of low-amplitude ventricular activity detectable on the body surface. These potentials are now mostly called "ventricular late potentials."

PATHOPHYSIOLOGIC BASIS FOR VENTRICULAR LATE POTENTIALS

Experimental and clinical studies have provided evidence that myocardial infarction may leave a zone of electrically abnormal ventricular myocardium that may be the site of origin of ventricular tachycardia.[15–17] This tissue is mostly located at the border zone of a previous myocardial infarction, and is characterized by islands of relatively viable muscle alternating with areas of necrosis and later fibrosis. Such tissue may result in fragmentation of the propagating electromotive forces with the consequent development of high-frequency components that can be recorded directly from these areas.[18–21] Gardner *et al.* were able to show that experimentally induced slow conduction alone did not cause fragmented activity.[19,20] Highly fractionated electrograms could only be recorded in preparations with chronic infarcts with interstitial fibrosis forming insulating boundaries between muscle bundles. The individual components of fragmented electrograms, therefore, most probably represent asynchronuous electrical activity in each of the separate bundles of surviving muscle under the electrode. The intrinsic asymmetry of cardiac activation due to fiber orientation (unisotropy) may be accentuated by infarction and may predispose to reentry.[19–21] The slow activation might result from conduction over circuitous pathways caused by the separation and distortion of the myocardial fiber bundles. The low amplitude of the electrograms from these regions probably results from the paucity of surviving muscle fibers under the electrode because of the large amounts of connective tissue, and not from depression of the action potentials. Therefore, the anatomic substrate for reentry seems to be present in regions where fragmented electrograms can be recorded which, thus, indicate slow inhomogenous conduction. (For a more detailed discussion, see Reference 22.)

Electrical recordings from these sites have demonstrated that the fractionated low-amplitude activity may extend beyond normal ventricular activation into the ST segment of the surface ECG. With conventional methods of ECG recording, these signals can normally not be registered on the body surface.

The areas from which ventricular late potentials arise have been considered as the arrhythmogenic electrophysiologic "substrate." A zone with arrhythmogenic properties may arise acutely (and be present only transiently) or it may exist chronically in form of myocardium interspersed with fibrosis after a previous myocardial infarction. The classical example of an acutely developing arrhythmogenic tissue leading to ventricular tachyarrhythmias is acute myocardial infarction that is frequently accompanied by ventricular fibrillation. The changes that occur in this situation are frequently transient in nature and may subside as soon as the tissue is completely necrotic. The electrophysiologic effects of acute ischemia are complex and may depend on the time after initiation and the situation under which they are studied. The ischemia-related direct electrophysiologic changes of the membrane potential are markedly influenced by an inhomogenous increase in extracellular potassium that may cause differences in resting membrane potential. In addition, the increase in sinus rate during ischemia may cause a marked increase in conduction delay in the ischemic zone. Regional activation of sympathetic nerves may cause heterogenous changes in refractory periods which, thus, increase the degree of dispersion of refractoriness.[23–25] Stimulation of beta receptors may increase the slow inward current and may cause facilitation of after depolarizations and of triggered activity.

There have been only few studies assessing the issue whether regions of delayed activation during a basic rhythm are the responsible arrhythmogenic substrate for reentry. El-Sherif *et al.* conducted a study in the four-day-old canine postinfarction model of reentry to determine if regions of delayed activation during a basic rhythm are the responsible arrhythmogenic substrate for reentry.[26,27] The signal-averaged ECG during basic rhythm at a cycle length of 400 to 500 mseconds detected late potentials that corresponded temporarily with the region of latest epicardial activation times. However, subsequent investigations revealed that sites of late potentials during basic rhythm were not always responsible for "early" potentials detected during reentrant activation. Regions showing marked conduction delay in a 1:1 pattern or showing Wenckebach or 2:1 conduction patterns during the basic rhythm usually blocked during a premature impulse and did not participate in the reentrant process. Their observations suggest a close association between myocardial zones showing a Wenckebach conduction pattern and the chance for development of spontaneous reentry. The presence of areas of 2:1 block also proved to be a strong marker for spontaneous reentry. They hypothesized that a body surface recording showing 2:1 or Wenckebach periodicity may represent a better electrophysiological marker for the propensity to develop reentrant arrhythmias than a recording that reflects primarily areas of conduction delays in a 1:1 pattern.

In areas of extensive fibrosis and disorganized myocardial fibers, fractionated and split electrograms are commonly recorded[28] similar to the ones recorded from chronic canine infarction.[19,20] However, it has never been shown that reentrant excitation occurs in areas of extensive fibrosis with disorganized, isolated, and uncoupled myocardial bundles in which very slow and possibly discontinuous conduction could be demonstrated.[26] According to El-Sherif *et al.*,[26] this is not surprising since very slow and circuitous conduction in such areas is usually too slow to participate in reentrant excitation. Therefore, they doubt the significance of these areas in the initiation and/or sustenance of clinical reentrant tachycardia. This issue obviously needs further attention in the future.

METHODOLOGICAL ASPECTS

Because of the low amplitude of the signals to be detected on the body surface, some means of noise reduction (FIGURE 1) is mandatory. Though noise reduction is the basic objective of signal averaging, the degree of noise reduction required to maximally detect low-amplitude signals on the body surface (such as ventricular late potentials) is unknown. The level to which noise that emerges from various sources[29] will be reduced by signal averaging depends not only upon the number of cycles averaged but also on the level of noise at the start of a study session. It is likely that this level of noise exhibits both intrapatient and interpatient variability. It may depend, e.g., on the anxiety of the patient which may induce muscular tremor.

Prior studies have used a fixed number of QRS complexes for performing signal averaging. Since the background noise level is variable, Steinberg and Bigger hypothesized that variable noise levels after signal-averaging could interfere with the detection of late potentials.[30] Therefore, they performed signal averaging to two prespecified noise endpoints. The first endpoint was 1.0 μV which has also been used previously as minimal residual noise level. The second was 0.3 μV which is a low level that generally can be obtained in less than 450 beats. The relative prevalence of late potentials was then evaluated in three groups of patients (26 patients with sustained ventricular tachyarrhythmias; 59 patients after myocardial infarction without ventricular tachyarrhythmias; 40 normal volunteers). The prevalence of late potentials was greater in the first and the second groups using the 0.3 point μV criteria whereas in normal volunteers, the prevalence of late potentials did not change. The greater chance of detecting late potentials within the 0.3 μV study was due to improved resolution of the terminal low-amplitude QRS segment. Therefore, using a lower noise level increased the sensitivity of detection of late potentials without a loss of specificity. Therefore, Steinberg and Bigger recommended performing signal-averaged ECGs to this prespecified low-noise endpoint.[30]

Initially, signal averaging was only performed in the time domain. This means that the signals of many cardiac cycles were analyzed for their voltage in relation to the timing of ventricular activation. Recently, additional approaches have been suggested such as signal averaging in the frequency-domain[12-14,31] as well as spatial averaging on a beat-to-beat basis[32-34] (TABLE 1).

Signal Averaging in the Time Domain

Signal averaging in the time domain (TABLE 2; FIGURES 2 and 3) has been most widely used since its introduction.[3-11] This approach is based on high-gain amplification and signal averaging of many identical beats to eliminate the remaining random noise and to improve the signal-to-noise ratio. Only identical beats should be averaged. Thus, one of the assumptions of the signal-averaging technique in the time domain is that the QRS morphology of the beats to be averaged is identical with respect to the presence and timing of any low-amplitude signal of potential interest. However, some degree of

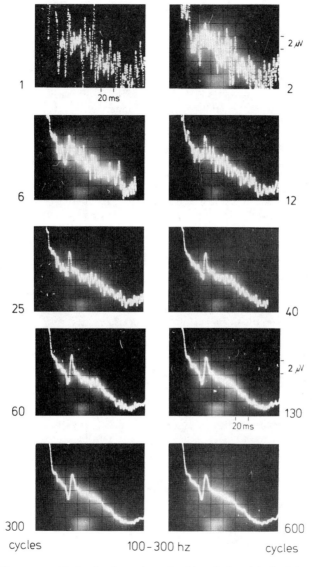

FIGURE 1. Improvement in the signal-to-noise ratio with evolution of the final signal during the averaging process with increasing number of cardiac cycles (from 1 to 600 cycles) in a patient with a left ventricular aneurysm and a history of sustained ventricular tachycardia. There was a circumscribed high frequency activity representing a late potential shortly after the QRS complex.

TABLE 1. High-resolution Electrocardiography

Signal averaging in the: ● Time domain ● Frequency domain ● Spectral mapping ● Spatial averaging (beat to beat)

beat-to-beat variation of the timing and configuration of ventricular late potentials may cause progressive attenuation of the low-amplitude tail of the highly amplified QRS complex during the averaging process. This may lead to cancellation of at least part or all of the signal to be recovered during the averaging process. Another problem is instability ("jitter") of the trigger point of the QRS complex. In case of significant jitter of the triggering point, major parts of the high-frequency signal may be attenuated. The frequency with which attenuation or cancellation of low-amplitude signals during the averaging process may occur is still not yet known.

For better identification of late potentials, high-pass filtering of the signal has to be performed if the time-domain approach is used. One problem with filter ringing of highly amplified signals is filtering after an abrupt transient, above all if sharp high-pass filters are used.[35] Elimination of low-frequency components of the signal is mandatory to prevent the ST segment saturating at the extremely high amplifications used for the detection of late potentials and to exclude respiratory movements. To prevent filter ringing either filters with flat characteristics have been used[5,6] or the signals have been analyzed retrogradely.[10] In the latter approach, a bidirectional filter was used that first analyzes the initial portion of the QRS complex and then retrogradely analyzes the signal backward in time.

Parameters to Analyze Signals in the Time Domain

Several parameters have been suggested to analyze signal-averaged recordings. These include the root-mean-square voltage in the terminal 40 mseconds of the QRS complex,[10] the duration of the terminal low-amplitude tail of the QRS complex,[36] and the time the terminal portion of the QRS complex stays below 40 μV.[37] Other parameters that have not proven to be of clinical significance include peak voltage of the terminal of the QRS complex or other voltage criteria.

Signal Averaging in the Frequency Domain

The second, more recent approach has been signal-averaging in the frequency domain (TABLE 3). This approach was suggested to avoid some major limitations of

TABLE 2. Signal Averaging in the Time Domain

● High-gain amplification ● Averaging of many identical beats to eliminate the remaining random noise and to improve the signal-to-noise ratio ● High-pass filtering

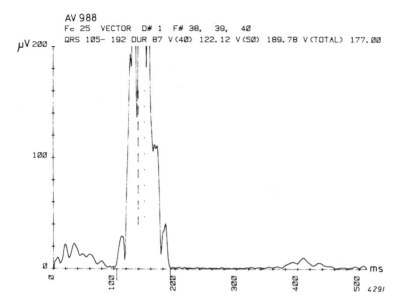

FIGURE 2. Signal-averaged and filtered recording of leads X, Y, Z (vector magnitude) using the software developed by M. Simson in a patient without a history of ventricular tachycardia and without structural heart disease. There is no low-amplitude activity at the end of the high-amplitude portion of the QRS complex. The voltage in the last 40 mseconds of QRS was 122.12 μV. The QRS duration was 87 mseconds.

time-domain analysis which includes the necessity for high-pass filtering that may disturb the character of the signals and may make a discrimination between noise and late potentials difficult. To overcome these limitations, Cain et al.[12,13] and Haberl et al.[14,38] developed methods to assess the frequency content in the otherwise low-frequent ST segment. Signals are processed for their frequency content (frequency domain) using fast Fourier transform analysis (FFTA) by analyzing all signals for higher sinusoidal components (harmonics) in relation to the sinusoidal component with the lowest frequency. All harmonics have frequencies that are integer multiples of the fundamental frequency. The use of FFTA for a discrete sample of a periodic waveform (e.g., the terminal portion of QRS) requires the assumption that the signal has a repetitive function and that the initial and final sample points are at a potential of zero. However, since this is not the case, a sharp-edged discontinuity will be introduced between the end of one cycle and the beginning of the next that will artefactually add both high and low frequencies to the original signal. To eliminate this source of harmonic error, time-domain samples are multiplied by a window function (e.g., a 4-term Blackman-Harris window)[12,13] that smoothes the initial and final sampling points to zero at the boundaries, allowing periodic extension of the finite signal. A major problem is that the results of FFTA when applied on limited segments of a periodic waveform critically depend on the duration and the position of this segment (window).

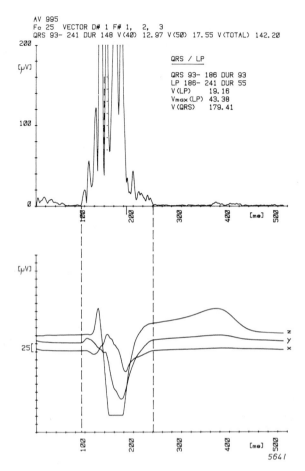

FIGURE 3. Signal-averaged and filtered recording of leads X, Y, Z (vector magnitude) using the software developed by M. Simson in a patient with ventricular tachycardia. QRS duration (DUR) in the highly amplified and filtered recording was 148 mseconds. The program automatically identified the end of the total QRS complex at 241 mseconds on the x axis. The amplitude in the terminal 40 mseconds was low (V(40) = 12.97 μV) extending into the ST segment of the surface ECG lower panel). The onset of low-amplitude activity that lasted for 55 mseconds was automatically identified at 186 mseconds by the automatic recognition program.[36]

TABLE 3. Signal Averaging in the Frequency Domain

- Analysis of the frequency content using fast Fourier transform analysis (FFTA)
- Assumptions: repetitive function; initial and final sample points are at a potential of zero
- Since this is not the case, a sharp-edged discontinuity will be introduced between the end of one cycle and the beginning of the next that will artefactually add both high and low frequencies to the original signal
- To eliminate this source of harmonic error, time-domain samples are multiplied by a window function

Spectral Mapping

Spectral mapping (TABLE 4) of the electrocardiogram with Fourier transform of multiple segments of the surface electrocardiogram during sinus rhythm after signal averaging is another modification of the signal-averaging technique.[38] In this approach, it was suggested to divide the ST segment into 25 segments; the first segment started 25 mseconds after the end of QRS with each segment having a size of 80 mseconds. The subsequent segment started progressively earlier in the ST segment in steps of 3 mseconds. Thus, the 25th segment started 25 mseconds inside the QRS complex. Similar to other approaches using FFT analysis, each segment is multiplied point by point with a window function to avoid edge discontinuities. The 25 frequency spectra are then combined into a three-dimensional plot. The frequency spectrum of segment 1 (which started far outside the QRS) was defined as a reference spectrum; the spectra of segments 2–25 are then compared with this reference spectrum by cross correlation in the frequency range 40 to 150 Hz. The similarity of spectra was indicated by the correlation coefficient from which a "factor of normality" was calculated. High-frequency content at the end of QRS which is absent far outside QRS causes the "factor of normality" to be low. A "factor of normality" below 30% was considered abnormal.[38]

The advantage of spectral mapping of the ST segment as suggested by Haberl *et*

TABLE 4. Spectral Mapping

- FFTA of multiple segments of the surface ECG after signal averaging
- Division of the ST segment into 25 segments
- The similarity of spectra is indicated by the correlation coefficient from which a "factor of normality" is calculated
- Advantages: does not require an exact definition of the onset and end of QRS; a single parameter ("factor of normality") is calculated; complex high-pass filtering is not necessary

---

al.[38] is that it does not require an exact definition of the onset and end of QRS which often are difficult to determine. Furthermore, a distinction between normal and abnormal is simpler and does not require more or less arbitrary criteria since the "factor of normality" is calculated as a single parameter. Complex high-pass filtering is not necessary, and a discussion about filter artefacts, signal distortion, and the choice of adequate cutoff frequencies is not necessary.[22] Finally, spectral mapping allows a discrimination between late potentials and noise which both have a typical spectral representation. Noise can easily be identified by spectral peaks that are present in all segments. Late potentials give rise to spectral peaks only in segments at the end of the QRS but not far outside the QRS-complex.

INCIDENCE OF LATE POTENTIALS IN PATIENTS WITH DOCUMENTED VENTRICULAR TACHYCARDIA

Ventricular late potentials (see TABLE 5) have rarely been detected in subjects with normal left ventricular function (FIGURE 2).[6–8,10,39–41] This is in contrast to patients with previously documented sustained ventricular tachycardia and/or fibrillation (outside the acute phase of myocardial infarction) in whom there is a high incidence of ventricular late potentials (FIGURE 3).[6,8,10,39,42-45] We previously reported that 45 out of 63 patients (71%) with documented sustained ventricular tachycardia/fibrillation had ventricular late potentials of any duration. The proportion of patients with late potentials increased to 37 of 47 patients (79%) if only patients with coronary artery disease were considered.[39] Simson, who was the first to use an algorithm for quantification of the terminal portion of the QRS complex, reported that patients with sustained ventricular tachycardia had a low-amplitude signal in the last 40 mseconds of the filtered QRS complex which was not detectable in the filtered output from patients without ventricular tachycardia.[9,10] He found that the voltage in the last 40 mseconds of the filtered QRS complex was able to discriminate well between patients with and without ventricular tachycardia. Patients with ventricular tachycardia had 15 ± 14.4 μV of high-frequency signal in this segment; in contrast, patients without ventricular tachycardia had 74 ± 77.7 μV ($p < 0.0001$). Twenty-five microvolts was the best threshold to discriminate patients with and without ventricular tachycardia.[10] Only three of 39 patients (8%) with ventricular tachycardia exceeded 25 μV. The filtered QRS voltage tended to be lower in patients with ventricular tachycardia than in those without (103 ± 30 versus 127 ± 43 μV; nonsignificant). The QRS duration was longer in patients with ventricular tachycardia (139 ± 26 versus 95 ± 10 mseconds; $p < 0.0001$). Freedman et al., who used a similar methodology, found late potentials in 33 of 53 patients (62%) with ventricular tachycardia.[43] Kanovsky et al. studied 174

TABLE 5. Various Definitions of Ventricular Late Potentials Recorded Noninvasively

---

1. Presence of low-amplitude signals in the last 40 mseconds of the filtered and averaged QRS complex (root-mean-square voltage) at a high-pass filter setting of 25 Hz: <25 μV.
2. Higher frequency content in the terminal 40 mseconds of the QRS-complex and ST-segment.
3. Duration of late potentials ≥ 40 mseconds.
4. Long QRS duration in the absence of bundle branch block (>120 mseconds).

---

patients after myocardial infarction,[45] 89 of these patients had recurrent sustained ventricular tachycardia. By multivariate logistic regression analyses, the signal-averaged ECG, peak premature ventricular contractions >100 per hour, and the presence of a left ventricular aneurysm were found to be independently significant. Patients with nonsustained ventricular tachycardia in whom sustained ventricular tachycardia can be induced by programmed ventricular stimulation have also been shown to have a significantly higher incidence of late potentials (67%) than patients without inducible sustained ventricular tachycardia (25%).[46] The filtered QRS duration was also longer (127 versus 100 mseconds).[46] Similar to patients with ventricular tachycardia after myocardial infarction, patients with congestive cardiomyopathy with a history of sustained ventricular tachycardia had a significantly greater incidence of late potentials and a longer QRS duration than those without ventricular tachycardia.[47]

Using fast Fourier transform analysis, it has been shown that patients with sustained ventricular tachycardia have a higher frequency content in their terminal QRS complex compared with normals.[12-14] Cain et al. demonstrated an increase in the amplitude of high-frequency components in the terminal QRS in 88% of patients with sustained ventricular tachycardia in contrast to 15% in patients without ventricular tachycardia.[12] In a subsequent report, these authors studied 87 patients (23 patients with and 53 patients without ventricular tachycardia after myocardial infarction as well as 11 normal subjects) in whom the terminal 40 mseconds of the QRS complex and the ST segment were analyzed as a single unit to enhance the frequency resolution.[13] The terminal QRS and ST segment from patients with sustained ventricular tachycardia contained 10- to 100-fold greater amplitudes of components in the 20 to 50 Hz range compared with corresponding electrocardiographic segments in patients without sustained ventricular tachycardia. There were no significant differences in the peak frequencies among the patient groups. However, the relative contribution of the magnitudes of these peak frequencies to the overall magnitude of the spectral plot differed significantly. No frequencies above 50 Hz contributed substantially to the energy spectra of the terminal QRS and ST segments in any group.

Similar results have been reported by Haberl *et al.* using spectral analysis of single beats.[48] The frequency content of the terminal QRS complex, expressed as area under the spectral plot, was significantly lower in patients with ventricular tachycardia compared with patients without any arrhythmias ($p < 0.01$). Additionally, the frequency content of the ST segment in the range 10–40 Hz was higher in patients with ventricular tachycardia than in patients without arrhythmias and in control subjects ($p < 0.01$). Thus, spectral analysis of single beat electrocardiograms may offer promise to identify noninvasively patients prone to sustained ventricular tachycardia in patients with coronary artery disease.

Presently, it remains unclear whether fast Fourier transform analysis is superior to signal averaging in the time domain. Only few comparative data exist. Both methods were assessed in 54 subjects comprising 26 patients with sustained ventricular tachycardia, 18 control patients with organic heart disease, but without sustained ventricular tachycardia, and 11 normal volunteers.[49] Time-domain analysis was performed with high-pass filtering of 25, 40, and 80 Hz and low-pass filtering of 250 Hz. Frequency-domain analysis was performed on the terminal 40 mseconds of the QRS complex, either alone or with 216 or 150 mseconds of the ST segment. Absolute summed energies of discrete frequency bands and band energy ratios were calculated. Frequency domain analysis was not considered as an improvement over time-domain analysis in differentiating patients with ventricular tachycardia from those without. This is in contrast to the results by Haberl *et al.*, who demonstrated superiority of frequency-domain analysis.[48] These differences in results may be due to different methodology and ask for further evaluation.

INCIDENCE OF LATE POTENTIALS IN PATIENTS WITH RECURRENT SYNCOPE

Syncope may result from many conditions[50] and has a variable prognosis.[51] Analysis of the high-frequency components of the terminal QRS complex using signal-averaged electrocardiography is a means to identify patients with a propensity to ventricular tachycardia after myocardial infarction,[52] especially in the presence of a left ventricular aneurysm[52-54] and in patients with arrhythmogenic right ventricular disease.[55] Therefore, signal averaging also might be useful to identify those patients with recurrent syncope in whom a ventricular tachyarrhythmia may be the underlying mechanism.

Gang *et al.* assessed the usefulness of signal averaging for detecting hitherto undocumented ventricular tachycardia in 24 patients with unexplained syncope.[53] Sustained ventricular tachycardia was documented in 9 patients (8 patients with inducible ventricular tachycardia and 1 with a spontaneous episode). The signal-averaged ECG contained a late potential and a filtered QRS complex longer than 120 mseconds in 8 of these 9 patients (sensitivity 89%). None of the remaining 15 patients had these electrocardiographic abnormalities.

We studied 40 patients (mean age 54 years) with syncope of unknown origin even after thorough medical and neurologic evaluation.[52] Twenty-two patients had late potentials (mean duration 34 ± 10.2 mseconds). In 18 of these 22 patients with late potentials, sustained ventricular tachycardia or fibrillation was inducible whereas only 8 of 18 patients without late potentials had inducible sustained ventricular tachycardia ($p < 0.05$).

A larger group of 150 consecutive patients presenting with syncope was studied by Kuchar et al.[54] Twenty-nine patients had late potentials, 107 patients had a normal signal-averaged ECG, and 14 patients had bundle branch block on the 12-lead ECG. The signal-averaged ECG identified late potentials in 16 of 22 patients with ventricular tachycardia and was normal in 101 of 114 patients in whom syncope was attributed to causes other than ventricular tachycardia or remained unexplained (sensitivity 73%; specificity 89%; predictive accuracy 54%). Absence of late potentials identified a group of patients with a very low incidence of ventricular tachycardia. During follow-up of 1 to 20 months (mean 11 months), 15 patients (10%) died, 6 of whom died suddenly. There was no significant difference in survival or recurrence of syncope between patients with or without late potentials.

These results suggest that signal averaging of the surface ECG may be a noninvasive test for detecting a high-risk subset of patients prone to lethal tachyarrhythmias.

PROGNOSTIC SIGNIFICANCE OF LATE POTENTIALS

During recent years, several studies have addressed the prognostic value of ventricular late potentials.[56-63] Our own experience is primarily based on two studies, both using signal averaging in the time domain. The first prospective trial was initiated at Düsseldorf University in 1980; it used the methodology for signal averaging that had been developed in our department between 1978 and 1979. This system was based on a hard-wired signal averager[5,6,39,56,57,64] which has subsequently also been used by other groups.[65,66] The second study was started in January 1983 (PILP study; post-infarction late potential study). It has recently been completed after inclusion of almost 800 patients. Data analysis has not yet been completed.

The results of the first prospective pilot study in 160 patients was reported in 1983.[56] Subsequently, another 788 patients without a history of sustained ventricular tachycardia or fibrillation outside the acute phase of myocardial infarction were studied. Mean duration of follow-up was 39 ± 15.0 months. A major arrhythmic event occurred in 35 patients (21 sudden deaths [3.3%]; 14 episodes [2.2%] of symptomatic spontaneous sustained ventricular tachycardia). The risk of major arrhythmic complications was 2.8 times greater in patients with late potentials of less than 40 mseconds duration compared to those without, and 9.3 times greater in those with a duration of 40 mseconds or more. The chance of sudden cardiac death within 1 hour was 3.3 and 5.4 times greater, respectively, whereas the chance for symptomatic sustained ventricular tachycardia was 2.0 and 17.4 times greater, respectively, depending on the duration of late potentials (less than 40 mseconds or greater). The chance of major arrhythmic complications such as sudden cardiac death or sustained symptomatic ventricular tachycardia was greatest in those patients who were studied within the first 4 to 8 weeks after their qualifying myocardial infarction.

These data are supported by other studies also using signal averaging in the time domain. Denniss et al. studied 110 patients 7 to 28 days after acute myocardial infarction.[59] Follow-up of these patients ranged between 2 to 12 months (mean: 5 months). There was a significant difference in the subsequent occurrence of symptomatic sustained ventricular tachycardia during follow-up in patients without late potentials (1.1%) compared to those with late potentials (17.4%). The incidence of sudden cardiac death was not reported in this study. In a more recent report, the same group presented the results of long-term observation in 403 clinically well survivors of transmural infarction who were 65 years old or younger,[59] 26% of the patients had late potentials. At 2 years, the probability of remaining free from cardiac death or nonfatal ventricular tachycardia or fibrillation was 0.73 for patients with late potentials and 0.95 for patients without. For patients with late potentials, the probability of remaining free from instantaneous death or nonfatal ventricular tachycardia or fibrillation was 0.85 at 1 year and 0.79 at 2 years, much lower than the corresponding figures of 0.98 ($p < 0.001$) and 0.96 ($p < 0.001$) for patients without late potentials.[59] Within the group of patients with late potentials, the patients who either died instantaneously or had nonfatal ventricular tachycardia or fibrillation had a longer mean ventricular activation time, a lower mean left ventricular ejection fraction, and a higher incidence of left ventricular aneurysms than patients who were event free.

Kacet et al. studied a population of 104 patients who were followed for 8.5 ± 4 months.[60] The incidence of subsequent symptomatic sustained ventricular tachycardia in patients without late potentials was 4.5% compared to 28.9% in patients with late potentials. None of the patients without late potentials died suddenly compared to 13% of patients with late potentials. In another study, Kuchar et al. reported the results of follow-up (3 to 12 months) of 123 patients who were studied 10 days (mean) after acute myocardial infarction.[61] The incidence of major arrhythmic complications such as sudden death or symptomatic sustained ventricular tachycardia was only 1.4% in patients without late potentials compared to 20.5% in patients with late potentials. In a study by Höpp et al., 50 patients were studied in the early postinfarction period.[62] These patients were followed for 24 ± 5 months; 12 of 30 patients who had late potentials (37%) died suddenly. In contrast, none of the 20 patients without late potentials died suddenly. The same authors studied another group of 200 patients with chronic, stable coronary artery disease.[62] Mean follow-up was 20 ± 5 months; 108 of 200 patients had ventricular late potentials; 15 of these patients (13.9%) died suddenly compared to 4 of 92 patients (4.3%) without late potentials ($p < 0.001$). Von Leitner et al. followed 518 patients who took part in a rehabilitation program after myocardial infarction.[63] These patients were studied between 6 and 8 weeks after onset of infarction. During a mean follow-up period of 10 months, cardiac mortality was 1.5% in patients without late potentials compared to 7.3% in patients with ventricular late potentials. Sudden cardiac death occurred in 0.9% of patients without late potentials compared to 3.6% of patients with late potentials. In none of these patients was symptomatic sustained ventricular tachycardia reported.

In contrast to this extensive information on the prognostic significance of signal averaging in the time domain, there has been no prospective large-scale study using signal averaging in the frequency domain.

CONCLUSIONS AND CLINICAL IMPLICATIONS

Based on these presently available prospective studies, the presence of ventricular late potentials obviously heralds an increased risk for subsequent occurrence of sudden cardiac death or symptomatic sustained ventricular tachycardia. This mainly applies to patients who are studied after recent myocardial infarction,[56,58,60–62] whereas patients who are included later and/or who are considered to be eligible for a cardiac rehabilitation program[63] obviously have a much lower incidence of arrhythmic events. Thus, the predictive value of the presence of ventricular late potentials largely depends on under which clinical circumstances they can be detected. Patients who have survived for a long period after their myocardial infarction have a much lower risk of subsequent development of sudden cardiac death or symptomatic sustained ventricular tachycardia. This is obviously based on a selection process as patients at greater risk might have died in the meanwhile. In addition, our results show that the duration of late potentials might be of prognostic significance. The chance for development of an arrhythmic event, mainly symptomatic sustained ventricular tachycardia, is proportional to the duration of the late potentials.

With regard to the complex mechanisms that may lead to sudden cardiac death, it cannot be expected that any single method will be able to predict the occurrence of sudden cardiac death with 100% sensitivity. Sudden cardiac death may be due to chronic electrophysiologic abnormalities as a consequence of regional slow conduction in the border zone of a previous myocardial infarction which is conventionally considered to be the electrophysiologic substrate for ventricular late potentials.

The presence of regional slow conduction is mostly not sufficient for the spontaneous occurrence of ventricular tachyarrhythmias. Instead, some trigger factor such as spontaneous ventricular ectopic beats is necessary to alter the electrophysiologic milieu in a way that tachycardia originates. However, most spontaneous ventricular arrhythmias detected during long-term ECG recording are not harmful to the patient as they obviously do not induce ventricular tachycardia. Instead, some change in, for instance, the coupling interval or the sequence of ectopic beats, including the occurrence of short runs, may alter the electrophysiologic milieu in a way such that the prerequisites for reentry are met. Such transient occurrence of complex ventricular arrhythmias acting as trigger factor might also be induced by short, regional episodes of ischemia induced by embolisation of platelet aggregates into the peripheral coronary system.[67]

Another mechanism that may lead to sudden cardiac death is the occurrence of more extensive ischemia due to reinfarction. There is no doubt that this may also lead to ventricular fibrillation and, thus, sudden cardiac death. Such a type of event, of course, cannot be predicted on the presence of preexisting indicators of regional slow conduction such as late potentials. However, it has been shown that preexisting myocardial damage increases the chance of ventricular fibrillation if regional ischemia occurs at a site remote from that of preexisting cardiac damage.[68]

Thus, with regard to the complex mechanisms that may lead to sudden cardiac death, only a combination of various parameters including late potentials, spontaneous ventricular arrhythmias during long-term ECG recording, results of programmed ventricular stimulation, extent of myocardial contractile disturbance (ejection fraction), and estimates of central nervous activity[69,70] might serve for further risk stratification in patients after recent myocardial infarction.

REFERENCES

1. STOPCZYK, M. J., J. KOPEC, R. J. ZOCHOWSKI, & M. PIENIAK. 1973. Surface recording of electrical heart activity during the P-R segment in man by computer averaging technique. Int. Res. Com. Syst. **11**(21,2): 73–78.
2. FLOWERS, N. C., V. SHVARTSMAN, L. G. HORAN, P. PALAKURTHY, G. S. SOHI & M. R. SRIDHARAN. 1983. Analysis of PR subintervals in normal subjects and early studies in patients with abnormalities of the conduction system using surface His bundle recordings. J. Am. Coll. Cardiol. **2**: 939.
3. FONTAINE, G., R. FRANK, F. GALLAIS-HAMONNO, I. ALLALI, H. PHAN-THUC & Y. GROSGOGEAT. 1978. Electrocardiographie des potentiels tardifs du syndrome de post-excitation. Arch. Mal. Coeur. **71**: 854–864.
4. BERBARI, E. J., B. J. SCHERLAG, R. R. HOPE & R. LAZZARA. 1978. Recording from the body

surface of arrhythmogenic ventricular activity during the ST-segment. Am. J. Cardiol. **41:** 697–702.

5. BREITHARDT, G., R. BECKER & L. SEIPEL. 1980. Non-invasive recording of late ventricular activation in man. (abstr.) Circulation **62:** III-320.

6. BREITHARDT, G., R. BECKER, L. SEIPEL, R. R. ABENDROTH & J. OSTERMEYER. 1981. Non-invasive detection of late potentials in man—a new marker for ventricular tachycardia. Eur. Heart J. **2:** 1–11.

7. HOMBACH, V., H. W. HOPP, V. BRAUN, D. W. BEHRENBECK, M. TAUCHERT & H. H. HILGER. 1980. Die Bedeutung von Nachpotentialen innerhalb des ST-Segmentes im Oberflächen-EKG bei Patienten mit koronarer Herzkrankheit. Dtsch. med. Wschr. **105:** 1457–1462.

8. ROZANSKI, J. J., D. MORTARA, R. J. MYERBURG, & A. CASTELLANOS. 1981. Body surface detection of delayed depolarizations in patients with recurrent ventricular tachycardia and left ventricular aneurysm. Circulation **63:** 1172–1178.

9. SIMSON, M., L. HOROWITZ, M. JOSEPHSON, E. NEIL MOORE & J. KASTOR. 1980. A marker for ventricular tachycardia after myocardial infarction. (abstr.) Circulation **62:** III-262.

10. SIMSON, M. B. 1981. Use of signals in the terminal QRS-complex to identify patients with ventricular tachycardia after myocardial infarction. Circulation **64:** 235–242.

11. UTHER, J. B., C. J. DENNETT & A. TAN. 1978. The detection of delayed activation signals of low amplitude in the vectorcardiogram of patients with recurrent ventricular tachycardia by signal averaging. In Management of Ventricular Tachycardia—Role of Mexiletine: 80–82. Excerpta Medica. Amsterdam & Oxford.

12. CAIN, M. E., D. AMBOS, F. X. WITKOWSKI & B. E. SOBEL. 1984. Fast-Fourier transform analysis of signal-averaged electrocardiograms for identification of patients prone to sustained ventricular tachycardia. Circulation **69:** 711–720.

13. CAIN, M. E., H. D. AMBOS, J. MARKHAM, A. E. FISCHER & B. E. SOBEL. 1985. Quantification of differences in frequency content of signal-averaged electrocardiograms in patients with compared to those without sustained ventricular tachycardia. Am. J. Cardiol. **55:** 1500–1505.

14. HABERL, R., E. HENGSTENBERG, R. PULTER & G. STEINBECK. 1986. Frequenzanalyse des Einzelschlag-Elektrokardiogrammes zur Diagnostik von Kammertachykardien. Z Kardiol. **75:** 659–665.

15. EL-SHERIF, N., B. J. SCHERLAG, R. LAZZARA & R. R. HOPE. 1977. Reentrant ventricular arrhythmias in the late myocardial infarction period. I. Conduction characteristics in the infarction zone. Circulation **55:** 686–702.

16. EL-SHERIF, N., B. J. SCHERLAG, R. LAZZARA & R. R. HOPE. 1977. Reentrant ventricular arrhythmias in the late myocardial infarction period. II. Patterns of initiation and termination of reentry. Circulation **55:** 702–719.

17. EL-SHERIF, N., R. LAZZARA, R. R. HOPE, & B. J. SCHERLAG. 1977. Reentrant arrhythmias in the late myocardial infarction period. III. Manifest and concealed extrasystolic grouping. Circulation **56:** 225–234.

18. FLOWERS, N. C., L. G. HORAN, J. R. THOMAS & W. J. TOLLESON. 1969. The anatomic basis for high frequency components in the electrocardiogram. Circulation **39:** 531–539.

19. GARDNER, P. I., P. C. URSELL, J. J. FENOGLIO & A. L. WIT. 1985. Electrophysiologic and anatomic basis for fractionated electrograms recorded from healed myocardial infarcts. Circulation **72:** 596–611.

20. GARDNER, P. I., P. C. URSELL, T. D. PHAM, J. J. FENOGLIO & A. L. WIT. 1984. Experimental chronic ventricular tachycardia: anatomic and electrophysiologic substrates. In M. E. Josephson & H. J. J. Wellens, Eds: 29–60. Tachycardias: Mechanisms, Diagnosis, Treatment. Lea and Febiger. Philadelphia, Pa.

21. RICHARDS, D. A., G. J. BLAKE, J. F. SPEAR & E. N. MOORE. 1984. Electrophysiologic substrate for ventricular tachycardia: correlation of properties in vivo and in vitro. Circulation **69:** 369–381.

22. BREITHARDT, G. & M. BORGGREFE. 1986. Pathophysiological mechanisms and clinical significance of ventricular late potentials. Eur. Heart J. **7:** 364–385.

23. PATTERSON, E., J. K. GIBSON & B. R. LUCCHESI. 1982. Electrophysiologic actions of

lidocaine in a canine model of chronic myocardial ischemic damage—arrhythmogenic actions of lidocaine. J. Cardiovasc. Pharmacol. **4:** 925–934.

24. SCHWARTZ, P. J. & A. ZAZA. 1986. The rational basis and the clinical value of selective cardiac sympathetic denervation in the prevention of malignant arrhythmias. Eur. Heart J. **7**(suppl. A): 107–118.

25. LOMBARDI, F. 1986. Acute myocardial ischaemia, neural reflexes and ventricular arrhythmias. Eur. Heart J. **7**(suppl. A): 91–97.

26. EL-SHERIF, N., W. B. GOUGH, M. RESTIVO, W. CRAELIUS & R. HENKIN. 1988. Electrophysiological basis of ventricular late potentials, *in* Progress in Clinical Pacing. M. Santini, M. Pistolese & A. Alliegro, Eds: 209–223. Excerpta Medica. Amsterdam, the Netherlands.

27. RESTIVO, M. 1986. J. Am. Coll. Cardiol. **7:** 85a.

28. KIENZLE, M. G., J. MILLER, R. FALCONE, A. HARKEN & M. E. JOSEPHSON. 1984. Intraoperative endocardial mapping during sinus rhythm: relationship to site of origin of ventricular tachycardia. Circulation **70:** 957–965.

29. SANTIPETRO, R. F. 1977. The origin and characterization of the primary signal, noise and interface sources in the high frequency electrocardiogram. IEEE Trans. Biomed. Eng. **65:** 707–713.

30. STEINBERG, J. S. & J. T. BIGGER JR. 1989. Importance of the endpoint of noise reduction in analysis of the signal-averaged electrocardiogram. Am. J. Cardiol. **63:** 556–560.

31. HABERL, R., M. WEBER, H. REICHENSPURNER, B. M. KEMKES, G. OSTERHOLZER, M. AUFHUBER & G. STEINBECK. 1987. Frequency analysis of the surface electrocardiogram for recognition of acute rejection after orthotopic cardiac transplantation. Circulation **76:** 101–108.

32. EL-SHERIF, N., R. MEHRA, J. A. C. GOMES & G. KELEN. 1983. Appraisal of a low noise electrocardiogram. J. Am. Coll. Cardiol. **1:** 456–467.

33. HOMBACH, V., V. KEBBEL, H. W. HÖPP, H. J. WINTER, V. BRAUN, H. DEUTSCH, H. HIRCHE & H. H. HILGER. 1982. Fortlaufende Registrierung von Mikropotentialen des menschlichen Herzens. Dtsch. Med. Wochenschr. **107:** 1951–1956.

34. HOMBACH, V., V. KEBBEL, H. W. HÖPP, V. WINTER & H. HIRCHE. 1984. Noninvasive beat-by-beat registration of ventricular late potentials using high resolution electrocardiography. Int. J. Cardiol. **6:** 167–183.

35. GRAENE, J. G., G. E. TOBEY & L. E. HUELSMAN. 1971. Operational Amplifiers. McGraw-Hill. New York, N.Y. 191.

36. KARBENN, U., G. BREITHARDT, M. BORGGREFE & M. B. SIMSON. 1985. Automatic identification of late potentials. J. Electrocardiol. **18:** 123–134.

37. DENES, P., P. SANTARELLI, R. G. HAUSER & E. F. URETZ. 1983. Quantitative analysis of the high frequency components of the terminal portion of the body surface QRS in normal subjects and in patients with ventricular tachycardia. Circulation **67:** 1129–1138.

38. HABERL, R., G. JILGE, R. PULTER & G. STEINBECK. 1989. Spectral mapping of the electrocardiogram with Fourier transform for identification of patients with sustained ventricular tachycardia and coronary artery disease. Eur. Heart J. **10:** 316–322.

39. BREITHARDT, G., M. BORGGREFE, U. KARBENN, R. R. ABENDROTH, H. L. YEH & L. SEIPEL. 1982. Prevalence of late potentials in patients with and without ventricular tachycardia: correlation to angiographic findings. Am. J. Cardiol. **49:** 1932–1937.

40. ABBOUD, S., B. BELHASSEN, S. LANIADO & D. SADEH. 1983. Non-invasive recording of late ventricular activity using an advanced method in patients with a damaged mass of ventricular tissue. J. Electrocardiol. **16:** 245.

41. KLEMPT, H. W. & W. WULSCHNER. 1983. Die Analyse des QRS-Komplexes sowie des ST-Abschnittes mit der Signalmittelungstechnik bei Herzgesunden. Z. Kardiol. **72:** 369.

42. KERTES, P. J., M. GLAUBUS, A. MURRAY, D. G. JULIAN & R. W. F. CAMPBELL. 1984. Delayed ventricular depolarization—correlation with ventricular activation and relevance to ventricular fibrillation in acute myocardial infarction. Eur. Heart J. **5:** 974–983.

43. FREEDMAN, R. A., A. M. GILLIS, A. KEREN, V. SODERHOLM-DIFATTE & J. W. MASON. 1984. Signal-averaged ECG late potentials correlate with clinical arrhythmia and electrophysiology study in patients with ventricular tachycardia or fibrillation. Circulation **70:** II-252.

44. HÖPP, H. W., V. HOMBACH, H. J. DEUTSCH, A. OSTERSPEY, U. WINTER & H. H. HILGER.

1983. Assessment of ventricular vulnerability by Holter ECG, programmed ventricular stimulation and recording of ventricular late potentials. *In* Cardiac Pacing: 625–632. Steinkopff Verlag, Darmstadt, FRG.

45. KANOVSKY, M. S., R. A. FALCONE, C. A. DRESDEN, M. E. JOSEPHSON & M. E. SIMSON. 1984. Identification of patients with ventricular tachycardia after myocardial infarction: signal-averaged electrocardiogram, Holter monitoring, and cardiac catheterization. Circulation **70:** 264–270.

46. BUXTON, A. E., M. B. SIMSON, R. FALCONE, *et al.* 1984. Signal averaged ECG in patients with nonsustained ventricular tachycardia: identification of patients with potential for sustained ventricular arrhythmias. (abstr.) J. Am. Coll. Cardiol. **3:** 495.

47. POLL, D. S., F. E. MARCHLINSKI, R. A. FALCONE & M. B. SIMSON. 1984. Abnormal signal averaged ECG in nonischemic congestive cardiomyopathy: relationship to sustained ventricular tachyarrhythmias. Circulation **70:** II-253.

48. HABERL, R., E. HOFFMANN & G. STEINBECK. 1985. Low-frequency components in patients with delayed ventricular activation. Circulation **72:** III-6.

49. MACHAC, J., A. WEISS, S. L. WINTERS, P. BARICCA & J. A. GOMEZ. 1988. A comparative study of frequency-domain and time-domain analysis of signal averaged electrocardiograms in patients with ventricular tachycardia. J. Am. Coll. Cardiol. **11:** 284–296.

50. WRIGHT, K. E. & H. D. MCINTOSCH. 1971. Syncope: a review of pathophysiologic mechanisms. Progr. Cardiovasc. Dis. **13:** 580–593.

51. SILVERSTEIN, M. B., D. E. SINGER, A. G. MULLEY, G. E. THIBAULT & G. O. BARNETT. 1982. Patients with syncope admitted to medical intensive units. JAMA **248:** 1185–1189.

52. BORGGREFE, M., U. KARBENN & G. BREITHARDT. 1986. Usefulness of Holter monitoring and non-invasive recording of late potentials in selection of patients for programmed ventricular stimulation. (abstr.) Circulation **74**(suppl. II): 745.

53. GANG, E. S., T. H. PETER, M. E. ROSENTHAL, W. J. MANDEL & Y. LASS. 1986. Detection of late potentials on the surface electrocardiogram in unexplained syncope. Am. J. Cardiol. **58:** 1014–1020.

54. KUCHAR, D. L., C. W. THORBURN & N. L. SAMMEL. 1986. Signal-averaged electrocardiogram for evaluation of recurrent syncope. Am. J. Cardiol. **58:** 949–953.

55. FONTAINE, G., G. GUIRAUDON & P. FRANK. 1978. Intramyocardial conduction defects in patients prone to ventricular tachycardia. III. The post-excitation syndrome in ventricular tachycardia. *In* Management of Ventricular Tachycardia—Role of Mexiletine. E. Sandoe, D. G. Julian & J. W. Bell, Eds.: 67–79. Excerpta Medica. Amsterdam, The Netherlands.

56. BREITHARDT, G., J. SCHWARZMAIER, M. BORGGREFE, K. HAERTEN & L. SEIPEL. 1983. Prognostic significance of ventricular late potentials after acute myocardial infarction. Eur. Heart J. **4:** 487–495.

57. BREITHARDT, G., M. BORGGREFE & K. HAERTEN. 1985. Role of programmed ventricular stimulation and noninvasive recording of ventricular late potentials for the identification of patients at risk of ventricular tachyarrhythmias after acute myocardial infarction. *In* Cardiac Electrophysiology and Arrhythmias. D. P. Zipes & J. Jaliffe, Eds.: 553–561. Grune and Stratton. New York, N.Y.

58. DENNISS, A. R., D. V. CODY, S. M. FENTON, D. A. RICHARDS, D. L. ROSS, P. A. RUSSELL, A. A. YOUNG & J. B. UTHER. 1983. Significance of delayed activation potentials in survivors of myocardial infarction. (abstr.) J. Am. Coll. Cardiol. **1:** 582.

59. DENNISS, A. R., D. A. RICHARDS, D. V. CODY, P. A. RUSSELL, A. A. YOUNG, M. J. COOPER, D. J. ROSS & J. B. UTHER. 1986. Prognostic significance of ventricular tachycardia and fibrillation induced at programmed stimulation and delayed potentials detected on the signal-averaged electrocardiogram of survivors of acute myocardial infarction. Circulation **74:** 731–745.

60. KACET, S., C. LIBERSA, J. CARON, B. BONDOUX D'HAUTE-FENILLE, X. MARCHAND, J. DAGANO & J. LEKIEFFRE. The prognostic value of averaged late potentials in patients suffering from coronary artery disease. (Personal communication.)

61. KUCHAR, D., C. THORBURN, & N. SAMMEL. 1985. Natural history and clinical significance of late potentials after myocardial infarction. Circulation **72:** III-477.

62. HÖPP, H. W., V. HOMBACH, A. OSTERSPEY, H. DEUTSCH, U. WINTER, D. W. BEHRENBECK,

M. TAUCHERT & H. H. HILGER. 1985. Clinical and prognostic significance of ventricular arrhythmias and ventricular late potentials in patients with coronary heart disease. *In* Holter Monitoring Technique. Technical Aspects and Clinical Applications. V. Hombach & H. H. Hilger, Eds.: 297–307. Schattauer. Stuttgart & New York.

63. VON LEITNER, E. R., M. OEFF, D. LOOCK, B. JAHNS & R. SCHRÖDER. 1983. Value of non invasively detected delayed ventricular depolarizations to predict prognosis in post myocardial infarction patients. Circulation 68: III-83.

64. BREITHARDT, G., M. BORGGREFE, B. QUANTIUS, U. KARBENN & L. SEIPEL. 1983. Ventricular vulnerability assessed by programmed ventricular stimulation in patients with and without late potentials. Circulation 68: 275–281.

65. JAUERNIG, R. A., J. SENGES, W. LANGFELDER, J. RIZOS, E. HOFFMANN, J. BRACHMANN & W. KÜBLER. 1983. Effect of antiarrhythmic drugs on ventricular late potentials at sinus rhythm and at constant heart rate. *In* Cardiac Pacing. D. Steinbach, D. Glogar, A. Laszkovics, W. Scheibelhofer & W. Weber, Eds.: 767–772. Steinkopff Verlag. Darmstadt, FRG.

66. OEFF, M., E. R. VON LEITNER, R. STHAPIT, G. BREITHARDT, M. BORGGREFE, U. KARBENN, T. MEINERTZ, R. ZOTZ & W. CLAS. 1983. Methods for non-invasive detection of ventricular late potentials—a comparative multicenter study. *In* Cardiac Pacing. K. Steinbach, D. Glogar, A. Laszkovics, W. Scheibelhofer & W. Weber, Eds.: 641–647. Steinkopff Verlag. Darmstadt, FRG.

67. DAVIES, M. J., F. R. C. PATH, A. C. THOMAS, M. R. C. PATH, P. A. KNAPMAN & J. R. HANGARTNER. 1986. Intramyocardial platelet aggregation in patients with instable angina pectoris suffering sudden ischemic cardiac death. Circulation 73: 418–427.

68. PATTERSON, E., K. HOLLAND, B. T. ELLER & B. R. LUCCHESI. 1982. Ventricular fibrillation resulting from ischemia at a site remote from previous myocardial infarction. A conscious canine model of sudden coronary death. Am. J. Cardiol. 50: 1414.

69. MALLIANI, A., P. J. SCHWARTZ & A. ZANCHETTI. 1980. Neural mechanisms in life-threatening arrhythmias. Am. Heart J. 100: 705–715.

70. TAVAZZI, L., A. M. ZOTTI & R. RONDANELLI. 1986. The role of psychologic stress in the genesis of lethal arrhythmias in patients with coronary artery disease. Eur. Heart J. 7(suppl. A): 99–106.

Spectral Estimation of the Electrocardiogram

EDWARD J. BERBARI,[a] DAVID E. ALBERT,[a]
AND PAUL LANDER[b]

University of Oklahoma Health Sciences Center
Department of Medicine
Division of Cardiology
and
Veterans Administration Medical Center
921 Northeast 13th Street
Oklahoma City, Oklahoma 73104

[b]Corazonix Corporation
4515 North Santa Fe
Oklahoma City, Oklahoma 73118

INTRODUCTION

Langner introduced the idea of a high fidelity electrocardiogram (ECG) using an oscilloscope display and a film recorder.[1] Subsequently, he examined this high resolution ECG in the context of myocardial infarction[2,3] and coronary artery disease[4] and concluded that slurs and notches within the QRS complex were strongly correlated with the presence of disease. This association was strengthened by Flowers *et al.* with correlation between QRS notching and anatomic identification of infarct scars.[5-7] Initial approaches for quantifying the spectrum of these notches and slurs in the QRS complex were done with narrow band analog filters in an attempt to characterize the frequency bands of normal and notched QRS complexes.[8,9] Subsequently, the use of digital computers gave rise to the discrete Fourier transform (DFT) method of spectral estimation.[10] These methods, for the most part, were applied to the QRS complex for analysis.

Two trends in cardiac electrophysiology gave rise to a reexamination of spectral estimation of the ECG. The first was the maturing of invasive cardiac electrophysiology and the study of arrhythmogenesis. Directly recorded cardiac electrograms identified arrhythmia substrates where slow conduction and nonuniform propagation occur. The second trend was the development of high resolution ECGs (HRECG) using computer implemented signal averaging to improve the signal-to-noise ratio of the ECG and allow the identification of very low level signals. The most common application of this methodology is the identification of signals after the QRS complex.[11-13] These "late potentials" have been extensively studied in various clinical populations and are assumed to originate from damaged or diseased regions of the ventricles such as the surviving border zones of myocardial infarction scars. Thus the notches and slurs identified in the earliest studies may likely originate in these regions and late potentials are those that occur latest in the cardiac cycle.

Goldberger *et al.* applied Fourier analysis to signal averaged ECGs but did not consider late potentials.[14,15] High pass filtering has been considered a necessary tool for

---

[a]Address correspondence to the VA medical center.

identifying late potentials in the signal averaged ECG.[11-13] However, these filters not only remove the low frequencies in the ST segment but can considerably alter the late potential signals as well. Cain *et al.* were the first to examine the region of late potential activation, i.e., the terminal QRS and ST segment, using the fast Fourier transform (FFT).[16] Frequency domain analysis has the advantage of not requiring high pass filters. A number of investigators[17-19] challenged this approach primarily from a technical point of view, demonstrating the overextension of the FFT method and its poor frequency resolution. However, there is still a strong rationale that regions of poor conduction would give rise to a higher frequency spectrum.

Spectral temporal mapping (STM) is a solution proposed to better estimate the spectral content of the ECG especially with regard to the fact that the ECG has a time varying spectrum.[20-22] Time becomes an added dimension in the display of the STM but, because of its use of the FFT, it still has many of the same limitations. This method is just now being applied to the ECG, and some examples are shown. The STM may improve on current methods for analyzing the HRECG and may open new avenues of investigation such as identifying late potentials in the presence of bundle branch block.[23]

THEORY

Biophysical Basis of High Frequencies in the ECG

This discussion will focus on ventricular activation and the frequency content of the QRS complex. The activation sequence of normal ventricles has been well studied and is characterized by uniform activation wavefronts which progress with relatively constant speed. Changes in the direction of wavefront propagation and the amount of tissue being activated give rise to the narrow and smooth appearance of the QRS complex. Some aspects of this appearance may be directly related to the bandwidth of the recording instruments as pointed out in the early studies cited previously.[1-4]

Myocardial infarction gives rise to well-known patterns in the ECG associated with the site of the infarct. (For this discussion we will ignore the QRS changes due to conduction system disorders.) Changes in the QRS are due to abrupt blockage in the activation sequence around the infarcted tissue. This gives rise to higher frequency QRS patterns. These are large changes in the QRS and are probably not the cause of slurs and notches observed in a high fidelity ECG. However, the presence of ischemic regions or infarct border zones gives rise to smaller regions of ventricular tissue with heterogeneous conduction properties. Such regions have been probed with both endocardial electrodes in man[24] and in many ventricular sites in animal infarction models.[25,26] The "fractionated" electrogram is an example of the complexity of the extracellular potentials generated by such heterogeneous regions. Two reasons why such regions develop multiphasic extracellular potentials are changes in conduction velocity and changes in the direction of activation. For example, a model study by Lesh *et al.* demonstrated that in a region of tissue with a zone of decreased conduction velocity it is possible to record a fractionated electrogram from a unipolar electrode.[27] Furthermore, activation under the electrode site did not necessarily correspond to the largest or most rapid deflection.

Changes in the direction of conduction can occur when a wavefront encounters a nonconducting region. We initially observed this in a model of the His-Purkinje system.[28] Simulating left anterior hemiblock as a nonconducting region of the fanlike left bundle produced body surface waveforms with very high frequency components compared to normal conduction. In fact, when such rapid changes in the net direction of activation occur the body surface manifestation may actually appear to be artifactual.

The rate at which conduction velocity changes or the direction of activation changes is directly linked to the high frequencies observed in extracellular or body surface recordings. Abrupt changes occurred in those models just described and hence produced very observable and quantifiable high frequency enrichment in the simulated signals.

High frequency components will also appear in the spectrum in proportion to the width of the QRS. An abnormal QRS complex is the product of some uniform activation and some nonuniform activation, i.e., slow and disordered conduction due to abrupt changes in the magnitude and direction of the activation wavefront in ischemic regions. High frequency components are also present with abnormal conduction due to these effects. The abnormal QRS complex is typically longer than the normal. This factor lowers high frequency content in proportion to the QRS width. Conduction disorders occur on macroscopic and microscopic scales. Examples of large scale conduction disorders are bundle branch block and big infarctions which produce major changes in the ECG waveform. Conduction disorders that may form a reentry substrate in ischemic zones are responsible for late potentials in the HRECG. This is a microscopic phenomenon since it usually involves small amounts of myocardium. Microscopic phenomena are not normally seen in the normal ECG. In this simple approach to determining the origins of high frequency content of the HRECG there are three contributing factors: (1) width of the QRS complex, (2) macroscopic patterns of ventricular activation, and (3) microscopic patterns of ventricular activation. The first two factors are almost certain to predominate in the HRECG spectrum due to the relatively small contribution of ischemic border zone activity. Late potentials are those microscopic potentials that occur at the end of and after the QRS complex. Earlier studies of the slurred and notched QRS may have examined the same phenomena, but due to the activation sequence the abnormal potentials occurred within the QRS.

Fourier Analysis

Mathematically, Fourier analysis derives the sinusoidal components that comprise a complex *periodic* waveform. (The best way to define these relationships is with the actual mathematical expressions, but for purposes of this discussion we will remain descriptive with the ECG as our focus. There are a number of texts on Fourier analysis and a good introductory text by Ramirez[27] is recommended. A more complete review of the application Fourier analysis to the ECG is in a paper by Lander *et al.*[22]) This Fourier series has sine and cosine waveforms which are mathematically defined from minus infinity to plus infinity. In practice we often do not have periodic waves nor do we analyze them for all time. Typically we analyze a pulse type waveform over a short window of time using the Fourier transform which is distinguished from the Fourier series. Digital methods only have samples of the original time domain signal, and this poses certain restrictions on the Fourier transform. The sampling theorem states that the rate of sampling, f_s, must be *at least* twice the highest frequency of interest, f_{max}. The maximum frequency in the transform is $f_s/2$. The time window of interest over which the waveform is transformed defines the resolution of the transform: $f_r = 1/T$ where f_r is the transform frequency resolution in Hertz and T is the duration, in seconds, of the transform window. Thus if a transform window is 0.5 second, f_r is 2 Hz. This ideal relationship is never achieved in practice because the time signal must be truncated using a window function. It is the duration of the signal itself that will define the frequency resolution and not an artificially widened window. The fast Fourier

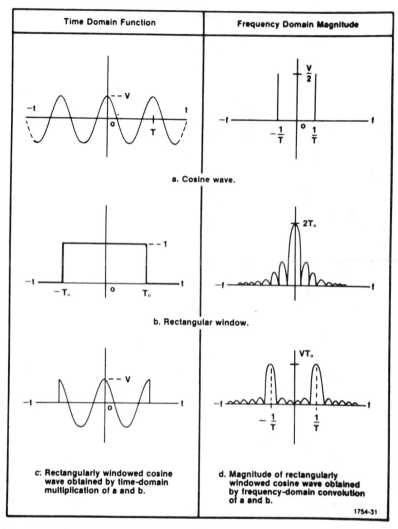

FIGURE 1. These are Fourier transform pairs of the time domain signals on the left and the frequency domain on the right. (Reprinted from Reference 29, with permission.)

transform (FFT) is a computationally efficient algorithm which requires that 2^n number of points, e.g., 32, 64, 128, etc., be transformed. Often the data to be transformed to meet this requirement and the data window can be artificially lengthened by adding zeros to the beginning or end of the data sequence. This is known as zero padding.

If a cosine wave of a fixed frequency with period T is Fourier transformed, the ideal magnitude transform will have a single value at $1/T$ and $-1/T$. FIGURE 1a shows this transform. Note that the sine wave extends to $\pm$ infinity. Before considering the case of the windowed cosine the spectral components of the rectangular pulse must be examined. The rectangular pulse and its magnitude transform are shown in FIGURE 1b. A short duration signal, such as the 2 cycles of the cosine function shown in FIGURE 1c, is obtained by multiplying the signal of interest by the rectangular pulse. Such a multiplication in the time domain is equivalent to convolving the two spectra in the frequency domain. Without regard to the mathematical formulation of convolution, the result is seen in FIGURE 1d. The frequency of the cosine wave can still be identified by the peaks of the two lobes at the frequency of $\pm 1/T$. However, the widening of the spectral distribution and the many side lobes have now introduced uncertainty and the Fourier analysis now provides an estimate of the spectrum. This spectral leakage is due to the windowing of data in the time domain. The sharp edges of the rectangular window account for the higher frequency side lobes. The time domain signal can be multiplied by other window functions with smoother edges to reduce this high frequency enrichment but usually at the cost of widening the main spectral lobe and further distortion of the signal spectrum.[30] For complex waveforms such as an ECG which has an unknown and changing spectrum it is impossible to specifically identify the signal spectrum compared to the spectrum of the window. Add this problem to the lack of frequency resolution in the transformed data and the results can often be confusing. It is probably impossible to distinguish between the high frequency spectral enrichment due to window function and those due to ventricular late potentials.

One solution to the problem of estimating the spectrum in a signal with a time varying spectrum is the spectrotemporal map (STM). These methods are used in many digital signal processing fields and a review by Cohen was recently published.[31] The STM uses a narrow window of data which is Fourier transformed. The transform window is then moved across the data window in an overlapping fashion. The central point in the Fourier transform window corresponds to a specific time in the signal. The result is a three-dimensional representation with each moment in time corresponding to a complete Fourier transform. This method is computationally expensive and the results still rely on the Fourier transform with the same limitations as outlined above. However, the addition of the time axis provides a visualization of the signal energy which may aid in identifying low level signals such as the ventricular late potentials.

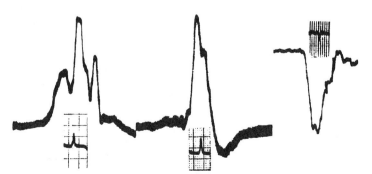

FIGURE 2. High fidelity QRS complexes from Langner. Next to each trace is a standard ECG recording. Of interest is the first trace where Langner comments on the post QRS notches. (Reprinted from Reference 4.)

Examples

FIGURE 2 is a figure from Langner demonstrating notching in three different QRS complexes.[4] Of some interest is his observation concerning the post-QRS notches seen in the first trace. He originally said it should be studied further, but there is no further evidence of this, and it is perhaps the first notion of ventricular late potentials in the literature.

FIGURE 3 shows a signal averaged ECG in the lower panel and three intervals are defined, T_1, T_2, and T_3. This ECG has late potentials that follow the QRS and are evident without the need of high pass filtering. The two panels above are examples of a rectangular window and a Blackman-Harris window. The mean value of the ECG data should be subtracted before windowing. This may leave a small residual dc component after windowing, but the ECG data are properly tapered to zero at the beginning and end of the window. However, if the windowed ECG data have a nonzero mean then subtracting this mean will create an abrupt transition between the first and last data points and the augmenting zeros. This is equivalent to superimposing upon the ECG data a rectangular pulse of the same length as the window, with a height equal to the subtracted mean value. The resulting spectrum will be the sum of the spectra due to the ECG data and the newly created pulse waveform.

FIGURE 4 illustrates the effects of dc removal, zero padding, and interval selection

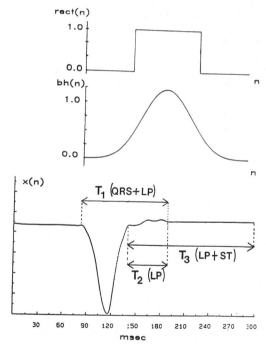

FIGURE 3. The lower trace is a signal averaged lead with evident late potentials following the QRS complex. Three intervals T_1, T_2, and T_3 are defined as the QRS plus late potentials, the late potentials only, and the late potentials plus the ST segment, respectively. Above the ECG is a rectangular and a Blackman-Harris window function.

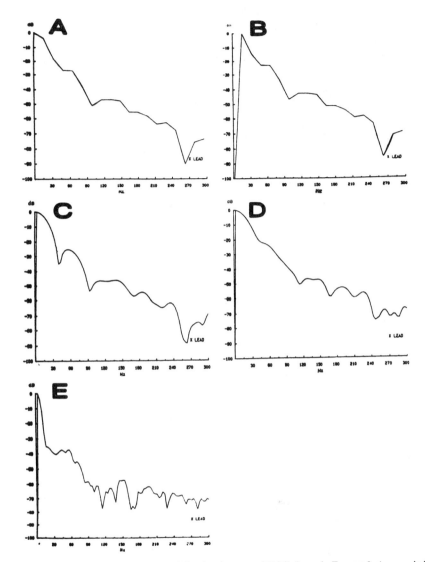

FIGURE 4. Power spectral estimates of the signal averaged ECG shown in FIGURE 3. A = period T_2, B = T_2 after DC removal, C = DC removal and zero padding, D = T_2 shifted back 6 mseconds, E = T_3.

on the power density spectrum of the signal averaged ECG of FIGURE 3. Panel A shows the power density spectrum (PDS), computed over interval T_2 (=60 mseconds), without dc removal or zero padding. Panel B shows the same spectrum with the dc component removed. Note that a fundamental harmonic component is always present. This is equal to the reciprocal of the observation interval, in this case, 1/60 mseconds = 16.7 Hz. This component must be taken into account when the spectrum is analyzed. Panel C shows the effect of zero padding. The fundamental harmonic occurs at a lower frequency and the spectrum has a smooth appearance. However, zero padding does not improve the resolution of the signal spectrum. Panel D shows the spectrum resulting from shifting the period T_2 6 mseconds back into the QRS complex. The shape of the spectrum is radically altered because of the prominence of QRS spectral characteristics. Panel E shows the spectrum resulting from the selection of interval T_3, i.e., the late potential spectral components are not improved at all by this extension of the observation interval. In addition the late potential spectrum is obscured due to the superposition of the spectral components of the ST segment.

Some of the limitations of the FFT can be overcome by using the spectrotemporal map. FIGURE 5 demonstrates the advantage of the STM over standard FFT ap-

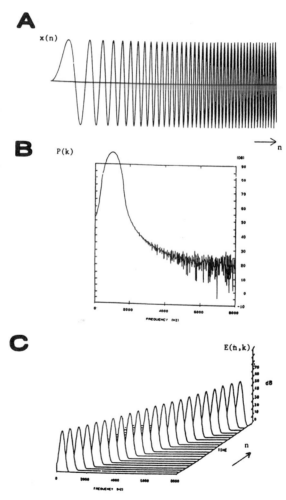

FIGURE 5. Panel A is a swept sine wave from DC to 8 KHz. Panel B is the power spectrum using a rectangular window and the FFT. Panel C is the spectrotemporal map of panel A.

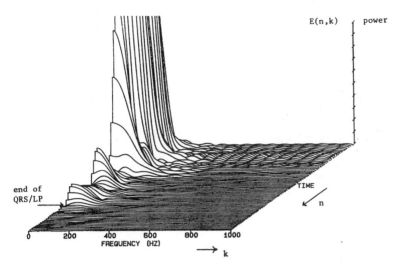

FIGURE 6. The STM of the ECG shown in FIGURE 3.

proaches. Panel A is a swept sine wave where the frequency of the sine wave increases linearly along the time axis. Panel B shows the power spectrum of the swept sine wave obtained with the FFT across the entire waveform. This spectrum gives no indication that the input was a swept sine wave. An STM is obtained by transforming a small window of data and shifting that small window across the entire data window.[21,22] FIGURE 5C shows the sequentially plotted spectra with spectral peaks demonstrating the linearly increasing frequency of the swept sine wave and the uniform distribution of signal power.

FIGURE 6 is an STM obtained from the signal averaged ECG in FIGURE 3. The large QRS energy is seen as the large waveforms that are clipped at the top of the figure. After the QRS ends there are spectral mounds which appear as "foothills" and represent the late potential signals. At present there are no quantitative measures of the STM that have been tested in a clinical population.

Currently, there are no time domain methods accepted for analyzing late potentials in the presence of bundle branch block. It is currently not possible to distinguish between low level signals from diseased regions that are activated late and low level signals from normal tissue that are activated late due to a conduction system disorder such as bundle branch block. The rationale for applying the STM to this problem is that normal tissue while activated late will still have uniform conduction wavefronts. Diseased regions will generate higher frequency signals for reasons discussed above. This hypothesis was tested in an animal model of late potentials and bundle branch block. Of interest in this discussion is the STM result and not the experimental details.

FIGURE 7 has data from two dogs. All panels were obtained with pacing induced left bundle branch block. Panels A and C are from one dog before and after coronary artery occlusion, respectively. Panels B and D are from another dog, also before and after coronary artery occlusion. The dog depicted in panels A and C did not have late potentials during sinus rhythm before or after coronary occlusion. The dog depicted in panels B and D had late potentials during sinus rhythm as a result of coronary occlusion. Each panel has a circle drawn on the STM in the same region. Only in panel

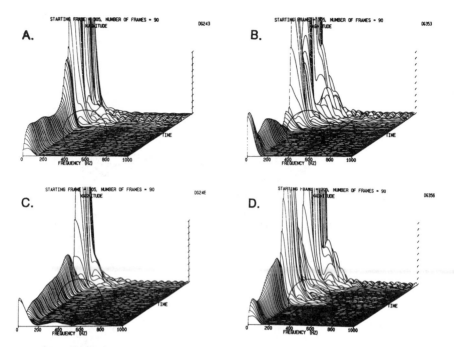

FIGURE 7. The STM from two dogs during pacing induced left bundle branch block. Panels A and C are from the same dog before and after coronary artery occlusion. No time domain late potentials were observed in this dog during normal sinus rhythm. Panels B and D are from the second dog that demonstrated late potentials (during normal sinus rhythm) before and after coronary occlusion, respectively. A circle is drawn on the STM to highlight the region of possible late potentials. Only Panel D has the late, higher frequency foothills associated with late potentials.

D, where late potentials are present during bundle branch block, is there evidence of higher frequency foothills. Further studies are needed to establish the value of STM in detecting late potentials during bundle branch block.

CONCLUSIONS

Frequency analysis of the ECG has many limitations. There is a strong rationale for spectral analysis based on biophysical principles. However, the ECG falls into a class of signals with a time varying spectrum. Traditional approaches are not adequate for identifying the spectrum and at best provides only estimates of the spectrum. Such estimates are not amenable to narrow band analysis as has been applied in earlier work.

The spectrotemporal map is an improvement over the fixed window Fourier transform. It retains the time domain information, but suffers many of the same frequency resolution problems because of its reliance on the Fourier transform. This method has yet to be tested on a large scale, and problems with quantification have yet to be overcome. Beyond the STM are other methods for spectral estimation that also await investigation.

REFERENCES

1. LANGNER, P. H. 1952. The value of high fidelity electrocardiography using the cathode ray oscillograph and an expanded time scale. Circulation **5:** 249.
2. LANGNER, P. H. & D. B. GESELOWITZ. 1960. Characteristics of the frequency spectrum in the normal electrocardiogram and in subjects following myocardial infarction. Circ. Res. **8:** 577.
3. LANGNER, P. H., D. B. GESELOWITZ & F. T. MANSURE. 1961. High-frequency components in the electrocardiograms of normal subjects and of patients with coronary heart disease. Am. Heart J. **62:** 746.
4. LANGNER, P. H. 1963. The value of high frequency electrocardiography. *In* Life Insurance Medicine, Professional Aspects. Board of Life Insurance Medicine. Philadelphia, Pa.
5. FLOWERS, N. C., L. G. HORAN, J. R. THOMAS & W. J. TOLLESON. 1969. The anatomic basis for high frequency components in the electrocardiogram. Circulation **39:** 531.
6. FLOWERS, N. C., L. G. HORAN, W. J. TOLLESON & J. R. THOMAS. 1969. Localization of the site of myocardial scarring in man by high-frequency components. Circulation **40:** 927.
7. FLOWERS, N. C. & L. G. HORAN. 1971. Diagnostic import of QRS notching in high frequency electrocardiogram of living subjects with heart disease. Circulation **44:** 605.
8. FRANKE, E. K., J. R. BRAUNSTEIN & D. C. ZELLNER. 1962. Study of high-frequency components in electrocardiogram by power spectrum analysis. Circ. Res. **10:** 870.
9. REYNOLDS, E. W., B. F. MULLER, M. C. CAPTAIN, G. J. ANDERSON & B. T. MULLER. 1967. High-frequency components in the electrocardiogram. A comparative study of normals and patients with myocardial disease. Circulation **35:** 195.
10. RIGGS, T., B. ISENSTEIN & C. THOMAS. 1979. Spectral analysis of the normal electrocardiogram in children and adults. J. Electrocardiol. **12:** 377.
11. BERBARI, E. J., B. J. SCHERLAG, R. R. HOPE & R. LAZZARA. 1978. Recording from the body surface of arrhythmogenic ventricular activity during the ST segment. Am. J. Cardiol. **41:** 697.
12. SIMSON, M. B. 1981. Use of signals in the terminal QRS complex to identify patients with ventricular tachycardia after myocardial infarction. Circulation **70:** 632–637.
13. BREITHARDT, G., J. SCHWARZMAIER, M. BOGGREFE, K. HAERTEN & L. SEIPEL. 1983. Prognostic significance of late ventricular potentials after acute myocardial infarction. Eur. Heart J. **4:** 487–495.
14. GOLDBERGER, A. L., V. BHARGAVA, V. FROELICHER, J. COVELL & D. MORTARA. 1980. Diminished peak-to-peak amplitude of the high frequency QRS in myocardial infarction. J. Electrocardiol. **13:** 367.
15. GOLDBERGER, A. L., V. BHARGAVA, V. FROELICHER & J. COVELL. 1981. Effect of myocardial infarction on high-frequency QRS potential. Circulation **64**(1): 34.
16. CAIN, M. E., H. D. AMBOS, F. X. WITKOWSKI & B. E. SOBEL. 1984. Fast-Fourier transform analysis of signal-averaged electrocardiograms for identification of patients prone to sustained ventricular tachycardia. Circulation **69:** 711.
17. KELEN, G. J., R. HENKIN, J. M. FONTAINE & N. EL-SHERIF. 1987. Effects of analyzed signal duration and phase on the results of fast Fourier transform analysis of the surface electrocardiogram in subjects with and without late potentials. Am. J. Cardiol. **60:** 1281–1289.
18. WORLEY, S. J., D. B. MARK, W. M. SMITH, P. WOLF, R. M. CALIFF, H. C. STRAUSS, M. G. MANWARING & R. E. IDEKER. 1988. Comparison of time domain and frequency domain variables from the signal-averaged electrocardiogram: a multivariable analysis. J. Am. Coll. Cardiol. **11:** 1041–1051.
19. HABERL, R., G. JILGE, R. PULTER & G. STEINBECK. 1988. Comparison of frequency and time domain analysis of the signal averaged electrocardiogram in patients with ventricular tachycardia and coronary artery disease: methodologic validation and clinical relevance. J. Am. Coll. Cardiol. **12:** 150–158.
20. LANDER, P., D. E. ALBERT & E. J. BERBARI. 1988. Spectro-temporal mapping: the next generation in late potential analysis. J. Am. Coll. Cardiol. **11:** 199A.
21. LANDER, P., D. E. ALBERT & E. J. BERBARI. 1990. Spectro-temporal analysis of ventricular late potentials. J. Electrocardiol. **23.** (In press.)

22. LANDER, P., D. ALBERT & E. J. BERBARI. Principles of frequency domain analysis. *In* High Resolution Electrocardiography. N. El-Sherif & V. Hombach, Eds. Futura Publishing Company. Mt. Kisco, N.Y. (In press.)

23. BERBARI, E. J., J. DYER, B. J. SCHERLAG & R. LAZZARA. 1989. Detecting late potentials in the presence of bundle branch block. PACE **12:** 638.

24. JOSEPHSON, M. E., L. N. HOROWITZ & A. FARSHIDI. 1978. Continuous local electrical activity: a mechanism of recurrent ventricular tachycardia. Circulation **57:** 658.

25. SCHERLAG, B. J., N. EL-SHERIF, R. R. HOPE & R. LAZZARA. 1974. Characterization and localization of ventricular arrhythmias due to myocardial ischemia and infarction. Circ. Res. **35:** 372–383.

26. EL-SHERIF, N., B. J. SCHERLAG, R. LAZZARA & R. R. HOPE. 1977. Reentrant ventricular arrhythmias in the late myocardial infarction period. I. Conduction characteristics in the infarction zone. Circulation **55:** 686–702.

27. LESH, M. D., J. F. SPEAR & M. B. SIMSON. 1988. A computer model of the electrocardiogram: What causes fractionation? J. Electrocardiol. (Suppl.): S69–S73.

28. BERBARI, E. J., S. M. COLLINS, Y. SALU & R. ARZBAECHER. 1983. Orthogonal surface lead recordings of His-Purkinje activity: comparison of actual and simulated waveforms. IEEE Trans. Biomed. Eng. **BME30**(3): 160.

29. RAMIREZ, R. W. 1985. the FFT Fundamentals and Concepts. Prentice-Hall. Englewood Cliffs, N.J.

30. HARRIS, F. J. 1978. On the use of windows for harmonic analysis with the discrete Fourier transform. Proc. IEEE **66:** 51–83.

31. COHEN, L. 1989. Time-frequency distributions. A Review. Proc. IEEE **77**(7): 941.

Autonomic Interactions in Cardiac Control[a]

MATTHEW N. LEVY

Department of Investigative Medicine
The Mt. Sinai Medical Center and
Case Western Reserve University
One Mt. Sinai Drive
Cleveland, Ohio 44106-4198

Most aspects of cardiac function are regulated by the autonomic nervous system. The effects of sympathetic activity are usually facilitatory, whereas the effects of tonic vagal activity are usually inhibitory. In healthy subjects at rest, both autonomic divisions are usually active. Under such conditions, the antagonistic effects of the two divisions on the heart summate nonlinearly. Such nonlinear summations, which are referred to as interactions, take place within the central nervous system and in the periphery. Only the peripheral interactions that influence the heart will be considered in this review.

EFFECTS ON HEART RATE

Rosenblueth and Simeone conducted the first quantitative studies of the cardiac autonomic interactions in 1934.[1] These investigators reported that a given level of vagal stimulation produced a greater reduction in heart rate in the presence than in the absence of tonic sympathetic stimulation. Other investigators have confirmed their results.[2,3] The augmented inhibitory response to vagal stimulation elicited by concomitant sympathetic activity has been termed *accentuated antagonism*.[4]

FIGURE 1 illustrates the accentuated antagonism that we observed when we stimulated the cardiac sympathetic and vagal nerves of anesthetized dogs at three combinations of frequencies.[2] The heart rate increased by 78 beats/minute when we stimulated the right stellate ganglion at 4 Hz (S = 4) in the absence of vagal stimulation (V = 0). Conversely, the heart rate decreased by 70 beats/minute when we stimulated the left vagus nerve at 8 Hz (V = 8) in the absence of sympathetic stimulation (S = 0). When we stimulated the sympathetic and vagal nerves simultaneously (S = 4, V = 8), however, the responses did not summate algebraically. The vagal effect was so dominant that the response to combined stimulation did not differ appreciably from the response to vagal stimulation alone.

FIGURE 2 shows the responses of this same animal to nine combinations of sympathetic and vagal stimulation frequencies.[2] As we progressively increased the sympathetic frequency in the absence of vagal stimulation (V = 0), the heart rate rose substantially. However, when we stimulated the vagus nerve at a frequency of 8 Hz (V = 8), changing the frequency of sympathetic stimulation had only a negligible effect. Changes in the frequency of sympathetic stimulation had an intermediate effect when we stimulated the vagus nerve at a frequency of 4 Hz (V = 4). The degree to which the curves in FIGURE 2 deviate from being parallel reflects the extent of the

[a]Supported by U.S. Public Health Service grants HL 10951 and HL 15758.

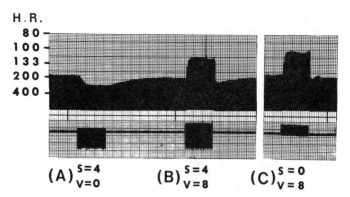

FIGURE 1. The changes in heart rate (H.R.) elicited by stimulating the right stellate ganglion (S) and left vagus nerve (V) simultaneously for 30 seconds at various frequency combinations (0, 4, and 8 Hz) in an anesthetized dog. (Modified from Reference 2.)

autonomic interaction. Interactions in the autonomic control of heart rate also prevail in animals with experimentally induced atrioventricular junctional rhythms,[5] but they are less pronounced.

EFFECTS ON ATRIOVENTRICULAR CONDUCTION

In contrast to the pronounced interactions that we observed in our studies of the regulation of heart rate (FIGURES 1 and 2), the autonomic interactions that prevailed in our studies of the control of AV conduction were negligible.[2,6] When we increased the frequency of vagal stimulation from 0 to 10 Hz (FIGURE 3), the AV conduction time significantly increased.[2] Also, as we increased the frequency of sympathetic stimulation from 0 to 6 Hz, the AV conduction time significantly diminished. The effect of any change in the sympathetic stimulation frequency was not influenced appreciably by the level of vagal activity. The apparently parallel courses of the three curves in FIGURE 3 reflect this negligible interaction.

Takahashi and Zipes[7] and Urthaler et al.,[8] however, did detect significant interactions in their experiments on the autonomic control of AV conduction. Their methods for detecting interactions may have been more sensitive than our techniques.[2,6] Nevertheless, because the interactions we observed in the control of heart rate were so pronounced (FIGURES 1 and 2) but were so inconspicuous in the control of AV conduction (FIGURE 3), we may conclude that such autonomic interactions are probably much more important in the regulation of cardiac automaticity than of AV conduction.

EFFECTS OF VENTRICULAR CONTRACTILITY

Hollenberg et al. provided the first convincing demonstration of an adrenergic-cholinergic interaction in the control of ventricular contractility in 1965.[9] They observed that left ventricular contractile force diminished only slightly when acetylcholine (ACh) was infused directly into a coronary artery of an anesthetized dog. However, when the same dose of ACh was infused during concurrent sympathetic nerve stimulation or while norepinephrine (NE) was being administered, that infusion of ACh now diminished ventricular contractile force substantially.

My collaborators and I observed that trains of vagal stimuli had effects on ventricular contraction[10] (FIGURE 4) that were similar to those produced by the ACh infusions in the experiments of Hollenberg *et al.*[9] As we progressively increased the volume of fluid in a balloon in the left ventricle (panels A, B, and C) in a dog on total heart-lung bypass, vagal stimulation decreased peak left ventricular pressure by 21%, regardless of the magnitude of the peak ventricular pressure. We then restored the fluid volume in the left ventricular balloon (panel D) to the volume that prevailed in panel A. Next, we stimulated the left stellate ganglion at a frequency of 2 Hz between the times denoted by event marks 1 and 3. Concurrently, we stimulated the vagus nerve (event mark D) at the same frequency that had been used to evoke the responses shown in panels A to C. During the tonic sympathetic stimulation, vagal stimulation decreased the peak left ventricular pressure by 35% (panel D). Hence, the increased level of sympathetic activity augmented substantially the negative inotropic effect of the vagal stimulation. Qualitatively similar sympathetic-vagal interactions have also been demonstrated in the atrial myocardium.[11]

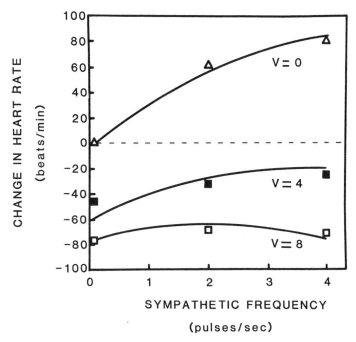

FIGURE 2. The changes in heart rate in an anesthetized dog, as a function of the frequency of right stellate ganglion stimulation. The responses to stellate stimulation were obtained during concomitant left vagal stimulation (V) at frequencies of 0, 4, and 8 Hz. The symbols represent the actual data; the curves were derived by regression analysis. (Modified from Reference 2.)

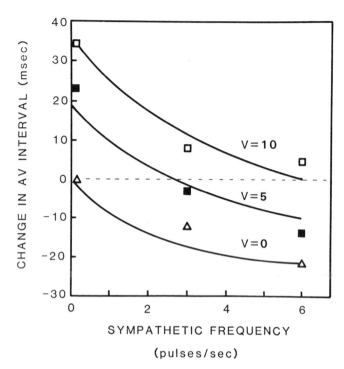

FIGURE 3. The changes in AV conduction time in an anesthetized dog, as a function of the frequency of right stellate ganglion stimulation. The responses to stellate stimulation were obtained during concomitant left vagal stimulation (V) at frequencies of 0, 5, and 10 Hz. The symbols represent the actual data; the curves were derived by regression analysis. (Modified from Reference 2.)

EFFECTS ON VENTRICULAR EXCITABILITY

Autonomic interactions are also involved in the control of ventricular excitability. Such interactions regulate the ventricular action potential duration, effective refractory period, fibrillation threshold, and repetitive extrasystole threshold.

Experiments on normally polarized Purkinje fibers disclosed that ACh by itself did not affect the action potential duration.[12] However, isoproterenol did decrease the action potential duration in these fibers, and ACh could partially reverse this action. Furthermore, when the resting transmembrane potential of other Purkinje fibers was diminished to about -50 mV by raising the external K^+ concentration, the excitability of the fibers was abolished.[12] Addition of isoproterenol restored excitability. This restoration of excitability could be abolished by a concentration of ACh that had no effect in the absence of isoproterenol.

In open chest, anesthetized dogs, the effective refractory period of the ventricular myocardium was slightly prolonged by vagal stimulation and slightly shortened by increased sympathetic activity.[13] When the vagal and sympathetic nerves were stimulated simultaneously, however, the effects did not summate algebraically; the vagal effects were mediated in part by antagonizing the prevailing sympathetic influences.

Similar interactions obtain in the regulation of ventricular excitability. In anesthetized dogs, "strength-interval curves" were derived by measuring the electrical stimulus strength that was just necessary to elicit a ventricular response at various times in early diastole.[14] Vagal stimulation caused the curves to be shifted in the direction that denoted a diminished ventricular excitability. Conversely, sympathetic stimulation caused the curves to be shifted in the opposite direction. After β-receptor blockade, however, vagal stimulation had no effect.[14] Therefore, the vagal effect appeared to be mediated principally by antagonizing the influence of the prevailing spontaneous level of sympathetic activity.

Sympathetic neural activity increases the ventricular vulnerability to fibrillation, and this effect can be neutralized by an increase in vagal activity.[15-18] In anesthetized dogs, stellate ganglion stimulation decreased the ventricular fibrillation threshold by about 60%, and norepinephrine (NE) infusions lowered the threshold by about 40%.[15] These effects of neurally released or of exogenous NE could be abolished by concurrent vagal stimulation, whereas vagal stimulation alone had no effect. A study from our laboratory showed that vagal stimulation and sympathetic stimulation, alone or combined, have effects on the repetitive extrasystole threshold[19] (FIGURE 5) that are analogous to those just described[15] for the fibrillation threshold.

Studies of chronically instrumented, unanesthetized dogs have revealed that those animals with relatively weak vagal baroreceptor reflexes are more susceptible to ventricular fibrillation when they are subjected to a regimen of exercise and acute coronary occlusion than are animals with stronger vagal reflexes.[18] Furthermore, if the more susceptible animals are subjected to an exercise program that strengthens their vagal baroreceptor reflexes, they then become much more resistant to ventricular fibrillation.

In anesthetized cats subjected to coronary artery occlusion and reperfusion, tonic vagal stimulation reduced substantially the incidence of ventricular fibrillation and ventricular tachycardia.[17] If the heart rate was held constant by ventricular pacing, vagal stimulation still decreased the incidence of ventricular fibrillation, but the effect was much less pronounced and not significant statistically. Vagal stimulation was substantially more effective in preventing ventricular tachycardia after reperfusion, and the effect prevailed regardless of whether heart rate was held constant or not.[17] The sympathetic nervous system plays an important role in the pathogenesis of reperfusion arrhythmias,[16] and the protective effects of vagal stimulation may be mediated by antagonizing these adrenergic influences.

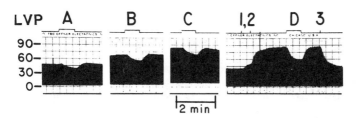

FIGURE 4. The effects of supramaximal vagal stimulation on left ventricular pressure (LVP, in mm Hg) in a canine isovolumic left ventricle preparation. During event marks A, B, C, and D, the right vagus nerve was stimulated at 20 Hz. After panels A and B, additional fluid was added to a balloon in the left ventricle in order to increase the diastolic pressure in the left ventricle. Between panels C and D, the balloon volume was restored to the level that obtained during panel A. Between event marks 2 and 3 in panel D, the left stellate ganglion was stimulated supramaximally at 2 Hz. (From Reference 10, with permission from the American Heart Association, Inc.)

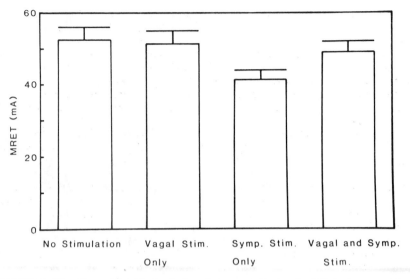

FIGURE 5. The effects of vagal stimulation alone, sympathetic stimulation alone, combined vagal and sympathetic stimulation, and the absence of neural stimulation on the multiple repetitive extrasystole threshold (MRET), in milliamperes, in a group of 12 anesthetized dogs. The bars represent mean ± standard error of the mean (SEM). (From Reference 19.)

INTERACTION MECHANISMS

The sympathetic and parasympathetic systems interact at prejunctional and postjunctional levels (FIGURE 6) of the autonomic neuroeffector junctions in the heart.[4,20–23] One prejunctional mechanism involves an inhibition of NE release from postganglionic sympathetic nerve terminals by the ACh released from nearby vagal fibers.[24–26] A second prejunctional mechanism involves the inhibition of ACh release from vagal endings by the NE[27] and neuropeptide Y[28] released from neighboring sympathetic terminals. The postjunctional interactions occur at the level of the cardiac effector cell membranes, and involve the adenylate cyclase system.[21,22]

Prejunctional Mechanisms

Postganglionic vagal and sympathetic fibers are often contiguous in the walls of the heart, and they may even be surrounded by a common Schwann sheath. Thus, transmitters released from nerve fibers of one autonomic division may be present in effective concentrations near the endings of the nerve fibers of the other autonomic division. In isolated atrial preparations, stimulation of vagal fibers diminishes the amount of NE that is released by concurrent sympathetic stimulation.[24] This inhibition of NE release appears to be mediated by muscarinic receptors that are located on the cell membranes of the postganglionic sympathetic nerve endings.[25]

Studies from our laboratory have revealed that such sympathetic-vagal interactions are not restricted to the atria; they also take place in the ventricles.[26] We measured the NE overflow into the coronary sinus blood of anesthetized dogs under control conditions, during cardiac sympathetic stimulation alone, and during combined sympathetic and vagal stimulation (FIGURE 7). During sympathetic stimulation alone, the NE overflows were 22 and 48 ng/minute during stimulation at 2 and 4 Hz, respectively. The NE overflows were diminished by 33% when the sympathetic and vagal nerves were stimulated concurrently. These vagally induced changes in NE overflow took place mainly in ventricular tissue, because more than 95% of the blood that drains into the coronary sinus has perfused ventricular tissue, and less than 5% has perfused atrial tissue.

Experiments on isolated atria have shown that the catecholamines, NE and epinephrine, inhibit the release of ACh from intramural vagal nerve endings.[27] This

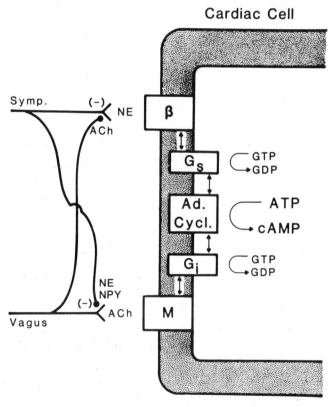

FIGURE 6. Mechanisms responsible for cardiac sympathetic-parasympathetic interactions. Prejunctionally, vagal activity inhibits ($-$) the release of norepinephrine (NE) from sympathetic nerve endings, whereas NE and neuropeptide Y (NPY) inhibit the release of acetylcholine (ACh) from vagal nerve endings. Postjunctionally, the norepinephrine released from sympathetic nerve endings occupies β-adrenergic receptors (β) on the cardiac cell surface. This process stimulates adenylate cyclase (Ad. Cycl.) to catalyze the formation of cyclic AMP (cAMP) from adenosine triphosphate (ATP). The β-adrenergic receptor (β) is coupled to adenylate cyclase through a stimulatory protein, G_s. Acetylcholine released from vagal endings occupies muscarinic receptors (M) on the cell surface. These receptors are coupled to adenylate cyclase through an inhibitory protein, G_i. (Modified from Reference 23.)

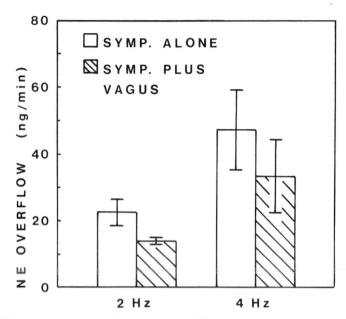

FIGURE 7. The mean overflows of norepinephrine (NE) into the coronary sinus blood (in excess of the control values) in a group of 7 anesthetized dogs during supramaximal sympathetic stimulation at 2 and 4 Hz and during combined stimulation of the sympathetic (2 and 4 Hz) and vagus (15 Hz) nerves. (Modified from Reference 26, with permission from the American Heart Association, Inc.)

constitutes a second type of prejunctional adrenergic-cholinergic interaction. The inhibition of ACh release appears to be mediated by α_1-adrenergic receptors on the vagal terminals. ACh release can be inhibited by various α_1-adrenergic agonists, such as methoxamine. However, it cannot be inhibited by α_2- or β-adrenergic agonists, such as clonidine or isoproterenol, respectively.[27]

A third type of prejunctional autonomic interaction involves the release of neuropeptide Y. This peptide, which is released along with NE from sympathetic nerve endings, attenuates the cardiac responses to vagal activity, probably by inhibiting the release of ACh.[28]

The effects of neurally released neuropeptide Y on the cardiac responses to vagal stimulation were first elucidated by Potter.[28] She observed that the chronotropic action of the vagus was inhibited after short periods of intense sympathetic stimulation (i.e., at frequencies greater than 16 Hz) for an average of 40 minutes in the anesthetized dog. The NE released during sympathetic stimulation was not responsible for the inhibition of the vagal actions on heart rate, because the inhibition remained after combined α- and β-adrenergic receptor blockade. Potter verified this by showing that exogenous NE did not inhibit the vagal responses as persistently as did sympathetic nerve stimulation. Exogenous neuropeptide Y mimicked the effects of intense sympathetic stimulation on the chronotropic responses to vagal stimulation. Exogenous neuropeptide Y did not, however, affect the negative chronotropic response to muscarinic agonists, such as methacholine. From these results Potter concluded that neuropeptide Y, released during intense sympathetic stimulation, inhibits the release of ACh from the vagal endings in the heart.[28]

Although NE and neuropeptide Y are released concomitantly upon direct sympathetic stimulation,[29] substantial evidence suggests that much higher stimulation frequencies are required to release detectable quantities of neuropeptide Y than of NE.[30] Consequently, Potter used relatively high stimulation frequencies in her experiments on the role of neuropeptide Y as a parasympathetic neuromodulator.[28]

In recent experiments performed in our laboratory, therefore, we sought to determine in more detail the stimulation conditions that release neuropeptide Y from cardiac sympathetic neurons.[31] We wished to determine whether appreciable effects ascribable to neuropeptide Y could be elicited by more physiological stimulation frequencies.

We used a protocol similar to Potter's to estimate indirectly the release of neuropeptide Y from the cardiac sympathetic nerve terminals in anesthetized dogs.[31] After 2 control vagal stimulations, we stimulated the ansae subclaviae at 10 Hz for 5 minutes. We then resumed the vagal stimulation every 2 minutes until the vagally induced chronotropic response returned to control. FIGURE 8 shows a representative response. Note that the vagally induced chronotropic responses were diminished immediately after the cessation of sympathetic stimulation, and they required about 40 minutes to return to control.

FIGURE 9 shows the recovery of the chronotropic responses to vagal stimulation after 5 minute trains of sympathetic stimulation delivered at frequencies of 5, 10, and 15 Hz in a representative animal.[31] Note that the magnitude and duration of the inhibitory effects increased as we raised the frequency of sympathetic stimulation. For example, after sympathetic stimulation at 5 Hz, the initial ($t = 2$ minutes) chronotropic response to vagal stimulation was inhibited by 53%, whereas after sympathetic stimulation at 15 Hz, the initial response was inhibited by 86%. The corresponding times for these responses to recover were 20 and 58 minutes, respectively.

The experiments depicted in FIGURE 10 disclose that the inhibitory effects imputed to neuropeptide Y are clearly discernible even when the sympathetic nerves are stimulated at frequencies as low as 2 Hz. Furthermore, these inhibitory effects are exaggerated when the α-adrenergic receptors are blocked.[31] The animals in these experiments were assigned randomly to a control, propranolol, or phentolamine group, and each experiment was subdivided into 2 observation periods. During the first period, 6 trains of stimulation (2 and 5 Hz, each for train durations of 1, 3, and 5 minutes) were delivered to the cardiac sympathetic nerves. We again used Potter's protocol[28] to estimate the release of neuropeptide Y. At the end of period 1, we administered saline, propranolol, or phentolamine to animals in the corresponding groups. During period 2, we repeated the 6 trains of sympathetic stimulation after a new randomization.

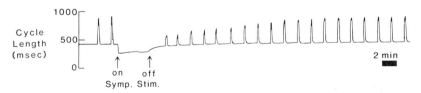

FIGURE 8. The effect of sympathetic stimulation (5 minutes, 10 Hz) on the changes in cardiac cycle length induced by 10 second trains of vagal stimulation delivered every 2 minutes in an anesthetized dog. (From Reference 31, with permission of the American Heart Association, Inc.)

During period 1 in the control and propranolol groups (FIGURE 10), the initial inhibitions observed after sympathetic stimulation were not significantly different from those obtained during period 2. In the group that received phentolamine, however, the initial inhibitions were significantly augmented by phentolamine (period 2). We concluded, therefore, that even low frequencies (2 to 5 Hz) of sympathetic stimulation can inhibit the chronotropic responses to vagal stimulation, and that α-blockade, but not β-blockade, significantly increases the magnitude and duration of the sympathetically induced inhibition of these chronotropic responses.[31]

Postjunctional Mechanisms

In the experiments of Hollenberg et al., cited above, the negative inotropic effects of ACh infusions on the ventricular myocardium were augmented by adrenergic interventions.[9] This accentuation of the ACh effects was induced not only by increased sympathetic neural activity, but also by the infusion of β-adrenergic agonists. Hence, the effects of ACh must not be mediated exclusively by the prejunctional inhibition of NE release from neighboring sympathetic nerve fibers (FIGURE 6). Part of the interaction must occur postjunctionally, at the surface of the cardiac effector cell itself.[4,20–22]

The mechanism for the postjunctional adrenergic-cholinergic interaction is depicted in FIGURE 6. The sympathetically released NE combines with β-adrenergic receptors (β) in the cell membrane. Occupation of the β-adrenergic receptors stimulates the membrane-bound enzyme, adenylate cyclase, which catalyzes the intracellular accumulation of cyclic AMP (cAMP) from ATP.[4,20–22] The stimulation of the adenylate cyclase by the β-adrenergic receptors is mediated by a stimulatory protein, G_s. This coupling by the G_s protein involves the hydrolysis of guanosine triphosphate (GTP) to guanosine diphosphate (GDP).

The first step in the antagonistic action of the ACh released from vagal nerve endings is the combination of the ACh with the muscarinic receptors (M) on the effector cell surface (FIGURE 6). The muscarinic receptors inhibit adenylate cyclase

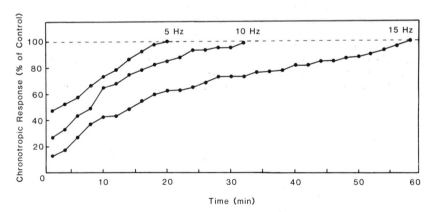

FIGURE 9. Recovery of the chronotropic responses to 10 second trains of vagal stimulation after 5 minute trains of sympathetic stimulation delivered at 5, 10, and 15 Hz in an anesthetized dog. Time zero is the time at which sympathetic stimulation was discontinued. (From Reference 31, with permission of the American Heart Association, Inc.)

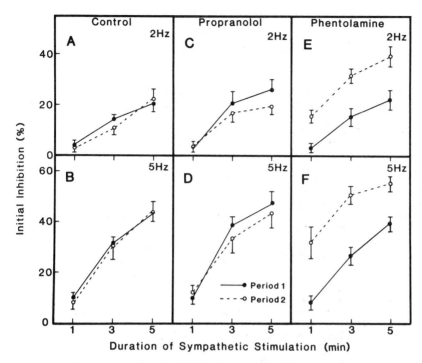

FIGURE 10. Effects of adrenergic receptor blockade on the sympathetically mediated inhibition of vagally induced chronotropic responses. In each panel, the change in the first chronotropic response (initial inhibition) after cessation of sympathetic stimulation is plotted versus the durations of sympathetic stimulation, in minutes. The animals were subdivided into a control group, a group that received propranolol, and a group that received phentolamine. In the latter two groups, the animals received the blocking drug between period 1 and period 2. In the phentolamine group only, the effects of sympathetic stimulation in period 2 were significantly different ($p < 0.001$) from the effects in period 1. Values are means ± SEM. (From Reference 31, with permission of the American Heart Association, Inc.)

through an inhibitory coupling protein, G_i. This inhibitory protein also catalyzes the hydrolysis of GTP to GDP.

The principal postjunctional adrenergic-cholinergic interaction thus operates through adenylate cyclase. The facilitatory effects of increased sympathetic activity are mediated by raising the intracellular levels of cAMP. The antagonistic effects of ACh released from postganglionic vagal endings is to inhibit adenylate cyclase, and thereby to attenuate the adrenergically induced rise in the intracellular concentration of cAMP.

REFERENCES

1. ROSENBLUETH, A. & F. A. SIMEONE. 1934. The interrelations of vagal and accelerator effects on the cardiac rate. Am. J. Physiol. **110:** 42–55.
2. LEVY, M. N. & H. ZIESKE. 1969. Autonomic control of cardiac pacemaker activity and atrioventricular transmission. J. Appl. Physiol. **27:** 465–470.

3. WARNER, H. R. & R. O. RUSSELL, JR. 1969. Effect of combined sympathetic and vagal stimulation on heart rate in the dog. Circ. Res. 24: 567–573.
4. LEVY, M. N. 1971. Sympathetic-parasympathetic interactions in the heart. Circ. Res. 29: 437–445.
5. WALLICK, D. W., D. FELDER & M. N. LEVY. 1978. Autonomic control of pacemaker activity in the atrioventricular junction of the dog. Am. J. Physiol. 235: H308–H313.
6. WALLICK, D. W., P. J. MARTIN, Y. MASUDA & M. N. LEVY. 1982. Effects of autonomic activity and changes in heart rate on atrioventricular conduction. Am. J. Physiol. 243: H523–H527.
7. TAKAHASHI, N. & D. R. ZIPES. 1983. Vagal modulation of adrenergic effects on canine sinus and atrioventricular nodes. Am. J. Physiol. 244: H775–H781.
8. URTHALER, F., B. H. NEELY, G. R. HAGEMAN & L. R. SMITH. 1986. Differential sympathetic-parasympathetic interactions in sinus node and AV junction. Am. J. Physiol. 250: H43–H51.
9. HOLLENBERG, M., S. CARRIERE & A. C. BARGER. 1965. Biphasic action of acetylcholine on ventricular myocardium. Circ. Res. 16: 527–536.
10. LEVY, M. N., M. NG, P. MARTIN & H. ZIESKE, JR. 1966. Sympathetic and parasympathetic interactions upon the left ventricle of the dog. Circ. Res. 19: 5–10.
11. STUESSE, S. L., D. W. WALLICK & M. N. LEVY. 1979. Autonomic control of right atrial contractile strength in the dog. Am. J. Physiol. 236: H860–H865.
12. BAILEY, J. C., A. M. WATANABE, H. R. BESCH, JR. & D. A. LATHROP. 1979. Acetylcholine antagonism of the electrophysiological effects of isoproterenol on canine cardiac Purkinje fibers. Circ. Res. 44: 378–383.
13. MARTINS, J. B. & D. P. ZIPES. 1980. Effects of sympathetic and vagal nerves on recovery properties of the endocardium and epicardium of the canine left ventricle. Circ. Res. 46: 100–110.
14. KOLMAN, B. S., R. L. VERRIER & B. LOWN. 1976. Effect of vagus nerve stimulation upon excitability of the canine ventricle. Am. J. Cardiol. 37: 1041–1045.
15. LOWN, B. & R. L. VERRIER. 1976. Neural activity and ventricular fibrillation. N. Engl. J. Med. 294: 1165–1170.
16. SHERIDAN, D. J., P. A. PENKOSKE, B. E. SOBEL & P. B. CORR. 1980. Alpha adrenergic contributions to dysrhythmia during myocardial ischemia and reperfusion in cats. J. Clin. Invest. 65: 161–171.
17. ZUANETTI, G., G. M. DE FERRARI, S. G. PRIORI & P. J. SCHWARTZ. 1987. Protective effect of vagal stimulation on reperfusion arrhythmias in cats. Circ. Res. 61: 429–435.
18. SCHWARTZ, P. J. & G. M. DE FERRARI. 1987. Influence of the autonomic nervous system on sudden cardiac death. Cardiology 74: 297–309.
19. FUREY, S. A., III & M. N. LEVY. 1983. The interactions among heart rate, autonomic activity, and arterial pressure upon the multiple repetitive extrasystole threshold in the dog. Am. Heart J. 106: 1112–1120.
20. LEVY, M. N. & P. J. MARTIN. 1979. Neural control of the heart. In Handbook of Physiology, Section 2, The Cardiovascular System. R. M. Berne & N. Sperelakis, Eds. 1: 581–620. American Physiological Society. Bethesda, Md.
21. STILES, G. L., M. G. CARON & R. J. LEFKOWITZ. 1984. β-Adrenergic receptors: biochemical mechanisms of physiological regulation. Physiol. Rev. 64: 661–743.
22. WATANABE, A. M., J. P. LINDEMANN & J. W. FLEMING. 1984. Mechanisms of muscarinic modulation of protein phosphorylation in intact ventricles. Fed. Proc. 43: 2618–2623.
23. LEVY, M. N. 1988. Sympathetic-parasympathetic interactions in the heart. In Neurocardiology. H. Kulbertus & G. Franck, Eds.: 85–98. Futura. New York, N.Y.
24. LOFFELHOLZ, K. & E. MUSCHOLL. 1970. Inhibition by parasympathetic nerve stimulation of the release of the adrenergic transmitter. Naunyn-Schmiedebergs Arch. Pharmakol. 267: 181–184.
25. MUSCHOLL, E. 1980. Peripheral muscarinic control of norepinephrine release in the cardiovascular system. Am. J. Physiol. 239: H713–H720.
26. LEVY, M. N. & B. BLATTBERG. 1976. Effect of vagal stimulation on the overflow of norepinephrine into the coronary sinus during cardiac sympathetic nerve stimulation in the dog. Circ. Res. 38: 81–85.

27. WETZEL, G. T., D. GOLDSTEIN & J. H. BROWN. 1985. Acetylcholine release from rat atria can be regulated through an alpha₁-adrenergic receptor. Circ. Res. **56:** 763–766.

28. POTTER, E. K. 1985. Prolonged non-adrenergic inhibition of cardiac vagal action following sympathetic stimulation: Neuromodulation by neuropeptide Y? Neurosci. Lett. **54:** 117–121.

29. PERNOW, J. 1988. Co-release and functional interactions of neuropeptide Y and noradrenaline in peripheral sympathetic vascular control. Acta Physiol. Scand. **133**(Suppl. 568): 1–56.

30. LUNDBERG, J. M., A. RUDEHILL, A. SOLLEVI, E. THEODORSSON-NORHEIM & B. HAMBERGER. 1986. Frequency- and reserpine-dependent chemical coding of sympathetic transmission: differential release of noradrenaline and neuropeptide Y from pig spleen. Neurosci. Lett. **63:** 96–100.

31. WARNER, M. R. & M. N. LEVY. 1989. Neuropeptide Y as a putative modulator of the vagal effects on heart rate. Circ. Res. **64:** 882–889.

Circadian Variations of Electrical Properties of the Heart[a]

JUAN CINCA, ANGEL MOYA, ALFREDO BARDAJI,
JORGE RIUS, AND JORGE SOLER-SOLER

Electrophysiology Laboratory
Cardiology Service
Valle de Hebrón General Hospital
08035 Barcelona, Spain

INTRODUCTION

Recent technical advances in intracardiac electrophysiology and dynamic electrocardiography led to the exploration of the influence of the circadian rhythms on some electrical properties of the human heart.[1-5] Using an appropriate electrocatheter technique we have been able to perform sequential bedside electrophysiologic testing over a period of 22 hours to investigate the existence of a possible daily variability in electrophysiologic parameters.[6-8] In this presentation we are going to compile our data on sequential 22-hour measurements of the refractory periods of the normal cardiac structures and accessory AV conduction pathways with special emphasis on the effects of a possible daily variability on electrical induction of reciprocating supraventricular tachycardia (SVT). Additionally, we will deal with some clinical aspects that remain to be investigated.

METHODS

Patients

Thirty-eight patients, 29 men and 9 women, with a mean age of 38 years (range 16 to 70 years) were studied to determine the mechanism of recurrent episodes of paroxysmal SVT in 25 or the origin of syncopal attacks in 13. All patients observed a normal nocturnal sleeping schedule and gave informed consent to participate in the study.

Sequential Electrophysiologic Testing

The first electrophysiologic study was performed at the laboratory between 11 AM and 2 PM in a nonsedated postabsortive state. Thereafter, the patients were transferred to a day-lit room to complete sequential bedside electrophysiologic measurements.

The electrocatheters were introduced percutaneously under local anesthesia with 2% mepivacaine hydrochloride. A quadripolar USCI no. 7F electrocatheter was inserted into the coronary sinus via the left subclavian vein. Two other electrocatheters, an octapolar and a bipolar USCI 7F probe, were introduced into the right femoral vein

[a]This work was supported by a grant from Fondo de Investigaciones Sanitarias de la Seguridad Social (86/1188).

and advanced into the right ventricular apex and right atrial wall, respectively. The octapolar catheter was designed in our laboratory to pace the right ventricle and to simultaneously record His bundle potentials with critically placed electrodes at 6 to 7 cm from the catheter tip.[8]

The effective refractory period (ERP) of the atria, AV node, right ventricle, Kent bundle, and accessory AV nodal pathways and the electrical induction of SVT were determined by programmed electrical stimulation (PES) at a basic cycle length of 600 mseconds. Location of the accessory AV pathway by mapping of the retrograde atrial activation during ventricular stimulation was evaluated using unipolar electrograms from the right atrium and coronary sinus.[7]

Recording of the intracavitary potentials and conventional ECG leads was done on an Elema Mingograf 82 ink-jet recorder at 100 mm/second paper speed. The stimulation protocol was carried out with a Medtronic 5325 stimulator delivering pulses of 2 msecond duration and twice the amplitude of the diastolic threshold. The recording system for bedside electrophysiologic monitoring was placed outside the patient's room to reduce the interference of the study protocol with the sleep periods.

Protocol

After completion of the first electrophysiologic study, the patients were transferred to an appropriate room for measurement of refractory periods and for induction of reciprocating SVT every 1 to 2 hours over a period of 22 hours. The bipolar right atrial catheter was withdrawn, whereas the coronary sinus probe and the right ventricular octapolar catheter were left in place and sutured to the skin to prevent displacements of the catheter tip. Intravenous sodium heparin, 5000 U every 4 hours, was given in all cases during the study protocol.

From 3 to 7 AM the protocol was purposely interrupted to avoid interference with the sleep rhythm. Meals were served up at 3 PM, 7 PM, and 7 AM.

Data Analysis

Values of the refractory periods were expressed as the mean ±1 standard deviation (SD), and the statistical significance of their 24-hour variability was assessed by analysis of variance (ANOVA) for repeated measurements. Electrical inducibility of SVT was expressed as the percentage of PES inducing at least one episode of SVT. The significance of arrhythmia inducibility was evaluated by the χ^2 analysis for trend. A p value <0.05 was considered significant.

RESULTS

An average of 9 bedside electrophysiologic studies (range 7 to 13) were completed in each patient and were followed by no complications.

Data from the first electrophysiologic exploration (TABLE 1) revealed the existence of an atrioventricular accessory pathway (Kent bundle) in 19 patients. In 8 out of the 19 cases the Kent bundle had bidirectional conduction whereas in the remaining 11 patients the accessory pathway disclosed exclusive retrograde conduction (latent Kent bundle). In 16 cases the Kent bundle was located at the left AV groove and in the other 3 patients it was found at the right cardiac side. In 6 out of the 38 cases a pattern of dual AV nodal pathways was observed during programmed atrial stimulation. Among

TABLE 1. Electrophysiologic Findings in 38 Patients

Bidirectional left-sided Kent bundle	5
Bidirectional right-sided Kent bundle	3
Latent left-sided Kent bundle	11
Dual AV nodal pathways	6
Prolonged AV nodal ERP	3
Normal electrophysiologic study	10
Total	38

the remaining 13 patients with syncopal attacks, 10 had normal electrophysiologic data and 3 showed a prolongation of the AV nodal refractory period.

Sequential Changes in Refractoriness

Normal Cardiac Structures

As illustrated in FIGURE 1, the effective refractory period (ERP) of the atria, AV node, and right ventricle followed a 22-hour variability with a range of 79 ± 65 mseconds for the AV node, 35 ± 14 mseconds for the atria, and 24 ± 10 mseconds for the right ventricle. The QT interval measured at fixed atrial pacing of 100 beats/minute showed a variability range of 27 ± 27 mseconds in the 30 patients without an ECG pattern of ventricular preexcitation.

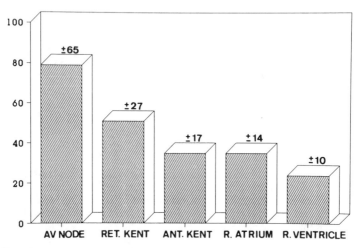

MEAN RANGE OF ERP
msec.

FIGURE 1. Twenty-two-hour effective refractory period (ERP) variability range of the AV node, antegrade and retrograde conduction through the Kent bundle, right atrium, and right ventricle.

Analysis of variance for the sequential ERP measurements showed a statistically significant variation during the 22-hour study period. As compared with the first electrophysiologic study during midnight and early morning there was a significant prolongation of the ERP of the atria ($p < 0.001$), AV node ($p = 0.002$), and right ventricle ($p < 0.001$) and a lengthening of the QT interval ($p < 0.008$) preceded by a transient shortening of these parameters between 7 to 8 PM (FIGURES 2 and 3). Measurements of the AV nodal ERP were only possible in 24 cases due to the existence of either a longer atrial ERP or a conduction through a Kent bundle. Patients with prolonged AV nodal ERP at baseline (3 cases) had a comparable daily variability to patients with normal AV nodal refractoriness.

The sinus node rate (RR interval) followed a significant prolongation at midnight, paralleling the changes in cardiac refractoriness (FIGURE 4).

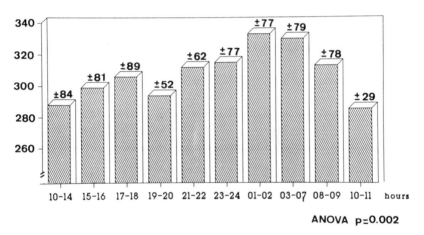

FIGURE 2. Sequential values of the AV nodal effective refractory period (ERP) during a period of 22 hours.

Accessory Conduction Pathways

The 22-hour variability range of Kent bundle ERP was 35 ± 17 mseconds for antegrade conduction and 51 ± 27 mseconds for retrograde conduction (FIGURE 5).

Sequential measurements evidenced a significant prolongation of retrograde Kent bundle ERP ($p < 0.005$) at midnight and early morning preceded by a transient shortening between 7 and 8 PM. Antegrade Kent bundle refractoriness, present in only 8 patients, tended to prolong at midnight but this change was not statistically significant (FIGURE 6).

In six patients with dual AV nodal pathways the ERP of the fast pathway experienced a lengthening at midnight and early morning preceded by a brief shortening at 7 to 8 PM (FIGURE 7). In contrast, the slow AV nodal pathway showed a different daily variability. In 5 patients two or more electrophysiologic testings evidenced

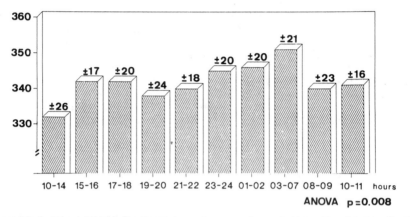

FIGURE 3. Sequential changes in QT interval measured at a fixed paced atrial rate of 100 beats/minute during a period of 22 hours.

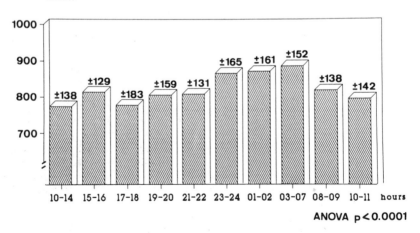

FIGURE 4. Sequential changes in sinus node rate during the 22-hour study protocol.

RETROGRADE KENT BUNDLE ERP
msec.

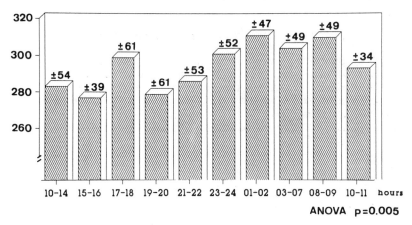

ANOVA p=0.005

FIGURE 5. Sequential changes in effective refractory period (ERP) of the retrograde conduction through the Kent bundle over a period of 22 hours.

ANTEGRADE KENT BUNDLE ERP
msec.

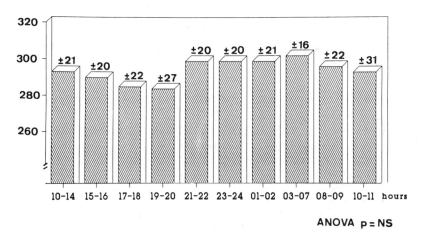

ANOVA p = NS

FIGURE 6. Sequential changes in effective refractory period (ERP) of the antegrade conduction through the Kent bundle during the 24 hour study protocol.

conduction block through the slow nodal pathway. This phenomenon was not related to the nocturnal part of the day but it tended to occur when ERP of the fast AV nodal pathway showed a concurrent shortening.

Sequential Changes in Electrical Induction of Reentrant Tachycardia

In 17 out of the 19 patients with Kent bundles, reciprocating tachycardia involving the accessory pathway was elicited by programmed electrical stimulation from either the apex of the right ventricle or the coronary sinus. However, the capacity to induce the arrhythmia varied throughout the study protocol. As illustrated in FIGURE 8 tachycardia induction expressed as the percentage of PES inducing the arrhythmia progressively decreased through the afternoon, showed a transient increase between 9

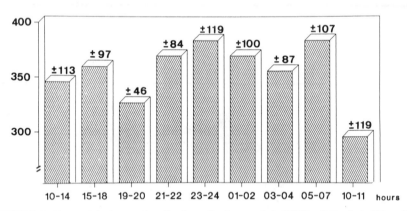

FIGURE 7. Sequential changes in effective refractory period (ERP) of the fast AV nodal accessory pathway over a period of 22 hours in six patients with dual AV nodal pathways.

and 10 PM, and finally reached the lowest values at midnight and early morning (from 75% to 42% at the coronary sinus, $p < 0.05$, and from 64% to 23% at the right ventricle, $p < 0.025$). The capacity to induce the arrhythmia from the coronary sinus tended to recover during the ensuing morning, but still remained within low values for the right ventricular stimulation. Although not significant, there was a tendency to observe a prolongation of the tachycardia cycle length at midnight whenever the arrhythmia was inducible. In 3 out of 6 patients with dual AV nodal pathways, a reentrant AV nodal tachycardia was inducible at the first electrophysiologic testing. However, in two cases the arrhythmia was no longer inducible at midnight and in the remaining patient the tachycardia had a longer cycle length at midnight (FIGURE 9) than at the diurnal part of the day.

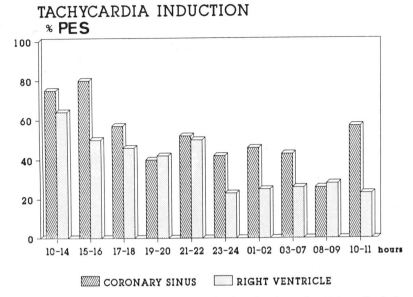

FIGURE 8. Sequential changes in electrical induction of reciprocating tachycardia during a period of 22 hours in 17 patients with Kent bundles.

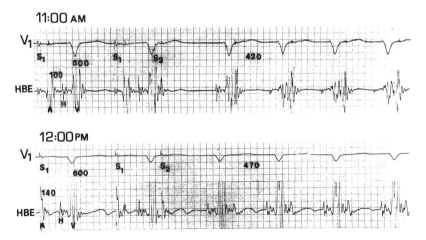

FIGURE 9. Prolongation of the tachycardia cycle length at midnight in a patient with reentrant AV nodal tachycardia using two AV nodal pathways.

DISCUSSION

Compiled data from this series of patients added new information to our previous studies based on a lower number of observations.[7,8]

22-Hour Variability in Cardiac Refractoriness

The maximal range of variability in the effective refractory period during an interval of 24 hours corresponded to the AV node and it was followed by that of retrograde and antegrade conduction through Kent bundles and, in a lesser degree, by refractoriness of the atrial and ventricular myocardium. These findings revealed that among the cardiac tissues explored in this study the AV node was the most sensitive to fluctuations in the autonomic nervous tone to the heart, but also noticeable was the observation that accessory atrioventricular muscle fibers (Kent bundles) were more sensitive to the autonomic nervous drive than the also muscular atrial and ventricular fibers. The AV node and Kent bundles would be, therefore, the most neurally dependent limbs of a reciprocating tachycardia encompassing the atria, AV node, ventricles, and Kent bundle fibers.

Daily variations in refractory period followed a well-defined pattern. Already known from our previous observations the effective refractory period of the atria, AV node, right ventricle, and that of conduction through Kent bundles showed a significant prolongation at midnight and early morning as compared with the baseline values obtained at midday.[7,8] However the current study demonstrated an unexpected brief shortening in refractoriness of the above cardiac structures between 8 and 10 PM, closely preceding the midnight prolongation. Lengthening of the AV nodal, atrial, ventricular, and Kent bundle refractory period is supposedly related to the presence of a heightened parasympathetic nerve tone normally occurring at midnight and early morning since hypervagotonia prolonged the refractory period of the AV node and ventricles in dogs,[9,10] whereas atropine and sympathetic stimulation shortened atrial refractoriness in humans[11] and in dogs[12] respectively, and also shortened the effective refractory period of the Kent bundle.[13] Accordingly, the brief shortening in cardiac refractoriness observed at the evening would reflect a lowered parasympathetic nerve drive or a transient sympatheticotonia. Whether the abrupt changes in cardiac refractoriness measured at the evening corresponded to spontaneous fluctuations in the autonomic nervous balance or were the result of external environmental stimuli influencing the neural tone to the heart, such as the postprandial period, pain, or mental stress, is difficult to ascertain from this study. However, although in our patients the refractory period shortening measured at the evening would correspond to the two-hour postdinner phase, similar changes were not detected after lunch. Patients were also free of pain or mental stress at this particular part of the day.

Even though our series of patients with dual AV nodal pathways is relatively small, collected data allowed us to draw new observations on 24-hour refractory period variability of both pathways. The fast AV nodal pathway followed a comparable brief shortening in refractoriness at the evening and a prolongation at midnight to patients with a normal AV nodal conduction pattern. In contrast, refractory period of the slow AV nodal pathway failed to show a comparable trend of changes. Conduction block through the slow AV nodal pathway was observed in several instances during the study protocol in 5 out of the 6 patients and in most of these circumstances there was a concurrent shortening in the fast AV nodal pathway refractoriness. These data appeared to support the concept that a requisite for the occurrence of a dual AV nodal conduction pattern was the existence of a certain degree of parasympatheticotonia which could maintain a relative prolongation of fast AV nodal pathway refractoriness. Conceivably, withdrawal of the vagal tone or increased sympathetic drive would produce a relatively nonuniform shortening of refractoriness on both AV nodal pathways rendering it difficult to be precise about at which moment a given programmed atrial stimulus is conducted through either the fast or the slow nodal pathways. In this situation conduction block through the slow pathway can be misleadingly diagnosed.

22-Hour Variability in Tachycardia Induction

We observed a concordance between the 22-hour refractory period variability and the capacity to electrically induce reciprocating tachycardia in patients with Kent bundles. Lengthening of the refractory period in tissues encompassed into the circuit of a reentrant tachycardia (atria, AV node, ventricles, and Kent bundles) occurring at midnight and early morning was associated with a significant reduction in electrical inducibility of the tachycardia, whereas shortening in refractory period of these cardiac structures transiently detected at the evening were accompanied by a transitory facility to induce the arrhythmia. This daily variability in tachycardia induction is in agreement with a recent study on the circadian occurrence of spontaneous symptomatic episodes of paroxysmal supraventricular tachycardia in 52 untreated patients.[4] These authors observed a maximal incidence of tachycardia at 6–8 PM and a corresponding minimum incidence at 4 AM. Induction of reciprocating tachycardia was more frequent from the coronary sinus than from the right ventricle. The presence of left-sided Kent bundles in the majority of our patients may be the reason for these differences in tachycardia inducibility. Arrhythmia induction from the coronary sinus is facilitated by the close relationship existing between the left atrial stimulation site (coronary sinus) and the atrial insertion of the left Kent bundle, as compared with the more distant position of the right ventricular pacing site from the left ventricular insertion of the left bypass tract.[14]

Reentrant intranodal tachycardia in three patients with dual AV nodal pathways was not inducible at midnight in two of the three cases and in the remaining patient the rate of the tachycardia decreased at that time of day.

Clinical Implications

The observation that circadian fluctuations in the autonomic nervous tone exerted a protection against reciprocating tachycardia at midnight and early morning but a facilitation of the arrhythmia at midday and late evening supports the hypothesis that antiarrhythmic drug therapy in patients with reciprocating tachycardia should be concentrated to these nonprotected parts of the day.

The 22-hour variability in cardiac refractory period and electrical induction of reciprocating tachycardia should be considered in studies assessing the effects of antiarrhythmic drugs on refractory periods and in those protocols testing the efficacy of drug regimes against electrical induction of tachycardia. Study protocols scheduled at midday would be more prone to induce tachycardia than those programmed early in the morning.

Our recording technique using the ventricular octapolar catheter reduced by one the number of electrocatheters required for an electrophysiologic study, and moreover, the procedure allowed prolonged bedside monitoring of the AV nodal conduction[6,8] and refractory periods of the AV conduction system and accessory AV pathways, as well as sequential assessment of electrical inducibility of supraventricular tachycardia. Therefore the procedure is of potential usefulness in chronic electrophysiologic and pharmacologic investigations.

Application of the protocol to our patients was followed by no complications and probably produced no significant alterations on the circadian pacemakers since the sinus node rate and the body temperature, considered by others as indirect indicators of a normal circadian rhythmicity,[15,16] followed a normal daily pattern in our patients.[7,8]

SUMMARY

Cardiac refractoriness and electrical inducibility of supraventricular tachycardia (SVT) were assessed at intervals of 1 to 2 hours over a period of 22 hours in 38 patients (25 with paroxysmal SVT). Daily variability of effective refractory period (ERP) had a mean range of 35 ± 14 mseconds for the atria, 79 ± 65 mseconds for the AV node, 24 ± 10 m seconds for the ventricles, 51 ± 27 mseconds for the retrograde Kent bundle, and 35 ± 17 mseconds for the antegrade Kent bundle. Between 11 PM and 8 AM there was a significant prolongation of the ERP of the atria (ANOVA, $p < 0.001$), AV node ($p = 0.002$), right ventricle ($p < 0.001$), and retrograde Kent bundle ($p = 0.005$), and a reduction in electrical induction of SVT from 75% to 42% ($p < 0.05$) with respect to the first electrophysiologic study. This nocturnal prolongation was preceded by ERP shortening of all explored cardiac sites and by increased tachycardia inducibility between 8 and 10 PM. Six patients with dual AV nodal pathways showed a prolongation of the fast pathway ERP at midnight, whereas conduction through the slow pathway followed an unpredictable daily variability. These data indicate a circadian influence on refractoriness of normal cardiac tissues and accessory pathways that exerted a midnight protection against electrical inducibility of reciprocating tachycardia but a transient arrhythmia facilitation at the evening.

REFERENCES

1. DE LEONARDIS, V., P. CINELLI, F. CAPPACI, M. DE SCALZI & S. CITI. 1983. Circadian rhythms in dynamic electrocardiography. J. Electrocardiol. **16:** 351.
2. BROWNE, K. F., E. N. PRYSTOWSKY, J. J. HEGER, D. A. CHILSON & D. P. ZIPES. 1983. Prolongation of the Q-T interval in man during sleep. Am. J. Cardiol. **52:** 55.
3. THORMANN, J., M. SCHLEPPER, & W. KRAMER. 1983. Diurnal changes and reproducibility of corrected sinus node recovery time. Catheterization Cardiovasc. Diagn. **9:** 439.
4. IRWIN, J. M., E. A. MCCARTHY, W. E. WILKINSON & E. L. C. PRITCHETT. 1988. Circadian occurrence of symptomatic paroxysmal supraventricular tachycardia in untreated patients. Circulation **77:** 298.
5. GILLIS, A. M., K. E. MACLEAN & C. GUILLEMINAULT. 1988. The QT interval during wake and sleep in patients with ventricular arrhythmias. Sleep **11:** 333.
6. CINCA, J., A. MOYA, J. FIGUERAS, F. ROMA & J. RIUS. 1986. Circadian variations in the electrical properties of the human heart assessed by sequential bedside electrophysiologic testing. Am. Heart J. **112:** 315.
7. CINCA, J., A. MOYA, A. BARDAJÍ, J. FIGUERAS & J. RIUS. 1987. Daily variability of electrically induced reciprocating tachycardia in patients with atrioventricular accessory pathways. Am. Heart J. **114:** 327.
8. CINCA, J., A. MOYA, A. BARDAJÍ, J. FIGUERAS & J. RIUS. 1988. Octapolar electrocatheter for His bundle recording and sequential bedside electrophysiologic testing. PACE **11:** 220.
9. SPEAR, J. F. & E. N. MOORE. 1973. Influence of brief vagal and stellate nerve stimulation on

pacemaker activity and conduction within the atrioventricular conduction system of the dog. Circ. Res. **32:** 27.

10. KOLMAN, B. S., R. L. VERRIER & B. LOWN. 1976. Effect of vagus nerve stimulation upon excitability of the canine ventricle: role of sympathetic-parasympathetic interactions. Am. J. Cardiol. **37:** 1041.

11. DHINGRA, R. C., F. AMAT-Y-LEON, C. WYNDHAM, P. DENES, D. WU, J. M. POUGET & K. M. ROSEN. 1976. Electrophysiologic effects of atropine on human sinus node and atrium. Am. J. Cardiol. **38:** 429.

12. KRALIOS, F. A. & C. K. MILLAR. 1981. Sympathetic neural effects on regional atrial properties and cardiac rhythm. Am. J. Physiol. **240:** H590.

13. WELLENS, H. J. J., P. BRUGADA, D. ROY, J. WEISS & F. W. BAR. 1982. Effect of isoproterenol on the antegrade refractory period of the accessory pathway in patients with the Wolff-Parkinson-White syndrome. Am. J. Cardiol. **50:** 180.

14. PRITCHETT, E. L. C., J. J. GALLAGHER & M. M. SCHEIMAN. 1978. Determinants of the echozone in patients with reciprocating tachycardia and the Wolff-Parkinson-White syndrome. Circulation **57:** 671.

15. MOORE-EDE, M. C., C. A. CZEISLER & G. S. RICHARDSON. 1983. Circadian timekeeping in health and disease. I. Basic properties of circadian pacemakers. N. Engl. J. Med. **309:** 469.

16. MOORE-EDE, M. C., C. A. CZEISLER & G. S. RICHARDSON. 1983. Circadian timekeeping in health and disease. II. Clinical implications of circadian rhythmicity. N. Engl. J. Med. **309:** 530.

Clinical Exploration of the Autonomic Nervous System by Means of Electrocardiography

ALBERTO MALLIANI, FEDERICO LOMBARDI,
MASSIMO PAGANI, AND SERGIO CERUTTI[a]
Cardiovascular Research Institute and
Cardiovascular Research Center, CNR;
Fidia Center
L. Sacco Hospital
Internal Medicine
University of Milan
via Grassi 74
20157 Milan, Italy

[a]*Electronics Department*
Milan Polytechnic Institute
20133 Milan, Italy

In his correspondence with Thomas Lewis, Einthoven wrote that the value of an instrument depends on what is done with it, not what might be possible.[1] He was obviously referring to electrocardiography. The present paper deals with an application that could not have been forseen by its inventor, a development that appears as the natural born child of another instrument, the computer.

A few premises seem necessary to introduce, from a methodological point of view, this new application: subsequently, some concrete examples will follow of what has been done up until now, and we will conclude with some thinking about what, hopefully, will be possible in the near future. In short, the merits of electrocardiography will be expanded to the exploration of the frequency domain, whatever the physiological and clinical relevance of this new approach will turn out to be.

NEURAL AND CARDIOVASCULAR RHYTHMS AS MARKERS OF FUNCTIONAL STATES

Rhythmicity is an intrinsic property of the nervous system. Various rhythms can be markers of normal events such as wakefulness or sleep and of abnormal conditions such as epilepsy. However, a rhythm is rarely unequivocally linked with a function: thus an atropinized cat can walk around with an electroencephalogram simulating placid sleep. On the other hand, circulation and respiration, strictly related transport functions, are both based on discontinuous events and oscillations of various orders characterize them, in particular cardiovascular variables. It has been a traditional endeavor of experimental physiology to describe such oscillations, to investigate their causes and, more recently, the links existing between neural and cardiovascular rhythms in view of a possible functional significance. Surely the oldest are the observations on rhythmic fluctuations of systemic arterial pressure as they started in 1733 with Reverend Stephen Hales' experiment during which oscillations of first and second order were

234

observed,[2] i.e., those related to cardiac cycle and respiration. As to the third order oscillations, i.e., those with a period apparently longer than the respiratory cycle, Koepchen has recently reviewed their history[3] and the various interpretations that have flourished around them: according to his conclusions we shall assume the waves described by Sigmund Mayer[4] and having a period of about 10 seconds as the prototype of the third order oscillations of arterial pressure. However, the period of this type of oscillation is highly variable.

With regard to the rhythms discernible in the discharge of the autonomic outflow, Adrian and coworkers were the first to record from sympathetic nerves an efferent impulse activity displaying a rhythm in phase with cardiac cycle and respiration.[5] Several decades had to elapse before Fernandez de Molina and Perl observed, in spinal cats, rhythmic increases in sympathetic discharge simultaneous to slow arterial pressure waves.[6] There has been much debate during the years on the origin of these neural rhythms, along two fundamental hypotheses. Indeed, they could depend either on afferent peripheral modulation or on autochthonous oscillating properties of the centers.[7] Concerning the oscillations of second order, Koepchen and coworkers suggested that two basic mechanisms are involved: a primary intracentral coupling with the generator of the cardiovascular-respiratory rhythm and a secondary reflex coupling.[8] For the third order fluctuations, Preiss and Polosa[9] and Polosa[10] maintained that it is the activity of a central oscillation, in part present at spinal level,[6] that produces the sympathetic rhythm and therefore the Mayer waves.

The experimental tool to distinguish between central origin and feedback mechanisms has been in most studies the surgical interruption of afferent pathways, mainly those impinging upon supraspinal structures. Thus, the finding of a cardiac rhythm in animals with sinoaortic denervation led to the suggestion that this rhythm represents an intrinsic oscillation of a brain stem network.[11] However, it should be realized that any deafferentation can only be partial: in fact it is practically impossible to interrupt all cardiovascular sympathetic afferent fibers[12] that constitute a huge and sparse afferent pathway transmitting to the spinal cord and higher centers many different types of rhythmic activities. Thus, the persistence of a sympathetic third order rhythm after stabilization of arterial pressure either mechanically or pharmacologically[10] appears as a particularly important additional finding in favor of a central oscillator.

Mayer waves are known to be increased by various manipulations such as hypotensive hemorrhage,[9] suggesting that they might reflect different functional states. As will be seen, the approach that we shall propose is largely based on the fact that numerous different conditions capable of inducing an increased sympathetic activity augment as well the third order rhythm discernible in several cardiovascular variables.

COMPUTER ANALYSIS OF HEART RATE VARIABILITY

The possibility recently offered by computer techniques of quantifying the small spontaneous beat by beat oscillations in cardiovascular variables and in particular in the electrocardiographic R-R interval, aroused a growing interest in view of the hypothesis that these rhythmical oscillations could provide some insight into the neural regulatory mechanisms operating in the intact organism under real life conditions.

Indeed, even somewhat crude analyses of the variability phenomena such as those offered by the use of standard deviation, frequency histograms, or simple filtering techniques provided important information on the course of pathophysiological processes such as diabetes[13] and myocardial infarction.[14]

However, the application of spectral techniques that were computationally efficient[15] offered the opportunity of assessing specifically the nonrandom components of heart rate variability thus quantifying the possible rhythmicity hidden in the signal. Sayers, for instance, employing the fast Fourier transform technique reported the existence in humans of three major components in R-R variability that he observed in specific bands of predetermined frequencies around 0.25, 0.10, and 0.03 Hz,[16] i.e., a component related to respiration (0.25 Hz) and two others at lower frequencies. Following this pioneering work, several other investigators applied this technique and, in spite of the consideration that the heart rate variability signal is not strictly periodical, as requested by the deterministic nature of the algorithm, it became clear that it could be used as a quantitative probe to assess heart rate fluctuations.[17]

As to the neural mechanisms underlying these fluctuations, vagal efferent activity appeared responsible for the higher frequencies, i.e., the component of heart rate variability related to respiration. This conclusion was based on the disappearance of this oscillation after vagotomy performed in experiments on decerebrate cats[18] or after muscarinic receptor blockade in conscious dogs[17] and man.[19] Both vagal and sympathetic outflows were considered to determine the lower frequency components, together with the hypothetical participation of other regulatory mechanisms such as those related to the renin-angiotensin system.[17]

METHODS

We shall briefly describe the methodology used in our laboratory (FIGURE 1). The electrocardiogram (ECG) is obtained with a standard AC amplifier and, after suitable amplification, it is fed through an A/D converter to the mass memory of a computer. Then the individual R waves with the peak as the fiducial point are sequentially recognized and thus the series of R-R intervals is stored in the memory as a function of the beat number. This series constitutes the tachogram. From sections of tachogram of 512 interval values, simple statistics (mean and variance) of the data are computed. This length of the tachogram has been selected as a best compromise between the need for a large time series, in order to achieve greater accuracy in the computation, and the need to obtain stationary recordings, which would be easier for short term periods. The computer program automatically calculates the autoregressive coefficients necessary to define the power spectral density estimate (see the Appendix in Reference 20). An important feature of the program is that it also calculates the model that provides the best statistical estimate and prints out the power and frequency of every spectral component. Each spectral component is presented in absolute units, as well as in normalized form, by dividing it by the total power less the DC component, if present, and multiplied by 100. This component can also be recognized in the graphs of the autospectra on the decaying part of the curve near the origin of the abscissa. Only components greater than 5% of the total power are considered significant.

It should be pointed out that in order to correctly apply spectral analysis techniques to a tachogram, the series must be stationary, a fact that can be assessed with the appropriate procedures. As a corollary, the very slow oscillations, i.e., those with a frequency of less than 0.02–0.03 Hz, which may contain significant physiological information and which on short time recordings appear as slow trends, cannot be properly assessed with this methodology, but require specific algorithms.[21]

Another important aspect is that with this methodology, which does not require any filtering or windowing of the data, the duration of the periodical phenomena in the variability signal is measured as a function of cardiac beats, rather than seconds. As an example, a four-beat periodical component is represented with a frequency of 1:4, i.e., 0.25 cycles/beat. However, this frequency is easily converted into hertz (Hz) by dividing it by the average R-R interval length. For instance, if the average R-R length were 1000 mseconds, this would correspond to 0.25 Hz Eq.

A recent development of the methodology refers to the possibility of analyzing long periods of analog recordings, by using a recursive version of the program of spectral analysis. For instance, Holter tapes, digitized at appropriate speed, can furnish a quantitative assessment of R-R variability throughout the 24 hour period of the

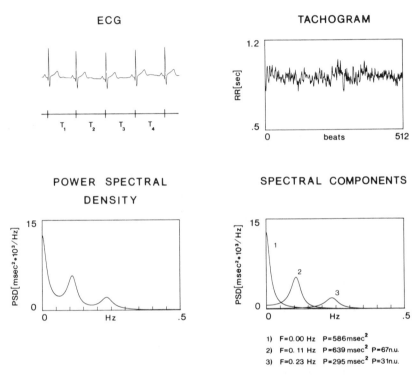

FIGURE 1. Schematic representation of the method employed for the spectral analysis of R-R variability. From the surface ECG (top left panel), the program computes the individual R-R intervals ($T_1 \ldots T_4$) and stores them in memory, as the tachogram. From the tachogram the power spectral density estimate is computed. Two major components (low frequency, LF; and high frequency, HF) are usually recognized, besides a large and variable fraction of very slow oscillations (below 0.03 Hz), which are not considered in the analysis. Notice that the computer program automatically recognizes and prints out for each component the center frequency and associated power (in absolute and normalized units NU). Power spectral ordinates should be multiplied by 10^3.

recording. From this signal a single ~100,000 intervals long tachogram is computed, from which approximately 250 spectra are derived, which describe the entire 24 hour period. These spectra can be presented in pseudotridimensional form in order to depict the different spectral patterns of heart rate variability throughout the day and night, continuously (FIGURE 6, right upper panel).

The spectral analysis in principle can be applied to any variability phenomena. In the case, for instance, of simultaneous measurements of heart rate and systemic arterial pressure variabilities, a similar procedure is used to compute the spectrum of the arterial pressure data for both systolic and diastolic values.

Further computations can be performed on the data, such as cross-spectral analysis, which can provide quantitative information on the coherence function, i.e., a measure of the statistical link between the two signals at any given frequency, and on the phase relationship.[20,22–24]

On the basis of this more complex analysis the continuous "closed-loop" relationship linking heart period and arterial pressure variabilities can be studied:[24] in our last attempt the closed-loop model includes also respiration.[25]

However, in the present context we shall only report data on heart rate variability extracted from the electrocardiographic signal.

THE GENERAL HYPOTHESIS

The neural regulation of circulatory functions is mainly effected through the interplay of the sympathetic and vagal outflows which are tonically and phasically modulated by means of the interaction of at least three major black boxes, the "central command," the reflex negative feedback and the reflex positive feedback peripheral mechanisms.[12] To study this whole interplay only through the action of single reflexes appears as an unsound illusion since the fragmented pieces of knowledge are difficult if not impossible to reassemble into a unitary regulatory system. Simplified but general hypotheses might be necessary. In this respect the sympathovagal interaction might be viewed as a push-pull or reciprocal relationship: that is to say that in most physiological conditions, as far as we know, the activation of either outflow is accompanied by the inhibition of the other.

It is the core hypothesis of this paper and of all of our work in this field that this interaction can be broadly explored in the frequency domain. In fact, we shall present data in support of the assumption that (1) the second order rhythm, i.e., the high frequency (HF) spectral component, is a marker of vagal activity (a fact well accepted by current literature); (2) the third order rhythm, i.e., the low frequency (LF) spectral component, is a marker of sympathetic activity (a hypothesis that we have introduced in the current research). A push-pull relationship will be shown to exist between the second and third order rhythms, which, in our opinion, parallels a similar functional relationship existing between the two neurovegetative outflows. In short, this exploration into the frequency domain is not motivated by serendipity but, on the contrary, by a very concrete aim to find new tools to interprete physiological and pathophysiological cardiovascular conditions.

RESULTS

As a premise, it should be pointed out that total spectral power, i.e., variance of the duration of the R-R interval, seems to be significantly correlated to age, variance decreasing with increasing age.[20] Variance alone does not provide a useful tool for interpreting the state of the sympathovagal interaction. In fact, although in several conditions of sympathetic activation variance decreases and, inversely, increases during vagal excitations, there are other instances in which a consistent change in sympathovagal balance is not signaled by changes in variance.[26] In addition, large differences often exist in the total power among individual spectra. It is mainly for this reason that spectral components will be presented both in absolute units, which also reflect the absolute value of variance, and in normalized units (NU, obtained as already explained in the Methods section), in order to better compare data obtained in various conditions and from different individuals. Moreover, normalized units are well indicative of the state of the sympathovagal balance.[20]

Experimental Alterations of the Sympathovagal Balance

In our studies in man, various maneuvers are used to shift the sympathovagal balance towards sympathetic predominance such as passive tilt to 90°,[20,26] light

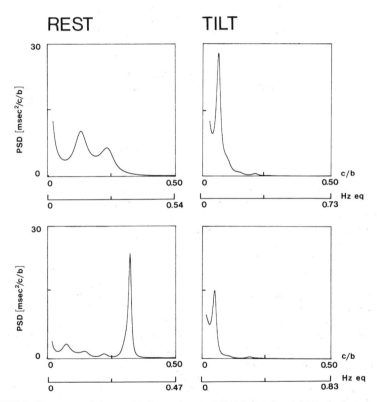

FIGURE 2. Representative example of autospectra of R-R interval variability during spontaneous breathing (top panels) and during controlled respiration, at 20/minute (bottom panels). Note that, with controlled respiration at rest, the relative power of the high frequency component becomes predominant. (From Reference 20 with permission.)

physical exercise,[24,27] mental stress.[28] Since the very initial attempts,[29] it appeared clearly that in normal conditions these maneuvers are always accompanied by a relative increase in the power of the LF component and in the LF/HF ratio, and by a decrease of the HF component (FIGURE 2, upper panels).[20] Vice versa, vagal predominance is mainly obtained with metronome breathing up to 20/minute.[20] In the case of FIGURE 2 (lower panels) it is clear that during metronome breathing there is, at rest, a predominant and narrow HF component, while during tilt the LF increase is less pronounced than during spontaneous breathing, all signs indicative of an enhanced vagal tone. Other maneuvers used to increase vagal tone include water immersion of the face and head down tilt.

In the conscious dog, sympathetic activation is obtained by moderate hypotension (produced by intravenous nitroglycerin infusion,[20,30] by nonhypotensive regional myocardial ischemia,[30] by physical exercise, by acute baroreceptor deactivation (Rimoldi et al., work in progress). Conversely, the normal predominance of vagal tone is further increased by baroreceptor stimulation (produced by phenylephrine infusion).[30]

An additional experimental approach includes the simultaneous power spectral analysis of the R-R and of the neural discharge directly recorded from the sympathetic cardiac nerves in the course of acute experiments on cats.[31]

Thus the methodological soundness of this simple attributive stage has been checked throughout quite numerous and different models: the collected data always fit the basic hypothesis that the HF rhythm is a marker of vagal tone, while the LF spectral component is a marker of sympathetic tone. As to the analysis of the neural mechanisms involved in the transmission of these rhythms to the various cardiovascular targets, an analysis that has absorbed much of our recent work, we have to refer to other articles.[20,30,32]

The Exploration of Various Pathophysiological States

In parallel the same approach has been applied to the study of pathophysiological conditions known to be accompanied by an altered neurovegetative regulation. In a noninvasive study using exclusively the spectral analysis of heart rate variability,[33] it was found that in hypertensive subjects LF was greater (LF = 68 ± 3 versus 54 ± 3 NU) and HF smaller (HF 24 ± 3 versus 33 ± 2 NU) than in normotensive age-matched controls. Additionally, passive tilt produced in hypertensive patients smaller increases in LF (LF 6.3 ± 3 versus 26 ± 2 NU) and decreases in HF (HF = −7.5 ± 2 versus −22 ± 2 NU) than in normotensive controls (FIGURE 3). Furthermore, the values of LF at rest and the altered effects of tilt on LF and HF were significantly correlated with the degree of the hypertensive state. In short, with this noninvasive approach it was possible to support Pickering's hypothesis of hypertension as an abnormal "quantity"[34] with the continuum in the markers of sympathetic activity found from normotension to hypertension. With a more sophisticated and invasive approach it was also possible to prove that in hypertensive patients the gain of the relationship between heart period and systolic arterial pressure was reduced, as an additional sign of enhanced sympathetic tone.[24]

Similarly, on the basis of a simple spectral analysis of heart rate variability, it was found that in a population of patients two weeks after myocardial infarction the LF component was significantly greater (LF = 69 ± 2 versus 53 ± 3 NU) and the HF component significantly smaller (HF = 17 ± 1 versus 35 ± 3 NU) than in age-matched control subjects:[26] thus there were clear signs of a sympathetic predominance (FIGURE 4). At the same time the LF component was not further increased by tilt. At 6 and 12 months after myocardial infarction there was a progressive decrease in the LF and a progressive increase in the HF component (FIGURE 4).

Evident signs of sympathetic activation as inferred from a sudden increase in LF and a decrease in HF were also noticed in the course of spontaneous asymptomatic transient myocardial ischemia (FIGURE 5) (Lombardi et al., work in progress), a finding also reported by other authors.[35] Thus it was possible to confirm in the clinical set the existence of an increased sympathetic activity likely to be reflexly initiated by myocardial ischemia. In experimental terms a cardiocardiac sympathetic reflex elicited by transient coronary occlusion was described 20 years ago:[36] subsequently it was proven that it was independent of baroreceptive mechanisms and, vice versa, mainly dependent on the excitation of the sympathetic cardiac afferent fibers.[37] During these years a similar reflex was also found by numerous other authors including those[38] who had previously negated its existence.[39] The possibility of monitoring with noninvasive

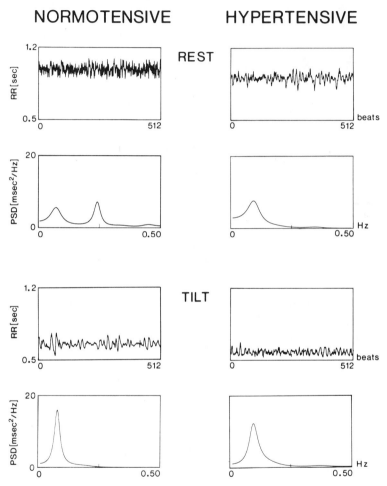

FIGURE 3. Spectral analysis of R-R interval variability in a normotensive (left panel) and a hypertensive subject (right panel), both at rest (top panels) and during tilt (bottom panels). Note the near absence of a high frequency component at rest in the hypertensive subject. (From Reference 33 with permission.)

techniques these indices of sympathovagal balance in conditions most often characterized by life-threatening arrhythmias, which in part depend on neural factors,[40] appears to open new perspectives in pathophysiological interpretation and therapy.

This noninvasive approach has also proven very useful in assessing the existence of peripheral neuropathies such as those occurring in diabetic patients. In a recent study,

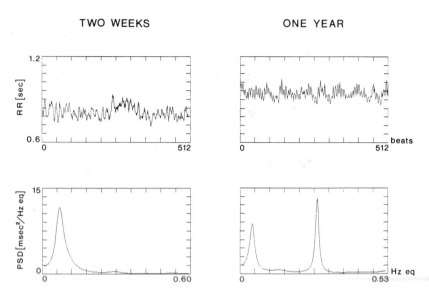

FIGURE 4. Tachogram (top) and autospectra (bottom) in a patient after acute myocardial infarction. At two weeks after the acute episode, there is a predominant low frequency component. At one year, two clearly separated low and high frequency components are present. (From Reference 26 with permission.)

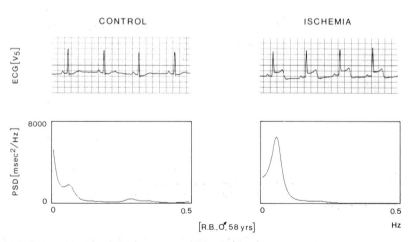

FIGURE 5. Example of the changes in R-R interval variability produced by an episode of spontaneous asymptomatic transient myocardial ischemia in a patient. Notice the large predominance of the low frequency component during the ischemic episode (From Lombardi *et al.*, work in progress.)

we found that patients with uncomplicated diabetes, as compared to controls, were characterized by a reduced R-R variance at rest,[41] as already reported by others,[42,43] and by an altered response to tilt of spectral indices of sympathetic activation and of vagal withdrawal.

The possible existence of a functional damage in the cardiac innervation has been similarly explored in patients with Chagas disease[44] and again clear signs were found of an altered response of spectral indices to an active orthostatic position.

Continuous Assessment of Sympathovagal Balance

As already mentioned in the Methods section, the spectral analysis can be carried out on Holter recordings for the 24 hour period. It becomes thus evident that the

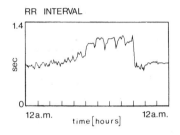

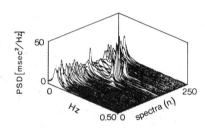

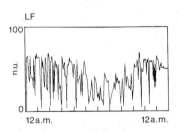

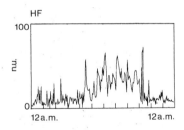

FIGURE 6. Spectral analysis of R-R interval variability in a normotensive subject during a 24 hour period. The R-R interval series (left) and all the autospectra (right) which describe the entire 24 hour period are displayed in the top panels. In the bottom panels the power of the LF and HF components is shown in normalized units.

sympathovagal balance changes a great deal during the 24 hours. In particular from the example of FIGURE 6 it can be appreciated that during the day there is a marked predominance of the LF component while, during the night, both components are evident, HF being predominant. The sympathovagal balance undergoes both a clear circadian rhythm and continuous fast oscillations (FIGURE 6, bottom panels) as revealed also by the assessment of the gain of the heart period–sytolic arterial pressure relationship.[24]

These changes in neurovegetative tone might obviously be of paramount importance in influencing the circadian variation of acute cardiovascular events.[45]

The Frequency Domain and the New Perspectives

The exploration in the frequency domain of the neurovegetative cardiovascular regulation, although based on indirect indices, seems to furnish a unitary vision which could not be provided by the assemblage of surely more specific but fragmented pieces of information. Such a unitiary evaluation might be crucial for the interpretation of still largely unknown territories such as those corresponding to the "autonomic disturbance" of the early phases of acute myocardial infarction[46] or to the moments preceding sudden cardiac death.[47] Prevention and therapy are likely to benefit from a more holistic interpretation.

REFERENCES

1. SNELLEN, H. A. 1984. History of Cardiology. Donker Academic Publications. Rotterdam, The Netherlands.
2. HALES, S. 1733. Statical Essays: Containing Haemastaticks. Innys, Manby and Woodward. London, England. (Volume 2).
3. KOEPCHEN, H. P. 1984. History of studies and concepts of blood pressure waves. In Mechanisms of Blood Pressure Waves. K. Miyakawa, H. P. Koepchen & C. Polosa, Eds.: 3–23. Japan Science Society Press. Tokyo, Japan.
4. MAYER, S. 1876. Studien zur Physiologie des Herzens und der Blutgefässe: 5. Abhandlung: Über spontane Blutdruckschwankungen. Sber. Akad. Wiss. Wien, 3. Abt. **74:** 281–307.
5. ADRIAN, E. D., D. W. BRONK & G. PHILLIPS. 1932. Discharges in mammalian sympathetic nerves. J. Physiol. **74:** 115–133.
6. FERNANDEZ DE MOLINA, A. & E. R. PERL. 1965. Sympathetic activity and the systemic circulation in the spinal cat. J. Physiol. **181:** 82–102.
7. LANGHORST, P., G. SCHULZ & M. LAMBERTZ. 1984. Oscillating neuronal network of the "common brainstem system." In Mechanisms of Blood Pressure Waves. K. Miyakawa, H. P. Koepchen & C. Polosa, Eds.: 257–275. Japan Science Society Press. Tokyo, Japan.
8. KOEPCHEN, H. P., D. KLÜSSENDORF & D. SOMMER. 1981. Neurophysiological background of central neural cardiovascular-respiratory coordination: basic remarks and experimental approach. J. Auton. Nerv. Syst. **3:** 335–368.
9. PREISS, G. & C. POLOSA. 1974. Patterns of sympathetic neuron activity associated with Mayer waves. Am. J. Physiol. **226:** 724–730.
10. POLOSA, C. 1984. Central nervous system origin of some types of Mayer waves. In Mechanisms of Blood Pressure Waves. K. Miyakawa, H. P. Koepchen & C. Polosa, Eds.: 277–292. Japan Science Society Press. Tokyo, Japan.
11. BARMAN, S. M. & G. L. GEBBER. 1980. Sympathetic nerve rhythm of brain stem origin. Am. J. Physiol. **239:** R42–R47.
12. MALLIANI, A. 1982. Cardiovascular sympathetic afferent fibers. Rev. Physiol. Biochem. Pharmacol. **94:** 11–74.
13. EWING, D. J., J. M. M. NEILSON & P. TRAVIS. 1984. New method for assessing cardiac parasympathetic activity using 24 hour electrocardiograms. Br. Heart J. **52:** 396–402.
14. KLEIGER, R. E., J. P. MILLER, J. T. BIGGER, A. J. MOSS and the Multicenter Postinfarction Research Group. 1987. Decreased heart rate variability and its association with increased mortality after acute myocardial infarction. Am. J. Cardiol. **59:** 256–262.
15. COOLEY, J. W. & J. W. TUKEY. 1965. An algorithm for the machine calculation of complex Fourier Series. Math. Comput. **19:** 297–301.
16. SAYERS, B. MCA. 1973. Analysis of heart rate variability. Ergonomics **16:** 17–32.
17. AKSELROD, S., D. GORDON, F. A. UBEL, D. C. SHANNON, A. C. BARGER & R. J. COHEN. 1981. Power spectrum analysis of heart rate fluctuation: a quantitative probe of beat-to-beat cardiovascular control. Science **213:** 220–222.
18. CHESS, G. F., R. M. K. TAM & F. R. CALARESU. 1975. Influence of cardiac neural inputs on rhythmic variations of heart period in the cat. Am. J. Physiol. **228:** 775–780.
19. POMERANZ, P., R. J. B. MACAULAY, M. A. CAUDIL, I. KUTZ, D. ADAM, D. GORDON, K. M.

KILBORN, A. C. BARGER, D. C. SHANNON, R. J. COHEN & H. BENSON. 1985. Assessment of autonomic function in humans by heart rate spectral analysis. Am. J. Physiol. **248:** H151–H153.

20. PAGANI, M., F. LOMBARDI, S. GUZZETTI, O. RIMOLDI, R. FURLAN, P. PIZZINELLI, G. SANDRONE, G. MALFATTO, S. DELL'ORTO, E. PICCALUGA, M. TURIEL, G. BASELLI, S. CERUTTI & A. MALLIANI. 1986. Power spectral analysis of heart rate and arterial pressure variabilities as a marker of sympathovagal interaction in man and conscious dog. Circ. Res. **59:** 178–193.

21. SAUL, J. P., P. ALBRECHT, R. D. BERGER & R. J. COHEN. 1987. Analysis of long term heart rate variability: methods, 1/f scaling and implications. *In* Computers in Cardiology: 419–422. IEEE Computer Society Press. Silver Spring, Md.

22. BASELLI, G., S. CERUTTI, S. CIVARDI, D. LIBERATI, F. LOMBARDI, A. MALLIANI & M. PAGANI. 1986. Spectral and cross-spectral analysis of heart rate and arterial blood pressure variability signals. Comput. Biomed. Res. **19:** 520–534.

23. CERUTTI, S., G. BASELLI, S. CIVARDI, R. FURLAN, F. LOMBARDI, A. MALLIANI, M. MERRI & M. PAGANI. 1987. Spectral analysis of heart rate and arterial blood pressure variability signals for physiological and clinical purposes. *In* Computers in Cardiology: 435–438. IEEE Computer Society Press. Washington D.C.

24. PAGANI, M., V. SOMERS, R. FURLAN, S. DELL'ORTO, J. CONWAY, G. BASELLI, S. CERUTTI, P. SLEIGHT & A. MALLIANI. 1988. Changes in autonomic regulation induced by physical training in mild hypertension. Hypertension **12:** 600–610.

25. BASELLI, G., S. CERUTTI, S. CIVARDI, A. MALLIANI & M. PAGANI. 1988. Cardiovascular variability signals: towards the identification of a closed-loop model of the neural control mechanisms. IEEE Trans. Biomed. Eng. **35:** 1033–1046.

26. LOMBARDI, F., G. SANDRONE, S. PERNPRUNER, R. SALA, M. GARIMOLDI, S. CERUTTI, G. BASELLI, M. PAGANI & A. MALLIANI. 1987. Heart rate variability as an index of sympathovagal interaction after acute myocardial infarction. Am. J. Cardiol. **60:** 1239–1245.

27. FURLAN, R., S. DELL'ORTO, W. CRIVELLARO, P. PIZZINELLI, S. CERUTTI, F. LOMBARDI, M. PAGANI, & A. MALLIANI. 1987. Effects of tilt and treadmill exercise on short-term variability in systolic arterial pressure in hypertensive men. J. Hypertens. **5:** S423–S425.

28. PAGANI M., R. FURLAN, P. PIZZINELLI, W. CRIVELLARO, S. CERUTTI & A. MALLIANI. 1989. Spectral analysis of R-R and arterial pressure variabilities to assess sympatho-vagal interaction during mental stress. J. Hypertens. 7(Suppl. 6): S14–S15.

29. BROVELLI, M., G. BASELLI, S. CERUTTI, S. GUZZETTI, D. LIBERATI, F. LOMBARDI, A. MALLIANI, M. PAGANI & P. PIZZINELLI. 1983. Computerized analysis of an experimental validation of neurophysiological models of heart rate control. *In* Computers in Cardiology: 205–208. IEEE Computer Society Press. Silver Spring, Md.

30. RIMOLDI, O., S. PIERINI, A. FERRARI, S. CERUTTI, M. PAGANI & A. MALLIANI. Analysis of the short term oscillations of RR and arterial pressure in conscious dogs. Am. J. Physiol. (In press.)

31. LOMBARDI, F., N. MONTANO, M. L. FINOCCHIARO, T. GNECCHI RUSCONE, G. BASELLI, S. CERUTTI & A. MALLIANI. Spectral analysis of sympathetic discharge in decerebrate cats. J. Auton. Nerv. Syst. (In press.)

32. MALLIANI, A., M. PAGANI, F. LOMBARDI & S. CERUTTI. Clinical and experimental evaluation of sympatho-vagal interaction: power spectral analysis of heart rate and arterial pressure variabilities *In* Reflex Control of the Circulation. I. H. Zucker & V. P. Gilmore, Eds.: The Telford Press. Caldwell, New Jersey. (In press.)

33. GUZZETTI, S., E. PICCALUGA, R. CASATI, S. CERUTTI, F. LOMBARDI, M. PAGANI & A. MALLIANI. 1988. Sympathetic predominance in essential hypertension: a study employing spectral analysis of heart rate variability. J. Hypertens. **6:** 711–717.

34. PICKERING, G. 1978. Normotension and hypertension: the mysterious variability of the false. Am. J. Med. **65:** 561–563.

35. BERNARDI, L., C. LUMINA, M. R. FERRARI, L. RICORDI, I. VANDEA, P. FRATINO, M. PIVA & G. FINARDI. 1988. Relationship between fluctuation in heart rate and asymptomatic nocturnal ischaemia. Int. J. Cardiol. **20:** 39–51.

36. MALLIANI, A., P. J. SCHWARTZ & A. ZANCHETTI. 1969. A sympathetic reflex elicited by experimental coronary occlusion. Am. J. Physiol. 217: 703–709.
37. LOMBARDI, F., C. CASALONE, P. DELLA BELLA, G. MALFATTO, M. PAGANI & A. MALLIANI. 1984. Global versus regional myocardial ischaemia: differences in cardiovascular and sympathetic responses in cats. Cardiovasc. Res. 18: 14–25.
38. MINISI, A. J., K. A. ELLENBOGEN & M. D. THAMES. 1988. Activation of cardiac sympathetic afferents during coronary occlusion: new insight into the mechanism of silent ischemia. Circulation 78(suppl. II): 701.
39. FELDER, R. B. & M. D. THAMES. 1981. The cardiocardiac sympathetic reflex during coronary occlusion in anesthetized dogs. Circ. Res. 48: 685–692.
40. MALLIANI, A., P. J. SCHWARTZ & A. ZANCHETTI. 1980. Neural mechanisms in life-threatening arrhythmias. Am. Heart J. 100: 705–715.
41. PAGANI, M., G. MALFATTO, S. PIERINI, R. CASATI, A. M. MASU, M. POLI, S. GUZZETTI, F. LOMBARDI, S. CERUTTI & A. MALLIANI. 1988. Spectral analysis of heart rate variability in the assessment of autonomic diabetic neuropathy. J. Autonom. Nerv. Syst. 23: 143–153.
42. KITNEY, R. I., S. BYRNE, M. E. EDMONDS, P. J. WATKINS & V. C. ROBERTS. 1982. Heart rate variability in the assessment of autonomic diabetic neuropathy. Automedica 4: 155–167.
43. LISHNER, M., S. AKSELROD, V. MOR AVI, O. OZ, M. DIVON & M. RAVID. 1987. Spectral analysis of heart rate fluctuations. A non-invasive, sensitive method for the early diagnosis of autonomic neuropathy in diabetes mellitus. J. Auton. Nerv. Syst. 19: 119–125.
44. GUZZETTI, S., D. JOSA, M. PECIS, L. BONURA, M. PROSDOCIMI & A. MALLIANI. Effects of sympathetic activation in heart rate variability in Chagas patients. J. Auton. Nerv. Syst. (In press.)
45. MULLER, J. E., G. H. TOFLER & P. H. STONE. 1989. Circadian variation and triggers of onset of acute cardiovascular disease. Circulation 79: 733–743.
46. WEBB, S. W., A. A. ADGEY & J. F. PANTRIDGE. 1972. Autonomic disturbance at onset of acute myocardial infarction. Br. Med. J. 3: 89–92.
47. LECLERCQ, J. F., P. MAISONBLANCHE, B. CAUCHEMEZ & P. COUMEL. 1988. Respective role of sympathetic tone and of cardiac pauses in the genesis of 62 cases of ventricular fibrillation recorded during Holter monitoring. Eur. Heart J. 9: 1276–1283.

Autonomic Nervous System and Arrhythmias[a]

GAETANO M. DE FERRARI AND PETER J. SCHWARTZ[b]

Arrhythmia Study Unit
Department of Medicine II
University of Milan
Milan, Italy

INTRODUCTION

Despite the recent trend toward a decline in cardiovascular mortality,[1] sudden cardiac death still represents a major health problem. The electrocardiogram may contain information helpful for the identification of individuals at greater risk, a key factor for an adequate preventive strategy. In this chapter we will examine the possibility that analysis of the autonomic control of heart rate may indeed provide such information and that it might also allow a better understanding of the mechanisms involved in arrhythmogenesis.

The evidence for a tight relationship between the autonomic nervous system and malignant arrhythmias has progressively increased over the past several years. As a consequence, targeted therapeutic approaches such as antiadrenergic interventions have been successfully utilized in the prevention of sudden death.

The limitations and shortcomings of a traditional approach with antiarrhythmic drugs in the management of patients affected by ischemic heart disease and cardiac arrhythmias have been dramatically highlighted in a recent report.[2,3] These results give further impulse to the exploitation of the influence of the autonomic nervous system on arrhytmias for the development of a more accurate prognosis and a more effective therapy.

The impact of sympathetic activity on arrhythmogenesis has been largely discussed in previous volumes of the Academy, both in terms of mechanisms and of therapeutic implications.[4-6] Here we will concentrate more on the relatively less explored relationship between the parasympathetic nervous system and malignant cardiac arrhythmias.

SYMPATHETIC HYPERACTIVITY AND SYMPATHETIC IMBALANCE

Clear evidence exists to indicate that an excessive sympathetic activity is detrimental in the setting of acute myocardial ischemia.[4,7-10] The negative effect is particularly evident if the release of norepinephrine is nonhomogeneous. Some degree of dishomogeneity occurs even in physiologic conditions due to the sparse distribution of sympathetic nerve terminals, and it is greatly enhanced if anatomic or functional dishomogeneity of innervation exists in parts of the ventricles. This has been shown to occur as a consequence of myocardial infarction[11] and may significantly contribute to the incidence of malignant arrhythmia in this time period.

[a]Supported in part by Grant HL 33727 from the National Institutes of Health.
[b]Author to whom correspondence should be addressed, at Clinica Medica II—Pad. Sacco, Via F. Sforza 35, 20122 Milano, Italy.

To test the potential efficacy of several pharmacologic interventions in the prevention of life-threatening arrhythmias we have utilized an acute, feline animal model that combines grossly inhomogeneous sympathetic activity (electrical stimulation of the left stellate ganglion after right stellectomy) and acute transient myocardial ischemia.[9, 12-14] The overall results are shown in FIGURE 1. Class I antiarrhythmic drugs have shown no beneficial effect in this preparation, whereas calcium antagonists and amiodarone have proved to be extremely effective. Beta adrenergic blockers have provided effective although incomplete protection against malignant arrhythmia; the addition of alpha blocking agents whenever beta blockade proved ineffective almost always provided complete protection. The specular observation was made in the more

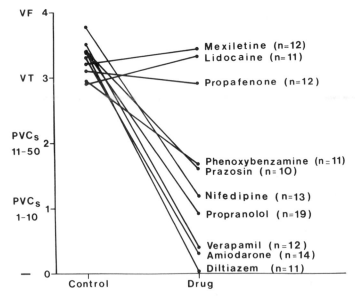

FIGURE 1. Effect of different drugs on the arrhythmias induced by coronary artery occlusion and left stellate ganglion stimulation in the acute feline model ($n = 125$). Ventricular arrhythmias are arbitrarily graded as follows: 0 = no premature ventricular contractions (PVCs); 1 = 1 to 10 PVCs; 2 = 11 to 50 PVCs; 3 = VT (defined as at least five consecutive PVCs); 4 = VF.

frequent condition of failure with alpha blockade alone. The efficacy of combined alpha and beta blockade underlines that the adverse influence of sympathetic hyperactivity is not solely beta mediated. This concept is also useful to explain the success of selective sympathetic denervation such as that achieved by high thoracic left sympathectomy after failure of medical therapy with beta-blockers.[6,10]

PARASYMPATHETIC ACTIVITY—EXPERIMENTAL BACKGROUND

Until the 70s it was largely thought that, in the setting of acute myocardial ischemia, vagal activity would be, if anything, detrimental. This was partly based on the incorrect assumption of a lack of parasympathetic innervation of the ventricles, and on the observation that very slow heart rates in nonischemic hearts would increase the dispersion of refractoriness and decrease ventricular fibrillation threshold.[15] However, several studies have subsequently shown that this is not the case in the setting of acute ischemia. Indeed, vagal stimulation was found to be beneficial in both canine and feline acute animal preparations.[16–18] More recently, we have shown that vagal stimulation reduces reperfusion-induced malignant arrhythmias, which are often refractory to most interventions.[19] The issue of vagal hyperactivity, however, received little attention for several years, and it was not clear whether these results were laboratory findings of mere research interest or had the potential for clinical application.

In the attempt to bridge this gap we explored the significance of vagal tone and reflexes in an animal model for sudden cardiac death that has provided during the last several years relevant pathophysiologic information.[20] In this experimental preparation conscious dogs with a healed anterior myocardial infarction undergo a submaximal exercise stress test coupled with a two-minute occlusion of the circumflex coronary artery.

This clinically relevant combination of transient myocardial ischemia at the time of physiologically elevated sympathetic activity results in ventricular fibrillation in approximately 55%–60% of the animals. The outcome during the exercise and ischemia test (ventricular fibrillation in "susceptible" animals, but not in "resistant" animals) is highly reproducible for up to three months, allowing internal control studies.

It was observed that the heart rate response to coronary artery occlusion was significantly different in susceptible and resistant dogs.[20,21] Whereas the susceptible dogs further increase an already physiologically elevated heart rate, the resistant tend to show a heart rate decrease. This decrease occurs despite continuation of exercise, is prevented by atropine, and suggests therefore the presence of dominant vagal reflexes.

Based on this finding, the hypothesis was made that the presence of strong vagal reflexes could be associated with a greater likelihood of survival during the exercise and ischemia test and that analysis of other autonomic, and primarily vagal, reflexes might contain information on the susceptibility to arrhythmia during acute myocardial ischemia. Accordingly, we chose to examine the relationship between baroreflex sensitivity (BRS) and susceptibility to sudden cardiac death in our animal model.[22] BRS was assessed, as described by Smyth et al.[23] Phenylephrine (10 μg/kg) was used to raise systolic arterial pressure by 30–50 mmHg; each R-R interval was plotted as a function of the preceding systolic pressure; a least-square-fit linear regression was performed, and BRS was expressed as the slope of the linear regression line.

Following the initial observations,[22] the results have been confirmed and extended and relate now to 192 dogs with a healed myocardial infarction.[24] BRS, evaluated few days before the exercise and ischemia test, was significantly lower among susceptible than resistant dogs (9.1 ± 6.0 vs. 17.7 ± 6.5 mseconds/mmHg, $p < 0.0001$). Analysis of the individual data, presented in FIGURE 2, allows the calculation of risk for sudden death with respect to BRS measured four weeks after myocardial infarction. The risk increased from 20% of dogs having a BRS >15 mseconds/mmHg to 91% for dogs having BRS <9 mseconds/mmHg. TABLE 1 provides details about the inverse relationship between BRS and risk of ventricular fibrillation in this large population of animals.

These experiments clearly indicate that analysis of the electrocardiogram during a simple reflex response, such as phenylephrine injection, allows the identification of a group of post–myocardial infarction animals at very high risk for ventricular fibrillation during a new ischemic episode.

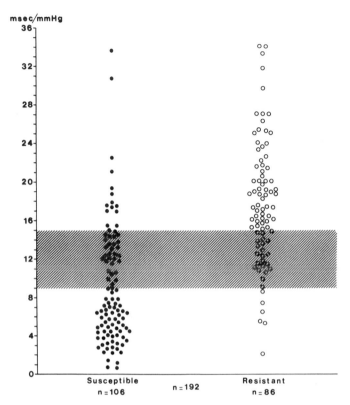

FIGURE 2. Plot of baroreflex sensitivity in 192 dogs after infarction and its relation with susceptibility to sudden death. Hatched area is an arbitrary gray zone. Less than 9 mseconds/mmHg, 91% of the dogs were susceptible to sudden death, whereas greater than 15 mseconds/mmHg, 80% of the dogs survived during the exercise and ischemia test. Note the large number of animals with baroreflex sensitivity less than 9 mseconds/mmHg. (From Reference 24 with permission of the American Heart Association, Inc.)

We also investigated whether the analysis of BRS in animals prior to myocardial infarction could provide predictive information about their outcome following either the infarction itself or the subsequent acute ischemia. For this purpose 23 susceptible dogs were analyzed together with 17 animals that died suddenly in the first four weeks after myocardial infarction and in which autopsy failed to show other cause than infarction. In this group of animals BRS before myocardial infarction was lower compared to the resistant dogs (16.2 ± 5.9 vs. 22.2 ± 6.2 mseconds/mmHg, $p < 0.001$). Thus, although considerable overlap exists among the two groups (FIGURE 3), it seems that analysis of BRS can identify high risk animals also *before* myocardial infarction.

The studies on BRS provided insights on vagal reflexes and raised the possibility that similar information might be acquired by analysis of markers of vagal tone. Heart rate variability (HRV), expressed as the standard deviation of the mean R-R interval, is a global index of vagal tone to the sinus node[25] quite suitable for research purposes and easily applied in the clinic. Therefore, we have assessed the predictive value of this measurement in our animal model.[26] In 17 susceptible dogs HRV, measured before the exercise test, was significantly lower than in an equal number of resistant dogs (141 ± 10 vs. 189 ± 15 mseconds, $p < 0.05$). On the other hand, no difference was seen between the two groups of animals, in the HRV measured *before* myocardial infarction. This finding, together with the baroreceptor data, suggests that after myocardial infarction both tonic vagal activity and vagal reflexes convey information on the susceptibility to malignant arrhythmias, whereas in healthy individuals it may be necessary to "stress" the system to obtain useful insights for risk stratification.

All these data, however, may only suggest a role for vagal tone and reflexes in the protection from lethal arrhythmia, but provide no direct evidence for this effect. Therefore, we have performed three different studies with this purpose.

In the first of these studies, atropine was given to a large series of resistant animals to test whether removal of muscarinic effects would induce ventricular arrhythmias.[27] Preliminary data indicate novel occurrence of arrhythmia or worsening of the pattern in 50% of the dogs, notably the occurrence of ventricular fibrillation in almost 25%. The animals in which atropine caused the appearance of ventricular fibrillation were characterized, in the control test, by a marked heart rate decrease which was absent in the other dogs. Therefore, in a significant minority of post–myocardial infarction animals undergoing transient myocardial ischemia, the presence of adequate vagal tone and reflexes does result in protection from sudden death.

In a further study we utilized a technique for direct electrical stimulation of the vagus nerve in the conscious state, recently developed in our laboratories.[28,29] Two groups of susceptible dogs were utilized. They underwent either a further exercise and ischemia test with no additional intervention (control group) or a trial in which right vagal stimulation was started few seconds after the beginning of the occlusion. Ventricular fibrillation occurred in 23/25 (92%) control animals but only in 3 of 15 (20%) vagally stimulated dogs.[30] An example of vagally mediated protection is shown in FIGURE 4. Vagal stimulation produced a mean reduction of 80 beats (b)/minute from 216 ± 33 to 136 ± 29 b/minute. Experiments performed with atrial and ventricular pacing indicate that the heart rate reduction played an important but not exclusive role in this protective effect. Therefore, electrically produced vagal hyperactivity is capable of drastically reducing the incidence of lethal arrhythmia in this conscious animal model.

Finally, we are performing studies with direct measurements of vagal activity through single fiber neural recording of efferent activity in the right cardiac vagal branch of anesthetized cats. We are, therefore, directly testing the hypothesis that animals that do not develop ventricular fibrillation during ischemia respond to both intravenous phenilephrine and ischemia itself, with a greater increase in cardiac vagal

TABLE 1. Baroreflex Sensitivity and Sudden Death in Dogs after Myocardial Infarction[a]

Baroreflex Sensitivity (mseconds/mm Hg)	Sudden death (n)	Percentage
>20	4/32	12
>15	15/73	20
9–15	28/50	56
<9	62/68	91
<4	23/24	96

[a]$n = 192$ dogs. (Reproduced from Reference 24 by permission of the American Heart Association, Inc.)

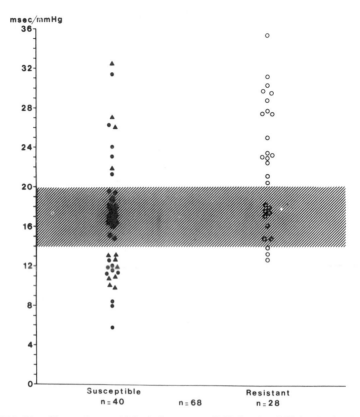

FIGURE 3. Plot of baroreflex sensitivity before myocardial infarction (MI) in 68 animals and its relation with susceptibility to sudden death after MI. In this case, the arbitrary grey zone extends from 14 to 20 mseconds/mmHg. Full circle = animals susceptible to sudden death during the exercise and ischemia test. Full triangle = animals that died suddenly during the first 4 weeks after MI. Open circle = Animals that survived during the exercise and ischemia test. Note how few animals have baroreflex sensitivity less than 9 mseconds/mmHg. (From Reference 24 with permission of the American Heart Association, Inc.)

nerve activity. A baroreceptor response is assessed, by intravenous phenylephrine, and the animals undergo left anterior descending coronary artery occlusion. FIGURE 5 shows an example of neural recording from a single cardiac vagal fiber and the relationship between activity and blood pressure curve. So far six cats survived the occlusion, whereas six cats died of ventricular fibrillation within the first few minutes of ischemia.[31] The two groups differed in their response to phenylephrine. For a similar blood pressure rise, vagal activity increased much more ($p < 0.05$) among survivors than among ventricular fibrillation cats (281% in the former, from 1.2 ± 0.2 to 4.1 ± 0.9 impulses/second, vs. 68% from 1.7 ± 0.3 to 2.7 ± 0.5 impulses/second in the latter), as shown in FIGURE 6. During coronary artery occlusion, vagal activity in the first two minutes did not change in ventricular fibrillation cats, while it increased in survivors by an average of 159% (from 2.1 ± 0.9 to 3.2 ± 1.1 impulses/second, $p < 0.05$). Therefore, whereas tonic vagal activity was similar in the two groups, the animals that survived coronary artery occlusion activated more powerful vagal reflexes in response to both blood pressure increases and acute myocardial ischemia. These converging findings on the protective role of vagal hyperactivity during acute myocardial ischemia suggest the opportunity to evaluate a different pharmacologic approach for the interaction with the autonomic nervous system, namely, direct muscarinic activation. Indeed, we are assessing the effects of the muscarinic agonist oxotremorine on the incidence of arrhythmias induced by the combination of transient myocardial ischemia and sympathetic hyperactivity in the acute feline animal model previously described (Reference 9 and FIGURE 1). Preliminary results[32] indicate that muscarinic activation is an effective antiarrhythmic approach in this model, one that affords a protection similar to propranolol. A beneficial effect is still present when the negative chronotropic effect is controlled by atrial pacing.

CLINICAL STUDIES

Do these experimental findings have a clinical counterpart? Most of the described studies are still in progress, so that several steps are still necessary before the suggested approaches can be potentially transferred to man. However, a few clinical investigations, which originate directly from the experimental studies, have been undertaken with the purpose of exploring possible clinical correlates and gathering new information for potentially direct application. Most of these studies deal with the value of information concerning the autonomic control of cardiac function and are directly

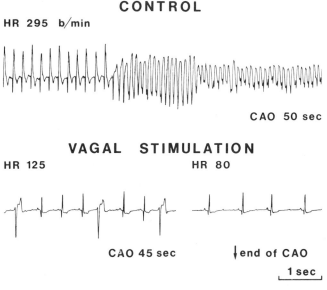

FIGURE 4. Vagally mediated protection from ventricular fibrillation. In the control test a ventricular tachycardia that degenerated into ventricular fibrillation occurred 50 seconds after the beginning of coronary artery occlusion (CAO). In the test with vagal stimulation only a few isolated premature ventricular contractions were observed.

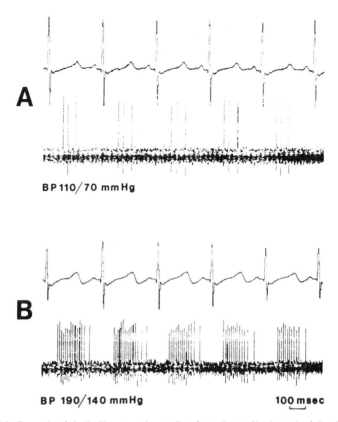

BP 110/70 mm Hg

BP 190/140 mm Hg   **100 msec**

FIGURE 5. Example of single fiber neural recording from the cardiac branch of the right vagus nerve in an anesthetized cat. Neural discharge is pulse synchronous and increases ar blood pressure (BP) increase.

obtained from surface electrocardiogram in the assessment of risk for cardiac death in patients with coronary artery disease.

One study[33] had the objective to examine the relationship between BRS, several clinical and hemodynamic variables, and mortality during a 24-month follow-up period of 78 patients who had suffered a first myocardial infarction 30 days before entering the study.[33] FIGURES 7 and 8 show two extreme examples of baroreflex sensitivity curves in these patients.

The BRS of the entire population was 7.8 ± 4.9 mseconds/mmHg. BRS was lower among patients with an inferior myocardial infarction (6.1 ± 3.3 vs. 8.9 ± 5.8 mseconds/mmHg, $p = 0.03$), with a three- versus a one-vessel disease (4.8 ± 2.7 vs. 7.1 ± 3.1 mseconds/mmHg, $p = 0.04$), and with episodes of ventricular tachycardia during 24 hour Holter recording or during an exercise stress test (5.1 ± 3.0 vs. 8.3 ± 5.1 msecond/mmHg, $p = 0.03$). There was no correlation between BRS and left ventricular ejection fraction or with mean pulmonary capillary wedge pressure at peak exercise.

During the two-year mean follow-up, there were seven cardiovascular deaths and four were sudden. The BRS of the deceased patients were strikingly lower than those of the survivors (2.5 ± 1.5 vs. 8.2 ± 4.8 mseconds/mmHg, $p = 0.004$). This is shown in FIGURE 9. The overall mortality, 9.2%, is rather low and this reflects the fact that all patients were below age 65, had had a first myocardial infarction, and had also been selected on the basis of their capability to perform a maximal exercise test without any supporting therapy. They were therefore already identified as a low-risk group. Nonetheless, analysis of BRS allowed the identification within this population of a subgroup at very high risk. When mortality was calculated in respect to the absence or presence of a markedly depressed BRS (<3.0 mseconds/mmHg), it was found to vary from 2.9% to 50%. Among patients with a reduced left ventricular ejection fraction, mortality increased from 10% (2 of 20) to 50% (3 of 6) according to the simultaneous absence or presence of a markedly reduced BRS (FIGURE 10).

This study provides the first in-depth analysis of the relationship between a specific autonomic reflex, such as baroreflex sensitivity, and several clinical variables of importance in the post–myocardial infarction risk stratification. Furthermore, it raises the possibility that analysis of the electrocardiogram during a baroreceptor reflex test in postinfarction patients may contribute to a more accurate identification of individuals at high risk for subsequent mortality.

The finding that a depressed BRS is associated with an increased risk does not allow us to conclude that a depressed BRS is an independent risk factor. Analyzing the characteristics of the deceased patients we may just speculate that, although the majority of patients with depressed BRS who subsequently died had also other traditional risk factors, it may be possible to identify by the presence of markedly depressed BRS some individuals at high risk who might otherwise go unrecognized.

A similar correlation with increased mortality as the one just described for poor vagal reflexes has been found for indexes of low vagal tone. Kleiger et al. have analyzed 24-hour heart rate variability in 808 patients a few days after myocardial infarction,

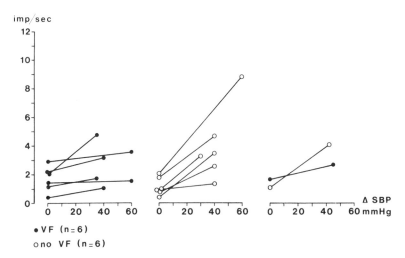

FIGURE 6. Vagal nerve activity in cats that develop ventricular fibrillation (VF) and that survive (noVF) during coronary artery occlusion. Individual values of nerve activity in impulses (imp)/second are expressed in the y axis, while blood pressure rise is expressed on the abscissa (D SBP). Mean values for the two groups of animals are plotted in the graph on the right.

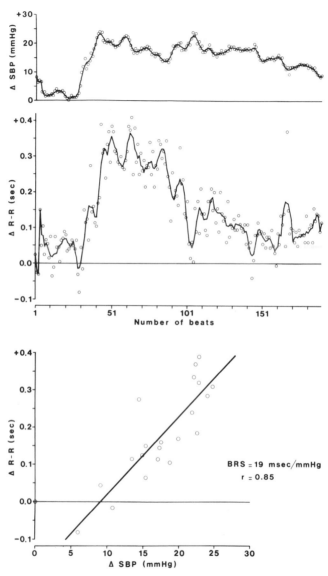

FIGURE 7. Retouched computer printout of a phenylephrine. Panels A and B: Beat-to-beat changes in systolic blood pressure (SBP) and in RR intervals compared with baseline values. Analysis is limited to the first major increase in blood pressure with the attendant changes in heart rate. These points are used (panel C) for calculation of the regression life. In this patient, phenylephrine produced a 25 mmHg increase in systolic blood pressure, which was accompanied by a marked increase in the RR intervals. Accordingly, the slope of the regression line expressing the baroreflex sensitivity (BRS) is rather high: 19 mseconds/mmHg. (From Reference 33 with permission of the American Heart Association, Inc.)

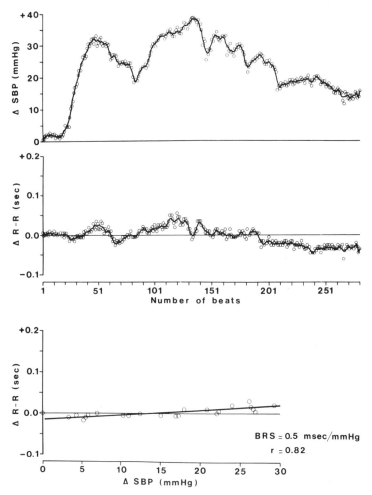

FIGURE 8. As in FIGURE 7. Heart rate in this patient did not change despite a clear-cut increase in systolic blood pressure (SBP). Accordingly, baroreflex sensitivity (BRS) is extremely depressed: 0.5 mseconds/mmHg. (From Reference 33 with permission of the American Heart Association, Inc.)

and followed the patients for a mean period of 31 months.[34] Of all Holter variables, HR variability had the strongest univariate (negative) correlation with mortality. The relative risk of mortality was 5.3 times higher in patients with standard deviation of the R-R intervals of less than 50 mseconds, compared to subjects with a value greater than 100 mseconds. Survival curves for the three different groups of patients are shown in FIGURE 11.

Rich *et al.* have extended the study of the correlation between heart rate variability and survival to patients without recent myocardial infarction.[35] They analyzed Holter recordings of 100 patients undergoing elective coronary angiography, and subsequently followed them for one year. Mortality was strikingly greater in the group of patients with heart rate variability <50 mseconds, compared to patients with a value greater than 50 mseconds (36% in the former, 2% in the latter, $p < 0.001$).

A more comprehensive approach to analyze heart rate variability, namely, power spectrum of R-R intervals, has been proposed, and utilized[36,37] in the assessment of sympathetic-parasympathetic interaction. This, as well as several other methods proposed by different authors, may potentially provide more careful evaluation of vagal activity to the heart and better correlation with prognosis.[38]

It is important to know whether information obtained by the analysis of vagal reflexes (as baroreflex sensitivity) may be predicted by the one gathered from the analysis of vagal tone (as heart rate variability). A study specifically designed to test this possibility indicates that the two methods have only a weak correlation and therefore are not redundant.[39]

To better define the potential role of the analysis of autonomic reflexes and autonomic tone in risk stratification after myocardial infarction, a multicenter trial has been organized. The ATRAMI study (Autonomic Tone and Reflexes after Myocardial Infarction) will enroll 1200 patients 10–20 days after myocardial infarction who will undergo BRS evaluation by the phenylephrine method and Holter recordings for the measurements of several different indexes of heart rate variability. Therefore, it will be possible to assess and compare the predictive efficacy of these different markers and to evaluate whether they may provide complementary information. Multivariate analysis

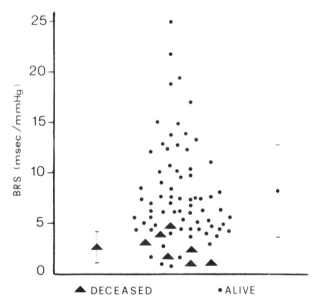

FIGURE 9. Relation between baroreflex sensitivity (BRS) and cardiovascular mortality. Besides the clear difference in BRS ($p < 0.005$) between the deceased patients and the survivors, it is worth noting that, while all deceased patients had a reduced BRS, four of them were in the extreme lower end of the distribution of BRS for the entire population.

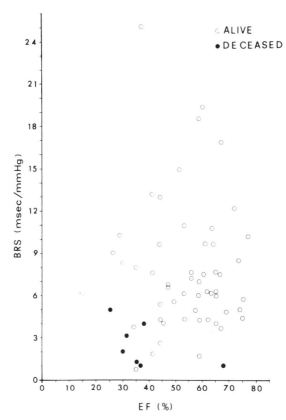

FIGURE 10. Relation between baroreflex sensitivity (BRS), left ventricular ejection fraction, and cardiovascular mortality. It is evident that among patients with depressed left ventricular function, the prediction of mortality is enhanced by the analysis of BRS.

will allow us to test the independence of their contribution to risk stratification from the variables already known to affect survival.

CONCLUSION

Experimental studies show that a sympathetic-parasympathetic balance with a parasympathetic dominance decreases the likelihood of malignant arrhythmia during myocardial ischemia. They suggest that manipulation of the autonomic nervous system according to this concept may be an effective measure against sudden death. They also indicate that electrocardiogram recordings may provide important indexes of autonomic state and notably of vagal tone and reflexes that correlate with survival.

The available clinical studies are in good agreement with the experimental data and demonstrate that relevant information on the autonomic balance can be gathered from patients with relatively simple techniques. A multicenter trial has been organized

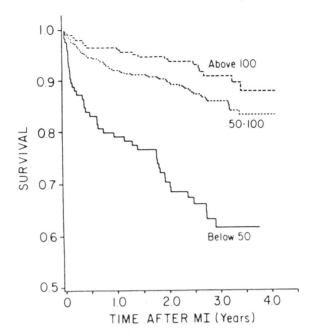

FIGURE 11. Cumulative survival over total follow-up period as a function of heart rate variability. By log-rank method, the patients that had a heart rate variability < 50 mseconds had a significantly ($p < 0.0001$) lower survival after myocardial infarction (MI), compared to the other two groups. (From Reference 34 with permission of the author and of the *American Journal of Cardiology.*)

to better define the role of these variables in risk stratification after myocardial infarction.

REFERENCES

1. GOLDBERG, R. J. 1989. Declining out-of-hospital sudden coronary death rates: additional pieces of the epidemiologic puzzle. Circulation **79:** 1369–1373.
2. The Cardiac Arrhythmia Suppression Trial (CAST) Investigators. 1989. Effect of encainide and flecainide on mortality in a randomized trial of arrhythmia suppression after myocardial infarction. N. Engl. J. Med. **321:** 406–412.
3. AKHTAR, M., G. BREITHARDT, A. J. CAMM, P. COUMEL, M. J. JANSE, R. LAZZARA, R. J. MYERBURG, P. J. SCHWARTZ, A. L. WALDO, H. J. J. WELLENS & D. P. ZIPES. 1990. CAST and beyond. Implications of the Cardiac Arrhythmia Suppression Trial. Circulation **81:** 1123–1127 & Eur. Heart J. **11:** 194–199.
4. SCHWARTZ, P. J. & H. L. STONE. 1982. The role of the autonomic nervous system in sudden coronary death. Ann. N.Y. Acad. Sci. **382:** 162–181.
5. HJALMARSON, A. 1984. Beta-blocker effectiveness post infarction: an antiarrhythmic or antiischemic effect. Ann NY Acad Sci **427:** 101–111.
6. SCHWARTZ, P. J. 1984. The rationale and the role of left stellectomy for the prevention of malignant arrhythmias. Ann. N.Y. Acad. Sci. **427:** 199–221.
7. LOWN, B. & R. L. VERRIER. 1976. Neural activity and ventricular fibrillation. N Engl. J. Med. **294:**1165–1170.

8. CORR, P. B., K. A. YAMADA & F. X. WITKOWSKI. 1986. Mechanisms controlling cardiac autonomic function and their relation to arrhythmogenesis. *In* The Heart and Cardiovascular System. H. A. Fozzard, E. Haber, R. B. Jennings, A. N. Katz & H. E. Morgan, Eds.: 1343–1403. Raven Press. New York, N.Y.

9. SCHWARTZ, P. J. & E. VANOLI. 1981. Cardiac arrhythmias elicited by interaction between acute myocardial ischemia and sympathetic hyperactivity: a new experimental model for the study of antiarrhythmic drugs. J. Cardiovasc. Pharmacol. **3:** 1251–1259.

10. SCHWARTZ, P. J. & S. G. PRIORI. Sympathetic nervous system and cardiac arrhythmias. *In* Cardiac Electrophysiology. From Cell to Bedside. D. P. Zipes & J. Jalife, Eds. W.B. Sunders Co. Philadelphia, Pa. (In press.)

11. BARBER, M. J., T. M. MUELLER, D. P. HENRY, S. Y. FELTEN & D. P. ZIPES. 1983. Transmural myocardial infarction in the dog produces sympathectomy in noninfarcted myocardium. Circulation **67:** 787–796.

12. SCHWARTZ, P. J., E. VANOLI, A. ZARA & G. ZUANETTI. 1985. The effect of antiarrhythmic drugs in life-threatening arrhythmias induced by the interaction between acute myocardial ischemia and sympathetic hyperactivity. Am. Heart J. **109:** 937–948.

13. PRIORI, S. G., G. ZUANETTI & P. J. SCHWARTZ. 1988. Ventricular fibrillation induced by the interaction between acute myocardial ischemia and sympathetic hyperactivity: effect of nifedipine. Am. Heart J. **116:** 37–45.

14. SCHWARTZ, P. J., S. G. PRIORI, E. VANOLI, A. ZAZA & G. ZUANETTI. 1986. Efficacy of diltiazem in two experimental models of sudden death. J. Am. Coll. Cardiol. **8:** 661–668.

15. HAN, J., D. MILLET, B. CHIZZONITTI & G. K. MOE. 1966. Temporal dispersion of recovery of excitability in atrium and ventricle as a function of heart rate. Am. Heart J. **71:** 481-487.

16. KENT, K. M., E. R. SMITH, D. R. REDWOOD & S. E. EPSTEIN. 1973. Electrical stability of acutely ischemic myocardium: influences of heart rate and vagal stimulation. Circulation **47:** 44–50.

17. CORR, P. B. & R. A. GILLIS. 1974. Role of the vagus nerves in the cardiovascular changes induced by coronary occlusion. Circulation **49:** 86–97.

18. VERRIER, R. L. 1980. Neural factors and ventricular electrical instability. *In* Sudden Death. H. E. Kulbertus & H. J. J. Wellens, Eds.: 137–155. Martinus Nijhoff. The Hague, the Netherlands.

19. ZUANETTI, G., G. M. DE FERRARI, S. G. PRIORI & P. J. SCHWARTZ. 1987. Protective effect of vagal stimulation on reperfusion arrhythmias in cats. Ciro. Res. **61:** 429–435.

20. SCHWARTZ, P. J., G. E. BILLMAN & H. L. STONE. 1984. Autonomic mechanisms in ventricular fibrillation induced by myocardial ischemia during exercise in dogs with healed myocardial infarction. An experimental preparation for sudden cardiac death. Circulation **69:** 790–800.

21. SCHWARTZ, P. J. & H. L. STONE. 1985. The analysis and modulation of autonomic reflexes in the prediction and prevention of sudden death. *In* Cardiac Arrhythmias: Mechanisms and Management. D. P. Zipes & J. Jalife, Eds.: 165–176. Grune and Stratton. New York, N.Y.

22. BILLMAN, G. E., P. J. SCHWARTZ & H. L. STONE. 1982. Baroreceptor reflex control of heart rate: a predictor of sudden cardiac death. Circulation **66:** 874–880.

23. SMYTH, H. S., P. SLEIGHT & G. W. PICKERING. 1969. Reflex regulation of arterial pressure during sleep in man: a quantitative method of assessing baroreflex sensitivity. Circ. Res. **24:** 109–121.

24. SCHWARTZ, P. J., E. VANOLI, M. STRAMBA-BADIALE, G. M. DE FERRARI, G. E. BILLMAN & R. D. FOREMAN. 1988. Autonomic mechanisms and sudden death. New insights from the analysis of baroreceptor reflexes in conscious dogs with and without a myocardial infarction. Circulation **78:** 969–979.

25. ECKBERG, D. W. 1980. Parasympathetic cardiovascular control in human disease: a critical review of methods and results. Am. J. Physiol. **239:** 581–593.

26. HULL, S. S., A. R. EVANS, E. VANOLI, M. STRAMBA-BADIALE, G. M. DE FERRARI, R.D FOREMAN & P. J. SCHWARTZ. 1988. Heart rate variability and sudden death in conscious dogs before and after myocardial infarction (abstr.) Circulation **78**(Suppl. II): 6.

27. STRAMBA-BADIALE, M., G. M. DE FERRARI, E. VANOLI, G. E. BILLMAN, S. S. HULL, D. R. FOREMAN & P. J. SCHWARTZ. 1988. Myocardial ischemia and ventricular fibrillation. Atropine and the role of vagal reflexes. (abstr.) Fed. Proc. **47:** A327.
28. STRAMBA-BADIALE, M., E. VANOLI, G. M. DE FERRARI & P. J. SCHWARTZ. 1987. Vagal stimulation in conscious dogs. (abstr.) Eur. Heart J. **8**(Suppl. 2): 186.
29. SCHWARTZ, P. J. 1987. Manipulation of the autonomic nervous system in the prevention of sudden cardiac death. *In* Twenty Years of Cardiac Electrophysiology. P. Brugada & H. J. J. Wellens, Eds.: 741–765. Futura Publishing Co. Mount Kisco, N.Y.
30. DE FERRARI, G. M., E. VANOLI, M. STRAMBA BADIALE, R. D. FOREMAN & P. J. SCHWARTZ. 1987. Vagal stimulation and sudden death in conscious dogs with a healed myocardial infarction. (abstr.) Circulation **76**(Suppl. IV): 107.
31. CERATI, D. & P. J. SCHWARTZ. 1989. Vagal reflexes and survival during acute myocardial ischemia in cats. (abstr.) Circulation **80**(Suppl. II): 552.
32. DE FERRARI, G. M., E. VANOLI, G. TOMMASINI, M. GROSSONI, G. UCKMAR, C. PATRONO & P. J. SCHWARTZ. 1989. Antiarrhythmic effect of muscarinic agonists during acute myocardial ischemia. (abstr.) Ciculation **80**(Suppl. II): 202.
33. LA ROVERE, M. T., G. SPECCHIA, A. MORTARA & P. J. SCHWARTZ. 1988. Baroreflex sensitivity, clinical correlates and cardiovascular mortality among patients with a first myocardial infarction: a prospective study. Circulation **78:** 816–824.
34. KLEIGER, R. E., J. P. MILLER, J. T. BIGGER, JR., A. J. MOSS & the Multicenter Postinfarction Research Group. 1987. Heart rate variability: a variable predicting mortality following acute myocardial infarction. Am. J. Cardiol. **59:** 256–262.
35. RICH, M. W., J. S. SAINI, R. E. KLEIGER, R. M. CARNEY, A. teVELDE & K. E. FREEDLAND. 1988. Correlation of heart rate variability with clinical and angiographic variable and late mortality after coronary angiography. Am. J. Cardiol. **62:** 714–717.
36. POMERANZ, B., R. J. B. MACAULAY, M. A. CAUDILL, I. KUTZ, D. ADAM, D. GORDON, K. M. KILBORN, A. C. BARGER, D. C. SHANNON, R. J. COHEN & H.BENSON. 1985. Assessment of autonomic function in humans by heart rate spectral analysis. Am. J. Physiol. **248:** H151–H153.
37. PAGANI, M., F. LOMBARDI, S. GUZZETTI, O. RIMOLDI, R. FURLAN, P. PIZZINELLI, G. SANDRONE, G. MALFATTO, S. DELL'ORTO, E. PICCALUGA, M. TURIEL, G. BASELLI, S. CERUTTI & A. MALLIANI. 1986. Power spectral analysis of heart rate and arterial pressure variabilities as a marker of sympathovagal interaction in man and conscious dog. Circ. Res. **59:** 178–193.
38. SINGER, D. H., G. J. MARTIN, N. MAGID, J. S. WEISS, EE&CS, J. W. SCHAAD, R. KEHOE, T. ZHEUTLIN, D. J. FINTEL, A. M. HSEIH & M. LESCH. 1988. Low heart rate variability and sudden cardiac death. J. Electrocardiogr. Suppl. I: S48–S55.
39. BIGGER, J. T., JR., M. T. LaROVERE, R. C. STEINMAN, J. L. FLEISS, J. N. ROTTMAN, L. M. ROLNITZKY & P. J. SCHWARTZ. 1989. Comparison of baroreflex sensitivity and heart period variability after myocardial infarction. J. Am. Coll. Cardiol. **14:** 1511–1518.

The Cellular Basis of Cardiac Arrhythmias[a]

A Matrical Perspective

MORTON F. ARNSDORF

Section of Cardiology
The University of Chicago
5841 South Maryland
Chicago, Illinois 60637

HISTORICAL INTRODUCTION

Two important streams of thought now converge and influence our thinking about the cellular basis of cardiac arrhythmias. The first flows from the work of investigators in the late 19th and early 20th centuries that led Wiggers in 1923 to venture a classification of cardiac arrhythmias based on "disturbances of impulse initiation" and "disturbances of impulse conduction."[1] Hoffman and Cranefield in 1964 related the phenomenologic classification of altered automaticity and impulse propagation to the electrophysiologic properties of single cardiac cells.[2] More recently, Wit and Rosen used the same classification and again updated the basic electrophysiologic work.[3]

The second stream concerns "irritability," the intrinsic ability or refractoriness of an excitable tissue to respond to an impulse or irritant; a concept that is now termed excitability.[4-6] Hodgkin, Huxley, and their coworkers developed new concepts and new techniques in the nerve.[7,8] In the 1950s and 1960s, Weidmann applied some of these concepts and developed others in his microelectrode studies of the heart and suggested that both active and passive cellular properties were important to cardiac excitability,[9-11] a concept supported by the theoretical work of Noble.[12] Hoffman and Cranefield pulled together much of this information in their influential book of 1960.[13]

In the early 1970s, Fozzard and Schoenberg[14] and Noble[15,16] advanced our fundamental understanding of excitability in their microelectrode studies on strength-duration relationships, threshold, and liminal length in cardiac tissues. In the early 1970s and into the 1980s, we published a series of papers that developed working experimental definitions of cardiac excitability, demonstrated the importance of passive properties and the interactions between active and passive properties in determining overall excitability in normal heart tissue and after arrhythmogenic and pharmacologic interventions; and most recently the development of a rapid one-line computer based data analysis system has led us to conclude that non–steady states of interactions were more the rule than the exception after an arrhythmogenic intervention, an antiarrhythmic drug, or a combination of both.[17-25]

In 1977, we suggested that altered excitability should be a third major division of arrhythmogenic mechanism because certain data, particularly those of Fozzard and his coworkers as well as our own, did not fit comfortably into the categories of altered automaticity or impulse propagation.[26] At about the same time, we introduced the

[a]Supported in part by U.S. Public Health Service grant 2 R37 HL 21788 (Merit Award) from the National Heart, Lung and Blood Institute.

concept of the electrophysiologic matrix in symposia, but it was not until 1984 that we wrote about the matrix as a simplifying intellectual construct in a clinical review.[27] The matrix consisted of active (sources) and passive cellular properties (sinks) that could be altered both by arrhythmogenic influences and by antiarrhythmic drugs. We suggested, "Reentry and automaticity in a real sense are descriptive of final common pathways; the determinants of which reside in perturbed matrices of cardiac excitability."[27] Subsequently, we further developed the theory and conducted experimental work designed to test the hypothesis of altered excitability in terms of the multidimensional mathematical model of active and passive properties that is the current version of the electrophysiologic matrix.[22–25,28–30]

This communication considers the cellular electrophysiologic mechanisms of cardiac arrhythmias from the perspective of the matrix which is quite different from the more traditional view as represented by the elegant review of Wit and Rosen mentioned above.[3] The perspectives, while different, are complementary.

THE NORMAL ELECTROPHYSIOLOGIC MATRIX

Cardiac excitability has an intuitive meaning which suggests the ease with which cardiac cells undergo individual and sequential regenerative depolarization and repolarization, communicate with each other, and propagate in a normal or abnormal manner. These events are strictly controlled to allow synchronized contraction and an effective cardiac output.

The first premise is that there is a matrix of electrophysiologic properties that determines normal cardiac excitability. These determinants include the resting potential and its determinants, active cellular properties, and passive cellular properties.

The Resting Potential and Its Determinants

The determinants of the resting potential (V_r) include the integrity of the membrane, the protein channels, and the energy-requiring pumps and other exchange mechanisms that maintain normal ionic activities and electrochemical gradients. Activity rather than concentration is the quantity of importance to the ability to carry current and to be pumped out of the cell. V_r is determined largely by intracellular and extracellular potassium activities (α_K^i and α_K^o, respectively) because the conductance of the membrane to potassium (g_K) is 20 to 100 times higher than for other conductances. FIGURE 1 illustrates the change in V_r as a function of α_K^o; a relationship that can be predicted by the Nernst equation. The equilibrium potential can be calculated from the Nernst equation and is defined as the potential required to oppose the concentration gradient.

Active Cellular Properties

Active properties are unique to excitable cells and include the voltage-, time-, and ligand-dependent mechanisms that control the ionic currents responsible for normal as well as abnormal depolarization, repolarization, and automaticity. The flow of an ionic species (i_{ion}) depends on the *driving force* (the difference between the transmembrane voltage, V_m, and the equilibrium potential which is approximately $+60$ mV for E_{Na}, -94 mV for E_K, and $+130$ mV for E_{Ca}) and the ease with which ions pass through the channels, the *membrane conductance* (g_{ion}). For the Na$^+$, K$^+$, and "slow inward" (primarily Ca^{++} under normal circumstances) ionic currents, the relationship becomes:

$$i_{ion} = g_K (V_m - E_K) + g_{Na} (V_m - E_{Na}) + g_{si} (V_m - E_{si}) + g_x (V_m - E_x) \quad (1)$$

This resembles Ohm's law, but the relationship is nonlinear rather than ohmic with the nonlinearities highly dependent on V_m and time.

The inrush of Na^+ current, i_{Na^+}, is responsible for the phase of rapid regenerative depolarization (phase 0) in the tissues of the atria, the Purkinje fibers of the specialized infranodal conduction system (fascicles, bundle branches, terminal Purkinje network), and ventricles. The maximal rate of rise of voltage ($\dot{V}_{max}$) when the sodium channel

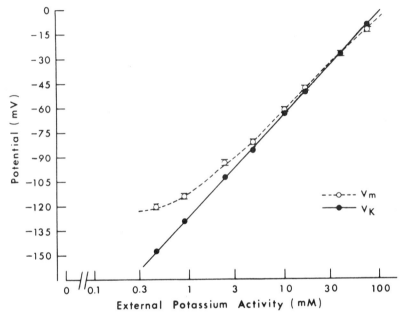

FIGURE 1. The resting membrane potential, V_r (unfilled circles, dashed line) in Purkinje fibers as a function of the external potassium activity in sodium-free superfusing solutions. The equilibrium potential for potassium, here termed V_K and represented by the filled circles and the solid line, was calculated from the measured α_K^i. Note the deviation from prediction at about 4 mM. (Reproduced with permission from Sheu *et al.*)[42]

opens and i_{Na} rushes into the cell is rapid, and, as a result, these tissues are often called *fast-response* tissues. Characteristics of fast-response tissues are summarized in TABLE 1. V_r and subthreshold conductance in fast response tissues are determined primarily by g_K. As the cell is depolarized from a V_r of about -90 mV to about -60 mV, the sodium channels open, and the response becomes regenerative and out of proportion to the stimulus. This point is often termed the *threshold voltage* (V_{th}). *Liminal length* is the more appropriate concept and is defined as the amount of tissue in which voltage rises above threshold (making the inward depolarizing current from one region greater than the repolarizing influences of the adjacent tissues) necessary to produce an action potential.[14] Liminal length, as will be seen, depends both on active and passive properties.

TABLE 1. Characteristics of "Fast" and "Slow" Response Cardiac Tissues[a]

	"Fast" Response Tissues	"Slow" Response Tissues
Geographic location	Working and specialized atrial tisues; infranodal specialized conduction system (Purkinje fibers); ventricular muscle; and accessory AV bypass tracts (Kent bundles, etc.)	SA and AV node; perhaps valves; coronary sinus; injured tissues in which i_{Na}-dependent converted to i_{si}-dependent phase 0
Passive membrane properties		
Normal resting potential (V_r)	Appx -80 to -95 mV	Appx -40 to -65 mV
Subthreshold membrane conductance	Primarily components of g_K, g_{K_1}	Probably a component of g_K
Active membrane properties		
"Threshold" voltage	Appx -60 to -75 mV	Appx -40 to -60 mV
Current responsible for phase 0 depolarization	i_{Na}	i_{si} (mixed current with both Ca^{++} and Na^+)
Activation and inactivation kinetics of channel responsible for phase 0 depolarization	Fast	Slow
Maximal rise velocity of Phase 0 (dV/dt_{max} or $\dot{V}_{max}$)	300–$1000+$ V/second	1–50 V/second
Peak overshoot	Appx $+20$ to $+40$ mV	-5 to $+20$ mV
Overall amplitude of action potential	Appx $+90$ to $+135$ mV	Appx -30 to $+70$ mV
Refractoriness and reactivation	Partial reactivation during phase 3; complete reactivation in normal tissue 10 to 50 mseconds after return to normal V_r.	Partial and complete reactivation returns after (>100 mseconds) attainment of V_r
Relationship of rate to:		
a. Action potential duration	Marked change	Slight change
b. Refractory period duration	Steep curve	"Flat" curve
c. Threshold	Independent	Varies directly with frequency
d. Conduction velocity	Independent	Decays with frequency
Supernormal excitability	Often present	Never seen
Conduction velocity	0.5 to 5 m/seconds	0.01 to 0.1 m/second
Safety factor	High	Low
Characteristics conducive to reentry	Only with inactivation of the sodium system	Present even in normally i_{si}-dependent tissues
Automaticity	Yes. Normally depends on decreasing i_{K_2} and/or increasing i_f.	Yes. Normally depends on increasing i_f.
Automaticity depressed by physiological increases in $[K^+]_o$	Yes	No

[a]Reproduced with permission from Arnsdorf.[5]

Repolarization is also a carefully regulated regenerative process. Phase 1 depends on the inactivation of g_{Na} and, in Purkinje fibers, perhaps on the activation of a calcium-activated K^+ current. Events during phase 2 or the plateau phase are complex. As V_m becomes less negative, the channel for i_{si}, mixed $Ca^{++}-Na^+$ or "slow inward" current, opens, and i_{si} helps maintain the plateau. An inward Na^+ current distinct from that active during phase 0, the "window" current, also contributes to the maintainance of the plateau. During the plateau, the driving force for the outward potassium ion $(V_m - E_K)$ increases and changes in g_K can produce large changes in ionic flow. At the V_m of the plateau, K^+ conductance decreases in the outward direction but increases in the inward direction, and this is termed rectification since current passes in one direction better than in another. The rectification is inward, so more K^+ enters than leaves the cell; a mechanism that maintains the plateau. During phase 3 repolarization (the rapid repolarization phase), there is a rapid return to V_r which results from inactivation of i_{si}, reversal of inward rectification, and activation of repolarizing outward K^+ currents. The increasing negativity of V_m produces a positive feedback system for these repolarizing processes. During phase 3, enough of the sodium system is normally reactivated that another action potential can be electrically induced.

FIGURE 2A diagramatically depicts the state of the Na^+ channel in the absence of a drug. The resting state (R) predominates in normally polarized fast-response tissues; the activated state (A) occurs transiently with opening of the Na^+ channel during phase 0; and the inactivated state (I) dominates at more positive V_m such as during the plateau or in tissues that have been depolarized due to injury, exposure to hyperkalemia, or other insult. The R, A, and O states correspond to resting, rapid depolarization (phase 0), and plateau phases (phase 3) of the action potential.

In some tissues, phase 0 of the action potential depends on i_{si}. The channel is distinct from the one that controls i_{Na}. This current is often called the calcium current since the channel preferentially carries Ca^{++}. Phase 0 in the sinoatrial and atrioventricular nodes normally depends on i_{si}, and depolarized fast-response tissues may switch over to action potentials dependent on i_{si}. These are often called *slow response tissues,* and some characteristics are summarized in TABLE 1. These tissues have a V_r of about -60 mV, a V_m at which the sodium system is essentially completely inactivated. The slow channel is voltage dependent and has resting, active, and inactivated phases. Inactivation depends both on voltage and time and extends into electrical diastole, a characteristic that limits the number of impulses that can transverse the atrioventricular node.

Passive Cellular Properties

Passive properties include the linear and nonlinear cable properties that determine the ionic leak through the membrane and the flow of ions between cells as well as in the extracellular space. The heart cell has a low resistance myoplasm surrounded by a membrane that has both capacitive elements and a high resistance, analogous to a telegraph cable with a low resistance core and a high resistance insulation. Equations were developed that were useful in describing transmission over telegraph cables. After modification, similar equations were found useful in describing electrical transmission experimental observations quite well in both nerve and later in heart.[9,17–25,29,31,32] Cells are connected and communicate with each other through gap junctions which normally have a low resistance to ionic flow. Injury increases gap junctional resistance and cells may uncouple, actions mediated by changes in pH and α_{Ca}^i (see reviews).[29,33] The membrane insulation is imperfect, so current leaks through. This current loss causes

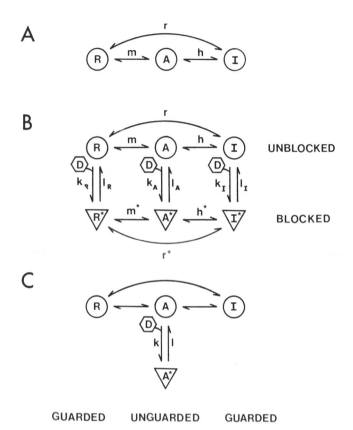

FIGURE 2. States of the sodium channel. States of the sodium channel in the absence of drug (panel A) and in the presence of drug according to the modulated receptor hypothesis (panel B) and one variation of a guarded receptor hypothesis (panel C). **Panel A,** absence of drug: The resting state (R) predominates in normally polarized tissues near E_K, at which time the sodium channel, according to the Hodgkin-Huxley scheme, is obstructed by the **m** gate. The activated or open state (A) occurs during the 2 mseconds or so during which the **m** element moves into a position and before the **h** element obstructs which allows the opening of the sodium channel. The inactivated state (I) is predominant at more positive potentials, particularly during the plateau when the sodium channel is obstructed by the **h** element. In actuality, there may be several closed states. Hodgkin-Huxley parameters are indicated by HH. **Panel B,** presence of drug according to the modulated receptor hypothesis: Drug molecules can associate (down arrow) or dissociate (up arrow) with the channels in all three states. The blocked drug–associated channels are R*, A*, and I*. Their Hodgkin-Huxley parameters are shifted to more positive potentials (m*, h*, r*) so the channels behave as if they are at a less negative transmembrane voltage than in the control. These actions are important in determining both an antiarrhythmic and proarrhythmic matrical configuration after an antiarrhythmic drug. **Panel C,** presence of drug according to one variation of the guarded receptor hypothesis: A drug can associate with a receptor only in the activated state (A) when both the **m** and **h** elements are not obstructing the channel, and this is the unguarded state. The receptor is guarded in both the R and I states in this example, at which time the drug cannot associate with the receptor but can diffuse off already occupied receptors.

less current to be available as a function of distance for the longitudinal flow of ions through the myoplasm and the gap junctions. The electrical analogue is shown in panel B of FIGURE 3. Panel C shows the dropoff in V_m as a function of distance, and the distance over which one cell may electronically influence another is contained in the length constant (λ) which in turn is a function of the square root of the resistances of the membranes (R_m) times the sum of the myoplasm and gap junctions (R_i).

Properties Dependent on Both Active and Passive Cellular Properties

Liminal length, as defined above, is directly proportional to the charge developed by the active cellular properties and inversely proportional to the membrane capacitance and the length constant (see Fozzard and Schoenberg for mathematical discussion).[14] If the liminal length requirements of element A-B in FIGURE 3B are not met, the electrotonic influence on neighboring element C-D will be insufficient to cause an action potential, and the current will decay exponentially. If, however, the electrotonic influence from membrane element A-B is sufficient for element C-D to attain threshold (or, more properly, to fulfill its liminal length requirements), regenerative depolarization and an action potential results in element C-D. The ability of a cell, then, to fulfill its liminal length requirements or reach threshold depends both on the current strength due to active cellular properties and on the sink of the tissue's cable properties. The longer the length constant, λ, the greater will be the electrotonic influence of one membrane element or one cell on neighboring elements or cells.

Impulse propagation also depends on both active and passive cellular properties. Once unit C-D is activated in FIGURE 3B, it may or may not fulfill the liminal length requirements of unit E-F. If it does, the action potential will propagate one unit further, and so on. If one looks at propagation in this manner, it is clear that it is inherently discontinuous. The discontinuities, however, are essentially negligible in the Purkinje cell cable, but are not when several bundles run together and there is transverse as well as longitudinal communication, when there is damage to the membrane or to individual cells, or when there are branches.[28] The *safety factor* for impulse propagation can also be defined in terms of the interaction between sources and sinks; that is, it represents the excess of current source over the drain due to passive properties, the sink, so that the liminal length requirements of one cell after another are met. A decrease in the intensity of the source generally reduces conduction velocity. But altered passive properties can also slow conduction velocity and cause asynchrony of activation. In a chronic canine model of myocardial infarction, for example, Ursell *et al.* found essentially normal action potentials in the area of fractionated activity on the electrogram, and concluded that the development of fibrosis after infarction progressively impedes transverse conduction, distorts the parallel orientation of fibers, and alters intercellular connections leading to slowed conduction despite normal action potential parameters.[34] Such findings suggest that alterations in passive properties may be more important determinants of abnormalities of conduction than are altered active properties.[29]

Normal *automaticity* also depends on the relationship among depolarizing inward currents, repolarizing outward currents, and the passive properties of the sink that determine electrotonic transmission and the successful or unsuccessful excitability of neighboring cells.

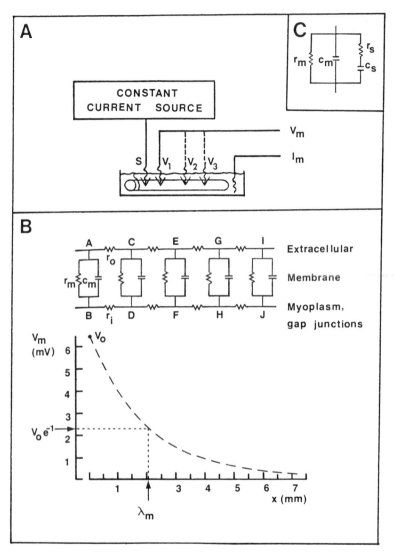

FIGURE 3. Panel A: Experimental arrangement for cable analysis. Constant current is injected intracellularly through a microelectrode positioned near the ligated end of a cardiac Purkinje fiber (S) allowing the assumption that all current will pass in one direction to the right. The response in V_m is recorded by microelectrodes impaled at several points along the cablelike preparation (V_1, V_2, V_3, etc.). The measurement of current (I) is obtained from the bath ground. **Panel B:** The electrical analogue of the passive properties of the extracellular space, membrane, and combined myoplasm–gap junctions is shown. Below, V_m is plotted as a function of the distance (x) of the stimulating from the recording microelectrodes. r_m, membrane resistance; c_m, membrane capacitance; r_i, internal or longitudinal resistance due to the myoplasm and gap junctions. The length constant, λ, is the distance at which V_m falls to $V_o e^{-1}$ of its value at the point of stimulation, V_o. **Panel C:** A more complex electrical analogue which includes series resistance and capacitance (r_s and c_s, respectively). (Reproduced with permission from Arnsdorf.)[30]

THE HYPOTHESIS OF ALTERED EXCITABILITY AND THE
PROARRHYTHMIC MATRICAL CONFIGURATION

The hypothesis of altered excitability states that excitability must be altered to produce abnormal excitability, a proarrhythmic matrical configuration, and cardiac arrhythmias. The implications of this hypothesis that are supported by experimental evidence include (1) arrhythmogenic influences and antiarrhythmic drugs affect one or more component of cardiac excitability, and net excitability depends on the balance and interrelationships between the determinants of excitability; (2) alterations in the determinants of excitability induced by an intervention change at different rates, suggesting that the non–steady state is of importance in the equivalent clinical situation; (3) certain matrical states are proarrhythmic while others are antiarrhythmic; (4) the traditionally described mechanisms of arrhythmogenesis such as reentry and abnormal automaticity are the end result of matrical perturbation; (5) similar arrhythmias may arise from different mechanisms; and (6) virtually identical final states of excitability result from different combinations of altered determinants.

Chronologically, our earliest observations on excitability dealt with the last-listed implication that identical final states of excitability result from different combinations of altered excitability. FIGURE 4 depicts strength-duration relationships before and after procainamide and lidocaine.[18,19] The index of excitability was the intracellularly applied current sufficient to produce an action potential (I_{th}). I_{th} as well as threshold voltage (V_{th}) were plotted as a function of current duration (t). Both drugs shifted the strength-duration curve upwards, that is, more current regardless of duration was required to fulfill the liminal length requirements after the drug. Classically, this shift indicates a less excitable membrane. The mechanisms, however, differed. Procainamide decreased excitability by rendering V_{th} less negative and by decreasing $\dot{V}_{max}$, terms dependent on g_{Na}, despite an actual increase in membrane R_m. Lidocaine decreased excitability by decreasing R_m in the subthreshold range without much affecting V_{th} or $\dot{V}_{max}$. Cable analysis showed that procainamide increased and lidocaine decreased λ.

FIGURE 5 shows a cartoon of the normal and perturbed electrophysiologic matrix. A few of the many determinants of excitability are included and the convention is explained in the figure legend. The bonds represent interactions and mutual dependencies. The normal state is depicted by the hexagon. As has been discussed, each of these six determinants has its own determinants which may be controlled by yet other factors. For example, g_{Na} depends on the R, A, and I states of the sodium channel. In truth, such complexity must be expressed by a multidimensional mathematical model, but the cartoon is useful for illustrative purposes. Experimentally, we exposed Purkinje fibers to lysophosphatidylcholine (LPC), a metabolite that increases in the ischemic myocardium and appears in the effluent of the ischemic myocardium.[21,23] LPC produced two types of matrical configuration: one increased and the other decreased excitability. As seen in the lower pathway of FIGURE 5, increased excitability resulted largely from an increase in R_m, which decreases the amount of current required to produce a given voltage change, and an increase in λ, which causes the source to electrotonically influence more cells at a distance. Excitability increased despite changes in V_r and V_{th} as well as an actual decrease in sodium g_{Na}. As seen in the upper pathway of FIGURE 5, LPC could also decrease excitability by decreasing g_{Na} and shifting V_{th} to a more positive value despite a persistently increased R_m and λ.

We have found that antiarrhythmic drugs act quite differently depending on the matrix encountered. Referring again to FIGURE 4, lidocaine affected the normal and perturbed matrices quite differently. Lidocaine had little effect on the matrical configuration in normal tissue (middle pathway). If the matrical configuration after

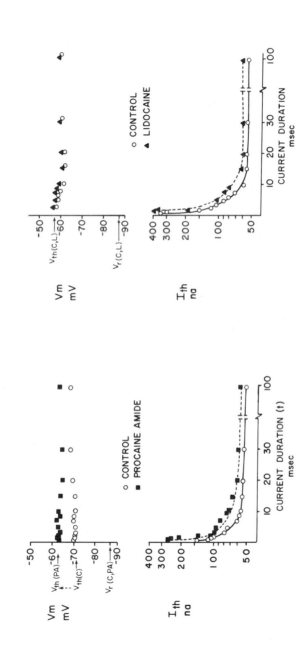

FIGURE 4. The effects of procainamide (panel A) and lidocaine (B) on strength-duration curves as assessed by the microelectrode technique of intracellular constant current application and transmembrane voltage recording in cardiac Purkinje fibers. In the upper portion of each panel, the threshold voltage (V_{th}) is plotted as a function of the current duration. In the lower panel, the strength-duration curve is depicted with the threshold current (I_{th}) plotted as a function of the current duration. As compared to the control, both procainamide and lidocaine shifted the strength-duration curve upward indicating that the threshold current requirement increased after the intervention. Neither drug affected V_r, but procainamide made V_{th} less negative while lidocaine little influenced V_{th}. Cable analysis and current-voltage analysis revealed that the drugs had opposite effects on membrane resistance at rest and in the subthreshold potential range. (Adapted and reproduced by permission from Arnsdorf and Bigger.)[18,19]

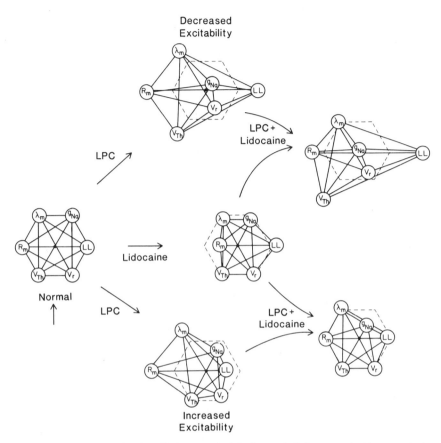

FIGURE 5. A cartoon of a simplified electrophysiologic matrix being perturbed by an arrhythmogenic intervention and an antiarrhythmic drug. The determinants depicted include the resting potential (V_r), threshold voltage (V_{th}), sodium conductance (g_{Na}), membrane resistance (R_m), the length constant (λ_m), and as a measure of overall excitability the liminal length (LL). Each in turn has its own determinants, as for example, the R, A, and I states of the sodium channel shown in FIGURE 2. Nevertheless, the depicted determinants contain broad descriptions of the resting potential and its several determinants; active cellular properties and the relevant gates; passive cellular properties which determine transmembrane and longitudinal current flow; and the net excitability. The bonds between the determinants suggest interactions and mutual dependencies. The normal state is depicted by the hexagon. A shift towards the center of the hexagon indicates a decrease in the quantity; a shift away from the center of the hexagon an increase in the quantity. After exposure to lysophosphatidylcholine (LPC), excitability may increase (lower pathway) due largely to an increase in R_m and λ despite a decrease in g_{Na} or decrease (upper pathway) due primarily to depression of g_{Na}. Lidocaine slightly decreases R_m in normal tissues (middle pathway). In the lower pathway, lidocaine decreases excitability and returns liminal length (LL) to nearly its normal value by decreasing R_m and λ despite some decrease in g_{Na}. Note that the effects on passive properties are primarily responsible for the near normalization of the matrix. In the upper pathway, lidocaine decreases excitability by further depressing g_{Na} and making V_{th} less negative rather than by affecting passive properties. (Reproduced with permission from Arnsdorf and Wasserstrom.)[28]

LPC increased excitability (lower pathway), lidocaine decreased excitability and returned liminal length towards normal primarily by countering LPC's effects on passive properties and by somewhat reducing g_{Na}. If the matrical configuration after LPC decreased excitability (upper pathway), lidocaine affected the matrix quite differently and further decreased excitability primarily by further depressing active generator properties (V_{th}, $\dot{V}_{max}$). Note the similarity in the matrical configurations of decreased excitability after LPC alone and after LPC with lidocaine. It is not surprising, then, that lidocaine and other antiarrhythmic drugs can produce proarrhythmic as well as antiarrhythmic matrical configurations. Often, the distinction between an antiarrhythmic and a proarrhythmic matrix is hazy.

It seems reasonable to suppose that our phenomenologic arrhythmogenic mechanisms result from matrical deformation of these types. Experimentally, we found that the state of decreased excitability was associated with a markedly depressed conduction velocity; presumably a proarrhythmic state that would favor the appearance of a reentrant rhythm. The state of increased excitability would be expected to respond more readily to boundary currents or to permit previously subthreshold automatic rhythms to attain threshold. As mentioned, Rosen and Wit have comprehensively reviewed recently the issue of abnormal impulse conduction and reentry.[3] In addition to the traditional discussion of depressed inward current leading to reentry, emphasis is placed on the manner in which altered passive properties, particularly cell to cell capacitive and ionic coupling, can slow conduction and create conditions conducive to reentry.

Changes in intracellular ionic activity are also of importance in arrhythmogenesis. LPC, antiarrhythmic drugs, and digitalis can alter intracellular ionic activities. Digitalis, for example, inhibits (Na^+, K^+)-ATPase which increases α^i_{Na}. The Na^+-Ca^{++} exchange mechanism then loads the cell with Ca^{++} leading to oscillatory calcium ion release from the sarcoplasmic reticulum, the development of a transient inward current, late afterpotentials which may lead to a sustained rhythm, and aftercontractions.

The perturbed matrix can affect repolarization leading to dispersion of refractoriness, tissues with two stable steady states, or, at times, the appearance of triggered arrhythmias.[35,36] FIGURE 6 shows the effect of lidocaine on triggered sustained rhythmic activity in a cardiac Purkinje fiber having an abnormality of repolarization.[35] In the control situations (panels A and B), the electrically induced action potential triggered oscillatory activity at a low membrane voltage which increased in amplitude and eventuated in nondriven sustained action potentials. The triggered sustained rhythmic activity persisted indefinitely until terminated by a hyperpolarizing intracellular current that permitted attainment of the repolarization threshold and a return to V_r (arrow in panel B). Lidocaine (panel C) caused attainment of the repolarization threshold and normalization of the action potential. After washout of lidocaine (panels D–F), the action potential duration prolonged and triggered sustained rhythmic activity rapidly reappeared. Abnormal Ca^{++} loading in such cells prolongs the action potential duration, thereby allowing sufficient time for calcium channels to cycle and produce early afterdepolarizations.[37] Shortening of the action potential duration or altering the V_m of the plateau will abort the recycling of the calcium channels and can be accomplished by pharmacologic means or by overdrive pacing.

THE NON-STEADY STATE, DISEQUILIBRIUM, BIFURCATIONS, AND CHAOS

Most studies on arrhythmogenesis and antiarrhythmic drugs have been conducted in the steady state; the Newtonian condition that presumes every event is determined

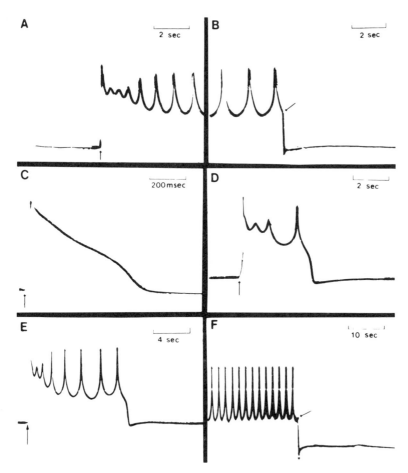

FIGURE 6. Failure of normal repolarization and the appearance of triggered sustained activity. **Panel A:** From a normal resting potential, an electrical stimulus induced an i_{Na}-dependent phase 0. The preparation failed to repolarize normally and the i_{Na}-dependent phase 0 triggered oscillatory activity. The oscillations increased in magnitude and resulted in nondriven sustained action potentials. Since sodium channels would be inactivated at this V_m, the oscillatory activity and subsequent sustained rhythmic activity must have depended on i_{si} for the inward current. **Panel B:** The triggered sustained rhythmic activity persisted indefinitely until terminated by a hyperpolarizing intracellular current that permitted attainment of the repolarization "threshold" and a return to V_r. **Panel C:** Lidocaine caused an almost immediate attainment of the repolarization threshold and a "normalization" of the action potential. **Panels D–F:** After washout of lidocaine, triggered sustained rhythmic activity rapidly reappeared. (Reproduced with permission from Arnsdorf.)[35]

by initial conditions and, if the techniques were sufficient, could be determined with precision. Our experiments with LPC, antiarrhythmic drugs, and other arrhythmogenic interventions have utilized rapid, on-line data analysis systems. In these studies, we have observed changes in excitability to occur in time that result from complex alterations in the rate of change of the passive and active cellular determinants. The milieu in ischemia is characterized by fluctuations within systems such as autonomic surges, changing electrolyte balance and oxygenation, and the accumulation of metabolites such as LPC. It is reasonable to assume that we are dealing with complex feedback systems in which the matrix is in constant change; a system in which equilibrium easily gives way to disequilibrium, nonlinear relationships are important or even paramount, and in which small and even stochastic perturbations may have profound sequelae.

Consider the bifurcation diagram in FIGURE 7. Beginning at point A, some condition changes and carries the system along the Y axis until point B is reached. At point B, feedback mechanisms fail to maintain the steady state and a transition occurs to a new equilibrium: in this case, C or D. For example, cardiac tissue has a steady-state resting potential and a relatively ohmic subthreshold current-voltage relationship until the liminal length requirements (1) are met resulting in an explosive transition to a new state or (2) are not met resulting in an exponential return of V_m to V_r. Our experiments with LPC can be considered similarly. LPC accumulation is the parameter that drives the reaction from left to right and, depending on the conditions encountered (e.g., $[K^+]_o$, pH, LPC metabolism) results in a matrical configuration that increases excitability (say C) or decreases excitability (say D).

The discussion thus far suggests that hierarchical classifications of antiarrhythmic drugs based on a predominant action should be fundamentally flawed, yet they have been empirically useful. How is this possible? In my view, this results from what is

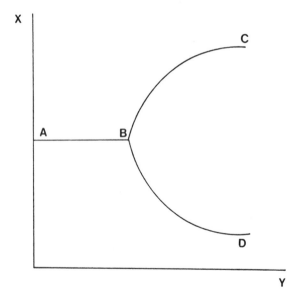

FIGURE 7. A symmetrical bifurcation diagram. At point A, the system is in a steady state, essentially in equilibrium. As the control parameter changes along the Y axis, the system remains essentially in equilibrium until point B is reached. At B, the system becomes unstable and bifurcates with two new stable steady states at C and D. So long as the control parameter increases in value or assumes a stationary value greater than the one that exists at point B, the value of X in large part will determine whether the system will equilibrate at new steady state C or D. If the value of X is near point A, chance may play a role in determining which steady state will be assumed.

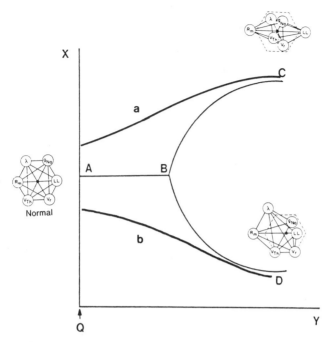

FIGURE 8. Quinidine, bifurcations, and assisted bifurcations based on data from Arnsdorf and Sawicki.[24] Quinidine superfusion of the Purkinje fiber is indicated by the arrow at Q. The system is driven from left to right, from A to B along the Y axis. At $[K^+]_o$ of 8.0 mM, either steady state C or D represented by the matrical configurations depicted can be chosen; the choice seemingly made at random. At a $[K^+]_o$ of 5.4 mM, the decision is assisted (path "b"), steady state D is preferred, and the matrical configuration increases cardiac excitability. At a $[K^+]_o$ of 12 mM, the decision is assisted (path "a"), steady state C is preferred, and the matrical configuration decreases excitability.

termed an assisted bifurcation. Given a choice of moving from B to C or D, the parameter along the X axis assists and determines the path taken. FIGURE 8 is based on our studies with quinidine.[24] In all experiments at $[K^+]_o$ of 5.4 mM, quinidine produced a matrical configuration that increased excitability, a change determined by a marked increase in membrane resistance and length constant that were more important to overall excitability than was the slight decrease in $\dot{V}_{max}$ that was used as an index for g_{Na}. At a $[K^+]_o$ of 8.0, quinidine could either increase or decrease excitability depending on whether the net excitability was determined primarily by the altered passive or active properties. We could not identify the reasons for the choice of pathway, and possibly it was random. At a $[K^+]_o$ of 12 mM, the matrical configuration that decreased excitability always occurred (pathway "a" to steady state C in FIGURE 8). In contrast, $[K^+]_o$ of 5.4 mM favored the matrical configuration that increased excitability (pathway "b" to steady state D in FIGURE 8). We postulate that during ischemia, elevated $[K^+]_o$ and perhaps pH changes cause an assisted bifurcation along path "a" resulting in a matrical configuration that decreases excitability. The so-called group I–type antiarrhythmic drug effect (depression of g_{Na} and decreased excitability) is predictably "predominant" in this particular and clinically often repeated situation.

The situation, however, may be quite different in hypokalemia due to diuretics where we would predict that path "b" would be followed, excitability would increase, and a classical Group I action would be meaningless.

For years, we have emphasized that normal excitability reflects strict control of ionic events and cell-to-cell communication. The result is that heterogeneous elements and events are coordinated to produce homogeneous, well-integrated cardiac functioning. Disruptions cause abnormal cardiac excitability. Other investigators have reached the same conclusion by following different paths. Glass and Mackey propose the existence of *dynamical diseases* which are characterized by abnormal temporal organization.[39] They, and others, have been analyzing normal and abnormal dynamical systems, including those involving the bioelectricity of the heart, mathematically in terms of nonlinear dynamics, fractal structure as exists in the Purkinje network, and chaos theory (see reviews).[38-40] The nonlinear dependence of the ionic conductances in Equation 1 on voltage changes and time has been used to model pacemakers which, in turn, have shown chaotic dynamics. Single impulse perturbations of pacemaker activity reset the phase of an ongoing rhythm. Periodic perturbations such as caused by pacemakers of the heart interact electrotonically resulting in mutual interdependencies, phase locking of rhythms, and entrainment. As elegantly summarized by Glass and Mackey,[39] spatial oscillations may produce abnormalities of impulse propagation in one dimension such as the Wenckebach phenomenon or reentry due to unidirectional block in anatomical or functional pathways; spiral wave propagation in two dimensions which perhaps underlies reentrant arrhythmias due to the leading circle mechanism proposed by Allessie et al.,[41] or scroll waves in three dimensions that may underlie ventricular fibrillation.

Looking ahead, I would hope to see the multidimensional mathematical model that is the matrix and the rigorous application of nonlinear dynamical theory inspiring new experimental approaches to understanding the processes of arrhythmogenesis and the actions of antiarrhythmic drugs; that is, as predicted, order may come out of chaos.

REFERENCES

1. WIGGERS, C. J. 1923. Modern Aspects of the Circulation in Health and Disease. Lea and Febiger. Philadelphia, Pa.
2. HOFFMAN, B. F. & P. C. CRANEFIELD. 1964. The physiological basis of cardiac arrhythmias. Am. J. Med. **37**: 670–684.
3. WIT, A. L. & M. R. ROSEN. 1989. Cellular electrophysiological mechanisms of cardiac arrhythmias. *In* Comprehensive Electrocardiology: Theory and Practice in Health and Disease. P. W. MacFarlane & T. D. Veitch, Lawrie, Eds. **2**: 801–841. Pergamon Press. New York, N.Y.
4. LEWIS, T. 1925. The Mechanism and Graphic Registration of the Heart Beat. 3rd edit. Shaw and Sons, Ltd. London, England.
5. BURRIDGE, W. 1932. Excitability: a Cardiac Study. Oxford University Press. London, England.
6. BROOKS, J. C. MC. C., B. F. HOFFMAN, E. E. SUCKLING, et al. 1955. The Excitability of the Heart. Grune & Stratton. New York, N.Y.
7. HODGKIN, A. L. & W. A. H. RUSHTON. 1946. The electrical constants of a crustacean nerve fibre. Proc. R. Soc. London Biol. **133**:444–479.
8. HODGKIN, A. L. & A. F. HUXLEY. 1952. A quantitative description of membrane current and its application to conduction and excitation in nerve. J. Physiol. London. **117**:500–544.
9. WEIDMANN, S. L. 1952. The electrical constants of Purkinje fibers. J. Physiol. London **118**: 348–360.

10. WEIDMANN, S. L. 1955. Effects of calcium ions and local anesthetics on electrical properties of Purkinje fibers. J. Physiol. London 129: 568–582.
11. WEIDMANN, S. L. 1970. The electrical constants of trabecular muscle from mammalian heart. J. Physiol. London 210: 1041–1053.
12. NOBLE, D. 1962. Modification of the Hodgkin-Huxley equations applicable to Purkinje fibre action and pacemaker potentials. J. Physiol. London 160: 317–352.
13. HOFFMAN, B. F. & P. C. CRANEFIELD. 1960. Electrophysiology of the Heart. McGraw Hill, New York, N.Y.
14. FOZZARD, H. A. & M. SCHOENBERG. 1972. Strength-duration curves in cardiac Purkinje fibres: effects of liminal length and charge distribution. J. Physiol. London 226: 593–618.
15. NOBLE, D. 1972. The relation of Rushton's "liminal length" for excitation to the resting and active conductances of excitable cells. J. Physiol. London 226: 573–591.
16. NOBLE, D. & R. B. STEIN. 1966. The threshold conditions for initiation of action potentials by excitable cells. J. Physiol. London 187: 129–162.
17. ARNSDORF, M. F. & J. T. BIGGER, JR. 1972. The effect of lidocaine hydrochloride on membrane conductance in mammalian cardiac Purkinje fibers. J. Clin. Invest. 51: 2252–2263.
18. ARNSDORF, M. F. & J. T. BIGGER, JR. 1975. The effect of lidocaine on components of excitability in long mammalian Purkinje fibers. J. Pharmacol. Expt. Ther. 195: 206–215.
19. ARNSDORF, M. F. & J. T. BIGGER, JR. 1976. The effect of procaine amide on components of excitability in long mammalian Purkinje fibers. Circ. Res. 38: 115–121.
20. ARNSDORF, M. F. & I. FRIEDLANDER. 1976. The electrophysiologic effects of tolamolol (UK-6558-01) on the passive membrane properties of mammalian cardiac Purkinje fibers. J. Pharmacol. Exp. Ther. 199: 601–610.
21. ARNSDORF, M. F. & G. J. SAWICKI. 1981. The effects of lysophosphatidylcholine, a toxic metabolite of ischemia, on the components of cardiac excitability in sheep Purkinje fibers. Circ. Res. 49: 16–30.
22. ARNSDORF, M. F., G. A. SCHMIDT & G. SAWICKI. 1985. The effects of encainide on the determinants of cardiac excitability in sheep Purkinje fibers. J. Pharmacol. Exp. Ther. 223: 40–48.
23. SAWICKI, G. J. & M. F. ARNSDORF. 1985. Electrophysiologic actions and interactions between lysophosphatidylcholine and lidocaine in the nonsteady state: the match between multiphasic arrhythmogenic mechanisms and multiple drug effects in cardiac Purkinje fibers. J. Pharmacol. Exp. Ther. 235: 829–838.
24. ARNSDORF, M. F. & G. J. SAWICKI. 1987. The effects of quinidine sulfate on the balance among active and passive cellular properties which comprise the electrophysiologic matrix and determine excitability in sheep Purkinje fibers: cardiac excitability and the electrophysiologic matrix. Circ. Res. 61: 244–255.
25. ARNSDORF, M. F. & G. J. SAWICKI. 1989. The effects of ethmozin on cardiac excitability and the electrophysiologic matrix in sheep Purkinje fibers. J. Pharmacol. Exp. Ther. 248(3): 1158–1166.
26. ARNSDORF, M. F. 1977. Membrane factors in arrhythmogenesis. Prog. Cardiovasc. Dis. 19(6): 413–429.
27. ARNSDORF, M. F. 1984. Basic understanding of the electrophysiologic actions of antiarrhythmic drugs: sources, sinks, and matrices of information. Med. Clin. North Am. 68: 1247–1280.
28. ARNSDORF, M. F. & J. A. WASSERSTROM. 1986. Mechanisms of action of antiarrhythmic drugs: a matrical approach. In The Heart and Cardiovascular System. H. A. Fozzard, E. Haber, R. B. Jennings, A. M. Katz & H. E. Morgan, Eds.: 1259–1316. Raven Press. New York, N.Y.
29. ARNSDORF, M. F. & J. A. WASSERSTROM. 1987. A matrical approach to the basic and clinical pharmacology of antiarrhythmic drugs. Rev. Clin. Basic Pharmacol. 6: 131–188.
30. ARNSDORF, M. F. 1989. A matrical perspective of cardiac excitability: cable properties and impulse propagation. In Function of the Heart in Normal and Pathological States. N. Sperelakis, Ed. 2nd edit.: 133–174. M. Nijhoff. Boston, Mass.
31. DOMINGUEZ, G. & H. A. FOZZARD. 1970. Influence of extracellular K^+ concentration on cable properties and excitability of sheep cardiac Purkinje fibers. Circ. Res. 26: 565–574.

32. PRESSLER, M. L., V. ELHARRAR & J. C. BAILEY. 1982. Effects of extracellular calcium ions, verapamil and lanthanum on active and passive properties of canine cardiac Purkinje fibers. Circ. Res. **51:** 637–651.
33. PAGE, E. & C. K. MANJUNATH. 1986. Communicating junctions between cardiac cells. *In* The Heart and Cardiovascular System. H. A. Fozzard, E. Haber, R. B. Jennings, A. M. Katz & H. E. Morgan, Eds.: 573–600. Raven Press. New York, N.Y.
34. URSELL, P. C., P. I. GARDNER, A. ALBALA, J. J. FENOGLIO, JR. & A. L. WIT. 1985. Structural and electrophysiological changes in the epicardial border zone of canine myocardial infarcts during infarct healing. Circ. Res. **56:** 436–451.
35. ARNSDORF, M. F. 1977. The effect of antiarrhythmic drugs on triggered sustained rhythmic activity in cardiac Purkinje fibers. J. Pharmacol. Exp. Ther. **201:** 689–700.
36. ARNSDORF, M. F. & D. J. MEHLMAN. 1978. Observations on the effects of selected antiarrhythmic drugs on mammalian cardiac Purkinje fibers with two levels of steady-state potential. J. Pharmacol. Exp. Ther. **207:** 983–991.
37. JANUARY, C. R. & J. M. RIDDLE. 1989. Early afterdepolarizations: mechanism of induction and block: a role for L-type Ca^{++} current. **64:** 977–990.
38. WINFREE, A. T. 1987. When Time Breaks Down: The Three-Dimensional Dynamics of Electrochemical Waves and Cardiac Arrhythmias. Princeton University Press. Princeton, N.J.
39. GLASS, L. & M. C. MACKEY. 1988. From Clocks to Chaos. Princeton University Press. Princeton, N.Y.
40. JALIFE, J. & D. C. MICHAELS. 1985. Phase-dependent interactions of cardiac pacemakers as mechanisms of control and synchronization in the heart. *In* Cardiac Electrophysiology and Arrhythmias. D. P. Zipes & J. Jalife, Eds.: 109–119. Grune & Stratton. Orlando, Fla.
41. ALLESSIE, M. A., F. I. M. BONKE & F. J. G. SCHOPMAN. 1977. Circus movement in rabbit atrial muscle as a mechanism of tachycardia. III. The "leading circle" concept: a new model of circus movement in cardiac tissue without the involvement of an anatomic obstacle. Circ. Res. **41:** 9–18.
42. SHEU, S-S., M. KORTH, D. A. LATHROP & H. A. FOZZARD. 1980. Intra- and extracellular K^+ and Na^+ activities and resting membrane potential in sheep cardiac Purkinje strands. Circ. Res. **47:** 692–700.

Irregular Dynamics of Excitation in Biologic and Mathematical Models of Cardiac Cells[a]

ALAIN VINET, DANTE R. CHIALVO, AND JOSE JALIFE[b]

Department of Pharmacology
State University of New York Health Science Center
Syracuse, New York 13210

INTRODUCTION

According to the original program, the title of this paper should have been "Computer Modeling of Cardiac Arrhythmias." However, we have decided to deal with a much more specific subject which is intimately related to that immensely broad field; i.e., the nonlinear dynamics of excitation of cardiac cells, and the analysis of such dynamics by means of simple unidimensional models. Moreover, although we are not yet prepared to discuss any direct implications of our studies in the understanding of clinical arrhythmias, we illustrate some peculiar behaviors of isolated cardiac tissues, and of computer models of cardiac cells, which may have some bearing on arrhythmias. The ultimate goal is, in fact, to provide clues about cellular dynamics and electrophysiology that would help the clinician in his efforts to disclose the secrets underlying the mechanisms of severe cardiac arrhythmias and sudden death.

THE CARDIAC CELL AS A DYNAMICAL SYSTEM

Cardiac cells are highly dimensional excitable systems which can undergo a transition from predictable to unpredictable behavior analogous to the transition from laminar to turbulent flow in a fluid.[1] In the past, the study of such transitions in cardiology has been purely descriptive and, except for few recent examples,[2-5] no rigorous experimental or theoretical approaches for the analysis of the underlying dynamics or mechanisms have yet been developed.

We firmly believe that, to us cardiac electrophysiologists, chaos theory offers some new and exciting tools for gaining a better insight into the complicated rhythms of the human heart. Therefore, we demonstrate here by example how one can use some of these tools to analyze experimental data and provide testable predictions about normal and abnormal heart behavior.

So, *What is Chaos?*

To the modern mathematician, physicist and biologist, chaos is a disordered behavior which may occur in nonlinear dynamical systems.[6] Dynamical system is defined as any system whose temporal evolution is determined by feedback processes among its intrinsic time-dependent variables.[6] When such a time dependence is nonlinear, the system can undergo either ordered or chaotic behavior.

[a] Supported by grants HL29439 and HL 40991 from the Heart, Lung and Blood Institute.
[b] Author to whom correspondence should be addressed.

Since excitable cells have several nonlinear time-dependent parameters, they can be considered as dynamical systems. Moreover, when these cells are stimulated electrically, complex patterns of excitation may occur at stimulus frequencies at which maximum nonlinearities are expected.[5,7–9]

OBJECTIVES OF THE STUDY

We have investigated the rate-dependent behavior of cardiac cells with the overall goal of providing accurate biological and theoretical background for the understanding of cardiac rhythm disturbances. Specifically, we aimed at three different objectives: Firstly, we wished to described the global rate-dependent behavior of these cells through a systematic exploration of their response to repetitive stimulation. Secondly, we wished to investigate the role of nonlinearity in the mechanism of this complex behavior. Finally, we wished to devise a mathematical model to explain and make predictions about rate-dependent cardiac cell activation on the basis of these nonlinear time-dependent parameters. Our studies are published in detail elsewhere[5,7–9] and here we give a brief review of those aspects that are relevant to the general theme of this volume.

We have used three different experimental approaches in our efforts to achieve our objectives: (1) we have done microelectrode experiments in Purkinje fibers; (2) we have used iteration techniques by means of a simple but powerful unidimensional model of cardiac excitation;[7] and (3) we have used a modified version of the Beeler and Reuter model[10] to test the predictions of the unidimensional model.

PURKINJE FIBER EXPERIMENTS

Microelectrode experiments were carried out in isolated sheep cardiac Purkinje fibers superfused with Tyrode solution containing two different potassium concentrations: 4 and 7 mM. Quiescent preparations were driven electrically through a suction pipette (see Reference 7 for details).

Repetitive stimulation of the fibers with depolarizing current pulses of critical magnitude and various cycle lengths led to a wide spectrum of rate-dependent excitation patterns which varied with the KCl concentration.

The simplest behavior occurred at 7 mM KCl. In FIGURE 1, panel A shows transmembrane potentials recorded from one of these fibers. The stimulus magnitude was constant at the level corresponding to threshold at a cycle length of 600 mseconds. Note that, as the cycle length was decreased, the number of dropped beats increased in a monotonic fashion. Panel B shows the results for the complete cycle length range. A plot of activation ratio (calculated as the number of action potentials over number of stimuli) versus stimulus cycle length shows a monotonic relationship. Clearly, as the stimulus basic cycle length (BCL) was decreased in small steps, there was a progressive and predictable decrease in the activation ratio. Intermediate Wenckebach patterns are detected between 1:1 and 2:1, and no irregular activity was observed. Indeed, in all the experiments in which recovery of excitability was monotonic as a result of high KCl superfusion,[7,11] the patterns of activation showed the characteristic staircase exemplified here. These data confirm theoretical predictions by other authors[2,3] in that the sequences of patterns that appeared as the BCL was accelerated followed the so-called arithmetic rule of Farey.[2,3,7] The rule predicts that in a given staircase, the widest step between $n{:}m$ and $N{:}M$ should always be $n + N{:}m + M$, where n and N are numbers of stimuli and m and M are numbers of responses.

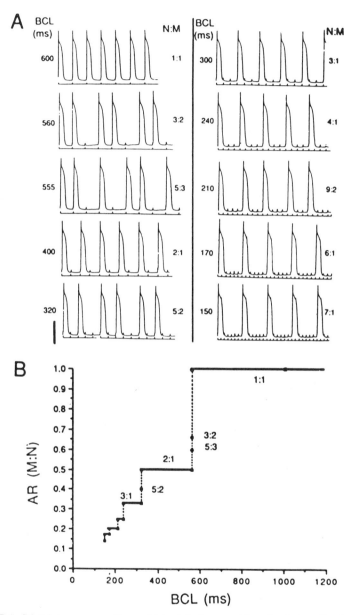

FIGURE 1. Stimulus:response patterns obtained during repetitive stimulation of a sheep Purkinje fiber at a KCl concentration of 7 mM: i.e., the strength-interval curve is monotonic. Panel A shows action potential recordings. For each BCL, the upper trace is of transmembrane potential and the lower trace is the stimulus monitor. Numbers to the right indicate the ratio (*N:M*) of stimuli (*N*) to responses (*M*). Calibration bars for transmembrane potentials indicate 40 mV. Panel B shows a so-called devil's staircase[2] in which the activation ratio (AR) is plotted vs. the BCL. AR is the reciprocal of the stimulus:response ratio (SRR). For clarity, the location of selected SRRs (1:1, 3:2, etc.) shown in panel A is indicated on the plot in panel B.

However, as shown in FIGURE 2, when similar measurements were repeated during exposure of the same fiber to 4 mM KCl Tyrode solution, a completely different picture emerged. There are three clearly apparent differences with respect to the previous case. First, decreasing the stimulation cycle length led to abrupt transitions between 1:1 and 2:1 as well as between 2:1 and 3:1 without any intermediate patterns. Second, at briefer cycle lengths the activation ratio increased and decreased over narrow ranges. And third, there are discontinuities in the plot corresponding to regions of irregular dynamics.

It is important to note that these irregular patterns were associated with supernormal excitability and occurred at intermediate ranges of current strength (FIGURE 3A). This corresponds to about 1.2 to 2.0 times diastolic threshold strength, which is used by most investigators in the study of cardiac excitation. In fact, repetitive stimulation within the range corresponding to current amplitude between the peak and dip of the supernormal phase (level II) brought about many types of regular and irregular cycle-length-dependent activation patterns, including the chaotic sequence shown in FIGURE 3B.

An example of irregular dynamics is presented in FIGURE 3B. This is a particular expression of chaotic activity with alternans in action potential duration and action potential amplitude. In this case, the magnitude of alternation during the successful 1:1 runs increases in a beat-to-beat manner, and a given pattern never repeats exactly, even after a sequence of 100 responses or more. Mathematical arguments suggest that the demonstration of this property of "amplification" of the initial "error" (in this case degree of alternation) and subsequent "reset" (i.e., activation failure) is essential for the establishment of deterministic chaos.[6]

As shown in FIGURE 4, a complete basic cycle length scan with repetitive stimuli of constant magnitude corresponding to the intermediate range (level II) may also lead the tissue through a series of bifurcations in its relevant parameters, in this case action potential amplitude (APA). At long BCLs, 1:1 activation is maintained and APA is constant. As BCL is gradually decreased, APA abbreviates progressively more until, at a critical BCL, a bifurcation occurs and APA alternans becomes manifest. This is replaced by 2:1 locking, followed by an additional bifurcation which leads to 3:1, and finally, to a very complex sequence in which APA changes on a beat-to-beat manner in pattern sequences that never repeat exactly.

We suggest that these behaviors are the result of the different modes of recovery of excitability and action potential duration at the two different KCl concentrations. FIGURE 5 shows recovery of excitability and action potential duration (APD) restitution curves measured in a fiber superfused with Tyrode solution containing two different KCl concentrations. When the KCl concentration was decreased from 7 to 4 mM, the excitability recovery function changed from monophasic (in panel A1) to triphasic (in panel B1), while the function describing action potential restitution remained monotonic (A2 and B2 for 7 and 4 mM KCl, respectively).

To summarize our findings thus far: at high potassium concentrations (i.e., when the recovery of excitability was monotonic), regardless of the stimulus amplitude, an increase in stimulation rate always induced a monotonic decrease in the activation ratio. On the other hand, during 4 mM KCl superfusion, the presence of supernormality allows the demonstration of two different kinds of behavior, depending on the stimulus strength. When strength was selected to be within range I or III, increases in stimulation rate led to monotonic decreases in the activation ratio. However, stimulation at increasing rates with pulses whose amplitude was within the critical range (range II) yields a nonmonotonic staircase with regular as well as irregular BCL-dependent activation patterns. Chaos was always found at these stimulus amplitudes.

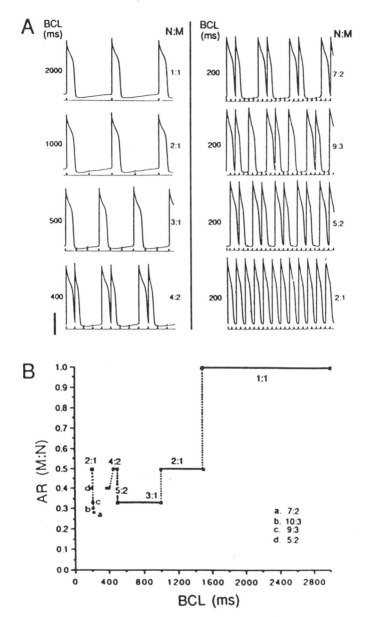

FIGURE 2. Stimulus:response patterns obtained under conditions of supernormality. Conditions were similar to those described for FIGURE 1, except that KCl concentration was 4 mM. For each BCL the upper trace is of transmembrane potential and the lower trace is the stimulus monitor. Numbers to the right indicate the ratio (*N:M*) of stimuli (*N*) to responses (*M*). The sequence of *N:M* ratios is markedly different from those obtained when the strength-interval curve is monotonic (cf. FIGURE 5). Calibration bars for transmembrane potentials indicate 40 mV. A plot of AR vs. BCL under these conditions (panel B) shows characteristic multiphasic increases and decreases in AR as BCL is shortened.

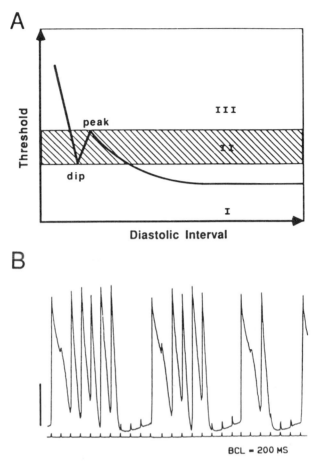

FIGURE 3. Panel A: Schematic representation of a nonmonotonic strength-interval curve with relative supernormality. Labels indicate those ranges (range I, range II, range III) of stimulus intensity in which different behaviors were observed experimentally during repetitive stimulation. **Panel B:** Chaotic activation sequence in a sheep Purkinje fiber driven repetitively at a BCL of 200 mseconds. Top trace, transmembrane potential recording; bottom trace, current pulse monitor. Note progressive increase in the magnitude of APD alternans during the successful 1:1 runs until failure and reset occur. A given sequence never repeats exactly. Vertical calibration bar = 35 mV.

THE DIFFERENCE-EQUATION MODEL

To explore analytically the dynamical consequences of these different modes of excitability recovery, we have devised a mathematical model which is based on three parameters: excitability, latency, and action potential duration as functions of the previous diastolic interval.

FIGURE 6 summarizes the model equations. In the top panel, we present the parameters used. S_n represents the first stimulus following a sudden BCL change, after which constant BCL is maintained. For beat $n + 1$, threshold, APD and latency are functions of the diastolic interval after beat n (DI_n). DI_n can be approximated as the BCL minus the APD_n minus L_n. The APD restitution, latency and threshold functions are determined experimentally, and their shapes will depend on the specific experimental circumstances (see FIGURE 5).

An iterative procedure is used to solve this set of equations in a personal computer. For a given BCL and stimulus magnitude, the calculated diastolic interval DI_n in each step determines the next latency, APD, and threshold. The values thus obtained are now used to establish the next diastolic interval (DI_{n+1}) and so on. The overall procedure is repeated iteratively until a steady-state response is obtained (see Reference 7 for further details about the model and its parameters).

The results of simulations in which we plotted the APA values obtained with the model as a function of BCL are summarized in FIGURE 7. In panel A, The APD restitution and excitability (threshold) functions used for this simulation were taken from the experiment at 7 mM KCl in which there was no supernormality. The current magnitude corresponds to threshold at an interval of 600 mseconds in the excitability curve. In this simulation, as the BCL is abbreviated, 1:1 activation is maintained with APA gradually being reduced until, after a brief bifurcation into a region of APA alternans, the pattern changes predictably to 2:1, then 3:1, 4:1, etc. In other words, just as in the experimental situation (see FIGURE 1), monotonic recovery leads to predictable locking patterns and APA values which follow Farey's arithmetic rule.

Panel B of FIGURE 7 shows data obtained in the presence of supernormal recovery of excitability. In this simulation, APD restitution and threshold values were obtained from the experiment in which 4 mM KCl was superfused. Current magnitude was at the critical range. Clearly, the model reproduces the experimentally obtained APA

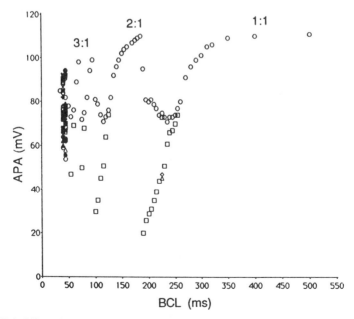

FIGURE 4. Bifurcation diagram of action potential amplitude (APA) as a function of basic cycle length (BCL). Data were obtained from a Purkinje fiber superfused with 4 mM KCl.

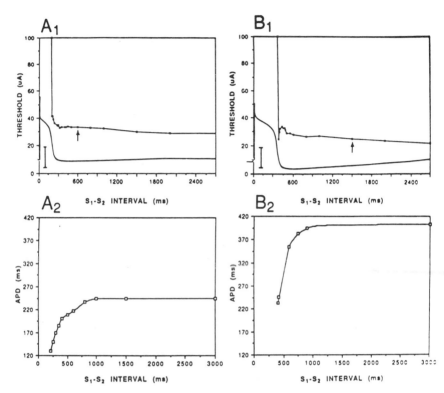

FIGURE 5. Strength-interval curves (A_1, B_1) and action potential duration (APD) restitution curves (A_2, B_2) obtained from a sheep Purkinje fiber preparation at a basic cycle length (S_1–S_1 of 3000 mseconds). In both (A_1 and B_1) an action potential is presented (lower left) to indicate the phase of membrane potential at which the test stimulus was applied. Calibration bars in A_1 and B_1 are for the action potentials and represent 30 mV. KCl concentration was 7 mM for panels A_1 and A_2 and 4 mM for panels B_1 and B_2. While no supernormality is present at the higher concentration (A_1), it becomes evident at the lower concentration (B_1). Arrows indicate the stimulus amplitude used during the repetitive stimulation shown in Figures 1 and 2.

data very well. As BCL is shortened, APA is gradually reduced within the 1:1 regime until a bifurcation occurs and APA begins to alternate on a beat-to-beat basis. This is followed by 2:1 locking and then by a series of bifurcations leading to chaotic activity which terminates abruptly and gives way to 3:1 block. Finally, an additional cascade of period doubling bifurcations reestablishes chaos, which is maintained until very short BCLs. These results provide quantitative support to our hypothesis that supernormality in the recovery of excitability may lead to complex patterns of excitation that fit the definition of chaotic regime.[1]

FIGURE 8 provides a summary of the results of large numbers of simulations with this model on the basis of experimental data obtained at high (panel A) and low (panel B) KCl concentrations. Wide ranges of cycle lengths (in the horizontal axes) and stimulation currents (vertical axes) were explored, and the resultant activation ratios were calculated. In panel A, when there is no supernormality, as the cycle length is shortened there is a boundary in which a transition from 1:1 to 2:1 occurs, then from 2:1 to 3:1, and so on. In other words, in the presence of monotonic recovery of excitability gradual changes in cycle length or stimulation amplitude yielded monotonic changes in the activation ratio.

When the supernormal recovery of excitability is incorporated into the model, the structure of the parameter plane change substantially, as presented in panel B. There are relatively low or high current strength ranges at which activation ratios change monotonically as the stimulation parameters are changed (see Reference 7 for details). However, at the intermediate range of current amplitude, changes in any of these parameters result in very complex (nonmonotonic) transitions in the activation ratio. Inside this range there are several small regions in which chaotic activation patterns are predicted.

From the results presented thus far, we can conclude the following:

1. Normal recovery of excitability leads to a monotonic change in the activation ratio during repetitive stimulation.
2. In the presence of supernormal excitability there are three different stimulation amplitude ranges which give rise to three different types of behavior:
   • Pulses of relatively low or high current strength at increasing pacing rates induce monotonic changes in the activation pattern.
   • Repetitive stimulation at intermediate current strengths yields very complex nonmonotonic changes in the activation ratio as a function of pacing rate, and can also lead to chaotic dynamics.

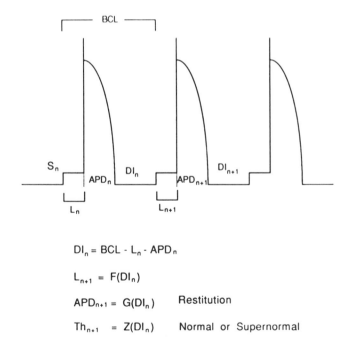

$$DI_n = BCL - L_n - APD_n$$

$$L_{n+1} = F(DI_n)$$

$$APD_{n+1} = G(DI_n) \quad \text{Restitution}$$

$$Th_{n+1} = Z(DI_n) \quad \text{Normal or Supernormal}$$

FIGURE 6. Parameters used in the formulation of the difference equation model. See text for details.

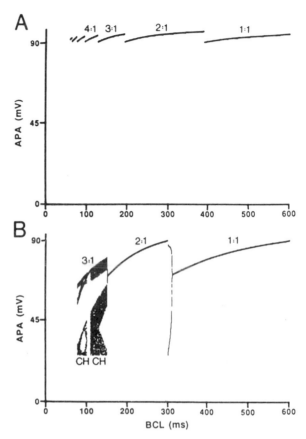

FIGURE 7. Bifurcation diagrams obtained by numerical solution of the difference equation model. For illustration, action potential amplitude (APA) is plotted as a function of BCL. In both cases, the strength-interval curve was nonmonotonic and the slope of APD restitution at early diastolic intervals was >1. **Panel A:** Current strength was constant within range I. Note monotonic changes in excitation patterns as BCL is gradually reduced. **Panel B:** Current strength was within the critical range (range II). Period doubling bifurcation and chaotic (CH) regions are apparent at the transitions between 2:1 and 3:1 and between 3:1 and 4:1. Note great similarity with experimental results in FIGURE 4.

THE MODIFIED BEELER AND REUTER MODEL

The demonstration of chaotic dynamics in isolated cardiac Purkinje fibers suggests the possibility of being able to explain mathematically cardiac conduction and rhythm disturbances. Moreover, our very simple difference equation model can reproduce a wide spectrum of Purkinje fiber behavior, and can provide testable predictions about the rate-dependent activation sequences that should be expected for a given set of experimental circumstances. Such predictions are accurate in spite of the fact that the unidimensional model has no regard whatsoever for underlying ionic mechanisms.

Nevertheless, recent work from our laboratory (Vinet *et al.*, submitted) indicates that a direct correspondence between the changes at the ionic level and the nonlinear parameters used in the difference equation model can indeed be made. Thus, as a first approximation to providing an ionic basis to complex excitation patterns in cardiac cells, we have tested the predictions of the difference equation model by determining the behavioral patterns of a highly dimensional ionic model in response to repetitive stimulation. We have used the Beeler and Reuter model[10] with modifications of the sodium current as proposed by Drouhard and Roberge.[12] The modified Beeler and Reuter (MBR) is a seven-dimensional, Hodgkin-Huxley[13] type model which includes the potential (V), the reversal potential of the calcium current (E_{si}) and five gating variables $(Y_i, i = 1,5)$. The model equations are as follows:

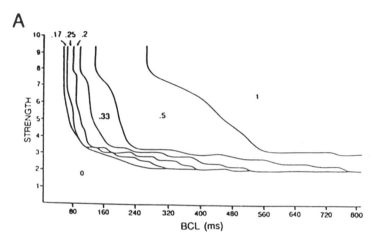

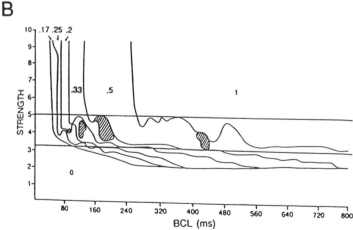

FIGURE 8. Parameter planes obtained by iteration of the model for monotonic (panel A) and nonmonotonic (panel B) modes of excitability recovery. The same APD restitution was used in both cases. See text for details.

$$\frac{dV}{dt} = -I_{ion} (V, E_{si}, Y_i, i = 1, 5) + I_{st}$$

$$I_{ion} = I_{na} (V, Y_1, Y_2) + I_{si} (V, Y_3, Y_4, E_{si}) + I_k (V, Y_5)$$

$$\frac{dY_i}{dt} = \frac{1}{\tau_i(V)} (Y_{i\infty} (V) - Y_i), i = 1, 5$$

$$\frac{dCa}{dt} = k_1 Y_3 Y_4 (V - E_{si}) - k_2 Ca$$

$$E_{si} = C \ln (Ca)$$

All functions and parameters can be found in Beeler and Reuter,[10] except for the sodium current (I_{na}) taken from Drouhard and Roberge.[12]

Simulated action potentials are presented in FIGURE 9. The data in panel A were obtained when depolarizing current pulses, 25 mseconds in duration and 3.3 $\mu A/cm^2$ in strength were applied at various cycle lengths. Progressive abbreviation of the stimulus cycle length yielded monotonic changes in the activation ratio from 1:1 through 2:1 and finally to 3:1. In panel B, at higher stimulus strength (3.7 $\mu A/cm^2$), abbreviation of the cycle length led the system from 1:1 activation (top trace) through a period doubling bifurcation into a 2:2 pattern with APD alternans (middle trace). Finally, at a still briefer cycle length (bottom trace) there was a complex sequence in which there was no periodicity in the response, as it was clear from the fact that a given pattern never repeated exactly, even after a run of 1500 cycle lengths.

To study rigorously these dynamics it is desirable to perform iterations with the

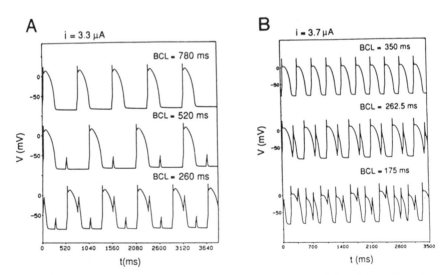

FIGURE 9. Stimulus:response patterns obtained during repetitive stimulation of the MBR model with depolarizing current pulses of 25 mseconds in duration at two different levels of current strength. Panel A shows a monotonic change in the activation ratio with period-adding sequences of 1:1, 2:1, and 3:1. Panel B shows sections of a period-doubling cascade toward irregular dynamics.

unidimensional difference equation model, and to compare the results with those obtained during long runs of repetitive stimulation of the MBR model. To this end, it was necessary to obtain from the latter the appropriate threshold and action potential duration functions through the application of premature stimulation techniques similar to those illustrated for the experimental situation (see FIGURE 5). In panel A of FIGURE 10 we have plotted recovery of excitability (i.e., threshold) and APD restitution curves constructed in the MBR model with 25 msecond pulses scanning the entire diastolic interval. It is clear that the threshold curve is nonmonotonic in the Beeler and Reuter model and shows a phase of supernormality at very early diastolic intervals. This nonlinearity is more strikingly illustrated if one applies pulses of relatively low but constant amplitude, as indicated by the horizontal line at 3.5 μA/cm^2. Panel B shows an example of supernormal excitability obtained under these conditions. The 12 superimposed tracings of membrane potential demonstrate that at this level of current there is a "silent range" of diastolic intervals bounded by two regions within which action potentials can be initiated.

The bifurcation diagram shown on the left of FIGURE 11 was obtained by iteration of the difference equation model with pulses of 25 mseconds and relatively high current strength. The data are plotted as predicted changes in action potential duration (i.e., G[DI]), as a function of BCL. On the right, a similar plot is presented for the MBR model. In this case it is possible to measure directly the changes in the ionic current at each particular BCL. Thus, maximum ionic current is plotted on the ordinate scale in terms of μA/cm^2. The predictions of the simple unidimensional model are surprisingly good. In both cases there are cascades of period doubling bifurcation, and sequences of irregular dynamics occur in both within the same range.

In fact, as shown in FIGURE 12, when the entire "parameter space" was plotted for large numbers of simulations at wide ranges of current magnitude (ordinate) and cycle length (abscissa), it became apparent that the individual regions of activation ratios were very similar for both models, and the transitions from one pattern to another occurred at very similar points. Moreover, in both cases there were three ranges of current amplitude in which the dynamics changed. At low levels of current strength, monotonic changes in activation ratio were seen in both; at intermediate levels, regions of unpredictable transitions were observed and finally at higher current levels, irregular dynamics were demonstrable at relatively wide ranges of BCL.

CONCLUSION

Whether or not the complex excitation patterns observed in the isolated Purkinje fiber as well as in the highly dimensional MBR model are the result of one or more ionic mechanisms remains to be determined. Yet, the demonstration of nonlinear dynamics and chaos in both systems suggests that it would be possible to use rigorous analytical techniques in the study of cardiac rhythm and conduction disturbances. Moreover, the applicability of simple unidimensional models derived from nonlinear mathematics to the electrophysiology of cardiac cells should help to improve our understanding of the transition from rhythmic to arrhythmic behavior. New theories may be developed by the study of bifurcation phenomena in cardiac tissues, which may lay the foundation for a more rigorous approach in "arrhythmology." Furthermore, such new theories may help to strengthen the ties between the basic scientist and the cardiologist by opening new research avenues which may lead to the disclosure of the fundamental mechanisms of severe cardiac arrhythmias and sudden death.

Thanks to currently available theoretical and experimental techniques it may be possible to answer some of the following questions in the not too distant future:

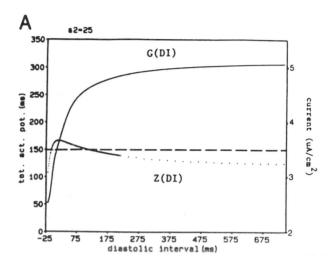

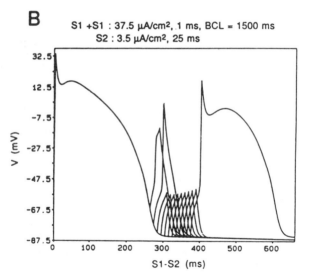

FIGURE 10. Panel A: Action potential restitution (G[DI] = APD[DI] + LAT[DI] no memory included) and threshold (Z[DI]) functions constructed from the MBR model for pulses of 25 mseconds in duration scanning the diastolic interval. Note the presence of supernormal excitability in the MBR model at relatively early intervals. These curves were used for iterations with the difference equation (DE) model and for construction of the maps shown in FIGURES 11 and 12. **Panel B:** Twelve superimposed transmembrane potential tracings illustrate the occurrence of a "silent" zone with subthreshold responses and supernormal excitability at relatively early intervals. Stimulus parameters are indicated on top of panel. Current strength corresponds to horizontal line in panel A.

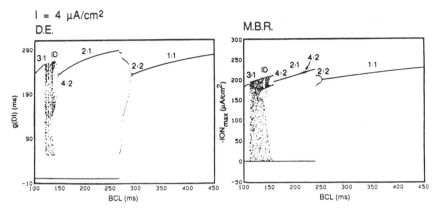

FIGURE 11. Bifurcation diagrams obtained with the difference equation (DE; left panel) and MBR (right panel) models for pulses of 25 mseconds at 4 μA/cm^2. For the DE model, data are plotted as beat-to-beat changes in action potential duration (G[DI]) as a function of basic cycle length (BCL). For the MBR model, data are presented as maximum ionic current ($-I_{ion\,max}$) as a function of BCL. Numbers on curves indicate the respective stimulus-response ratios. ID indicates those regions in which irregular dynamics were manifest. In the DE model, such dynamics were demonstrated to be truly chaotic.

1. What are the cellular and subcellular mechanisms associated with the nonlinear dynamics of heart-rate-dependent conduction abnormalities?
2. What are the dynamics of the transition from rhythmic to arrhythmic cardiac excitation.
3. Is supernormality important in determining vulnerability to cardiac arrhythmias in the clinical situation?
4. Is sensitivity to initial conditions important for the establishment of functional dispersion of refractoriness and to the establishment of reentry?
5. Is the transition from rhythmic to fibrillatory activity associated with chaotic dynamics?

In fact, answers to some of these questions are already under way. Supernormality is intimately related to the development of chaotic dynamics of excitation in experiments and computer simulations of cardiac cells.[5,7-9] The demonstration of such a relationship at the cellular level opens new possibilities in terms of propagation at the tissue and organ levels which may be readily explored.

One of the hallmarks for the demonstration of chaotic dynamics in deterministic system is that such dynamics are exquisitely sensitive to changes in the initial conditions.[1] Sensitivity to initial conditions is a property of rate-dependent excitation of cardiac cells.[7] Indeed, iterations of the unidimensional difference equation have shown that under the appropriate conditions for irregular dynamics, a 10-microsecond difference in the initial diastolic interval of two otherwise identical simulation runs is sufficient to lead to a huge divergence of the individual solutions, and to markedly different excitation patterns.[7] Because of this very high sensitivity to initial conditions, a premature stimulus might be able to initiate a highly irregular arrhythmia in a very small group of cells having identical electrophysiological properties and just a tiny difference in their respective activation times.

Finally, the issue of whether fibrillation is really chaotic or not is a matter of intense

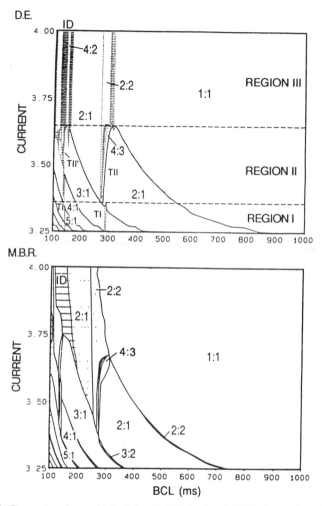

FIGURE 12. Parameter planes obtained for the DE (top) and MBR (bottom) models during repetitive stimulation with 25 msecond pulses at wide ranges of current strength and basic cycle length (BCL). The numbers in each plot indicate the activation ratios, and the curves mark the individual boundaries between those ratios; i.e., those BCL and current amplitudes where changes occur in the activation ratio or in the number of stimulations in the periodic sequence. Data for the DE model are more complete because of the extremely high computer time needed for the MBR simulations. However, the global structure is very similar for both models. In both, there are three general regions of current strength (see horizontal broken lines on top panel). In region I (low current strength), monotonic changes with successive n:1 ratios are seen, with narrow zones of transition (TI) to Wenckebach-like patterns (i.e., 3:2, 4:3, etc.). In region II (intermediate current strength), transitional regions (TII) to more complex sequences with period doubling begin to appear. In region III (high current strength) relatively wide regions of period doubling (e.g., 1:1, 2:2, 4:4, etc.) and irregular dynamics (ID) become clearly manifest.

controversy.[14,15] Yet, there is no doubt that the theory of dynamical systems has already provided important insight into the behavior of cardiac cells in response to repetitive stimulation. One question that remains, however, is whether we can use the theory of dynamical systems to further our understanding of the transition from rhythmic to fibrillatory activity. An increasing number of laboratories are beginning to address this important question which, in our opinion, opens a new avenue of systematic and rigorous research which may lead to a unifying theory of the dynamics and ionic mechanisms of sudden cardiac death.

SUMMARY

Excitation and impulse propagation in cardiac tissues are dependent on the heart rate and can occur in extremely complex patterns. In this chapter we present the results of Purkinje fiber experiments and of computer simulations using an ionic (Beeler & Reuter) model for the ventricular cell. We have studied the global rate-dependent behavior of cardiac cells through a systematic analysis of their response to single as well as repetitive depolarizing stimuli, and determined the role of nonlinearity in the mechanism(s) of their behaviors. To this end, we devised an analytical difference equation model of cardiac cell excitation which could be used to predict simple as well as chaotic behavior of both the Purkinje fiber and the Beeler & Reuter cell, depending on the stimulation rate. Both experimental and modeling results suggest that the presence of supernormal recovery in cell excitability establishes sufficient nonlinearity so that, during repetitive stimulation, the dynamics of cell response may be regular and predictable when the stimulus magnitude is either very small or very large, or they may be chaotic and very unpredictable when the stimulus magnitude is intermediate. The overall results suggest that the application of nonlinear systems theory to electrophysiology may have importance in the understanding of cardiac rhythm and conduction disturbances, and may have clinical implications as well.

REFERENCES

1. BERGE, P., Y. POMEAU, & C. VIDAL. 1984. Order within Chaos. Towards a Deterministic Approach to Turbulence. John Wiley & Sons. New York, N.Y.
2. GUEVARA, M. R., A. SCHIER, & L. GLASS. 1988. Phase-locked rhythms in periodically stimulated heart cell aggregates. Am. J. Physiol. **254** (Heart Circ. Physiol. **23**): H1–H10.
3. KEENER, J. P. 1981. On cardiac arrhythmias: AV conduction block. J. Math. Biol. **12**: 215–225.
4. SHRIER, A., H. DUBARSKY, M. ROSENGARTEN, M. R. GUEVARA, S. NATTEL, & L. GLASS. 1987. Prediction of complex atrioventricular conduction rhythms in humans with use of the atrioventricular nodal recovery curve. Circulation **76**: 1196–1205.
5. CHIALVO, D. R. & J. JALIFE. 1987. Non-linear dynamics of cardiac excitation and impulse propagation. Nature **330**: 749–752.
6. THOMPSON, J. M. T. & H. B. STEWART. 1986. Nonlinear Dynamics and Chaos. John Wiley and Sons. New York, N.Y.
7. CHIALVO, D. R., D. MICHAELS & J. JALIFE. 1990. Supernormal excitability as a mechanism of chaotic dynamics of activation in cardiac Purkinje fibers. Circ. Res. **66**: 525–545.
8. CHIALVO, D. R., R. F. GILMOUR, JR. & J. JALIFE. 1990. Low dimensional chaos in cardiac tissue. Nature. **343**: 653–657.
9. VINET, A., D. R. CHIALVO, D. C. MICHAELS & J. JALIFE. Nonlinear dynamics of rate-dependent activation in models of single cardiac cells. (Submitted.)
10. BEELER, G. W. & H. REUTER. 1977. Reconstruction of the action potential of ventricular myocardial fibres. J. Physiol. London **268**: 177–210.

11. SPEAR, J. F., & E. N. MOORE. 1974. The effect of changes in rate and rhythm on supernormal excitability in the isolated Purkinje system of the dog. Circ. Res. **50:** 1144–1149.
12. DROUHARD, J. P. & F. A. ROBERGE. 1987. Revised formulation of the Hodgkin-Huxley representation of the sodium current in cardiac cells. Comp. Biomed. Res. **20:** 333–350.
13. HODGKIN, A. L. & A. F. HUXLEY. 1952. A quantitative description of membrane current and its application to conduction and excitation in nerve. J. Physiol. London **117:** 500–544.
14. KAPLAN, D. T. 1989. The dynamics of cardiac electrical instability. PhD thesis. Harvard University. Cambridge, Mass.
15. SAVINO, V. G., L. ROMANELLI, GONZALEZ, O. PIRO & M. E. VALENTINUZZI. 1989. Evidence for chaotic behavior in driven ventricles. Biophys. J. **56:** 273–280.

Modulation of Arrhythmia Substrate[a]

MICHIEL J. JANSE AND HANS SPEKHORST

Department of Clinical and Experimental Cardiology
Academic Medical Center
University of Amsterdam
Meibergdreef 9
1105 AZ Amsterdam ZO, the Netherlands
and
Interuniversity Cardiology Institute of the Netherlands

INTRODUCTION

Most arrhythmias occurring in man appear to be based on a reentrant mechanism. Evidence for reentry in man is largely circumstantial. However, when a tachycardia is initiated by a premature stimulus, an inverse relationship between the coupling interval of the premature stimulus and the interval between premature response and first complex of the tachycardia (the echo interval) speaks in favor of reentry.[1,2] On the basis of this criterion, tachycardias (both supraventricular and ventricular) were reentrant by nature in 417 of 425 patients in whom tachycardias could reproducibly be induced.[1]

In this paper, therefore, we will limit our discussion on arrhythmia substrate to the various forms of reentry. We will emphasize the concept of wavelength to indicate in which ways the substrate for reentry can be modulated. Finally, we shall describe a body surface mapping technique, and its application in 25 patients, by which some of the modulations may be detected by man.

THE WAVELENGTH CONCEPT

Two basic types of reentrant circuits may be distinguished, an anatomical and a functional circuit.[3,4] Anatomical circuits may be formed by the bundle branches of the specialized conduction system, by the route atria—AV conducting system—ventricles, and accessory AV connections in patients with the Wolff-Parkinson-White syndrome, by the tissue around the orifices of the venae cavae, or that around the ostium of the coronary sinus, or by isolated bundles of surviving myocardium within a healed infarct. During a reentrant tachycardia, the impulse circulates in the pathway indicated around a central, anatomically defined obstacle. In contrast, in a functional reentrant circuit there is no central inexcitable obstacle and the circuit is defined by the functional characteristics of the tissue involved. For example, in an area where local differences in refractory period exist, a premature impulse may be blocked transiently in the regions with the longest refractory periods, slowly conducted through other regions, and eventually return to the initial area of block after this has recovered its excitability to reexcite it. In each type of reentrant circuit, the conduction time of the impulse traveling around the area of block must be long enough to allow elements proximal to the zone of block to recover their excitability. The significance of the wavelength for circus movement was recognized by early investigators such as *Mines*[5] and later formulated as the distance traveled by the depolarization wave during the

[a]This study was supported by the Netherlands Heart Foundation, grant no. 85.027.

duration of the refractory period: wavelength = conduction velocity × refractory period.[6] In a reentrant circuit with an anatomical obstacle, the wavelength may be less than the path length and part of the circuit is therefore fully excitable during circus movement tachycardia. In a functional circuit of the leading circle type, an excitable gap may not exist because the impulse travels in the smallest pathway available. For every type of reentry, the general rule holds that the shorter the wavelength, the greater the chance for the establishment of a reentrant rhythm. Wavelength can be altered by changing conduction velocity, refractory period, or both.

In a recent study, wavelength in the atria of conscious dogs was manipulated by a variety of compounds. Wavelength was found to be a reliable index predicting inducibility of various atrial arrhythmias by programmed electrical stimulation: at wavelengths shorter than 7.8 cm, atrial fibrillation was induced in 82% of cases by premature stimuli; atrial flutter was produced in 73% of cases at wavelengths between 7.8 and 9.7 cm; at wavelengths between 9.7 and 12.3 cm only a short series of repetitive responses was obtained in 65% of attempts; whereas premature stimuli were unable to induce any arrhythmia in 80% of cases when wavelength was longer than 12.3 cm. The refractory period duration and conduction velocity each were poor parameters to predict the occurrence of these arrhythmias.[7] Thus, a drug that slowed conduction, which in principle is a proarrhythmic effect, might prolong the refractory period to such an extent that wavelength remained unchanged.

The electrocardiographic detection of changes in wavelength that enhance the likelihood for reentrant arrhythmias is far from easy. Analysis of the QRS complex may yield information concerning conduction velocity, and we will come back to this later. The QT interval may be used as an index of the ventricular refractory period, as "it appears reasonable to assume that the end of the T wave closely approximates the longest duration of ventricular repolarization."[8] However, a prolonged QT interval is also indicative of a marked asynchrony of repolarization.[8,9] This may be due to a greater dispersion of refractory periods or to a greater dispersion of activation times.[9] Both types of inhomogeneity are arrhythmogenic in the sense that the chance for occurrence of unidirectional block, one of the prerequisites for reentry, is enhanced.

In the presence of increased dispersion in recovery of excitability, premature impulses or a mere increase in heart rate may lead to unidirectional block and the initiation of a reentrant arrhythmia. One example where inhomogeneity in recovery of excitability is "unmasked" by an increase in heart rate, resulting in ventricular fibrillation, is shown in FIGURE 1. Four transmembrane potentials were simultaneously recorded from the ischemic segment of the left ventricle of a pig heart, four minutes after occlusion of a coronary artery. During regular pacing of the right atrium at a cycle length of 400 mseconds the four cells recorded from were activated in a reasonably synchronous way. Upon decreasing the pacing cycle to 300 mseconds this synchronicity was lost: the alternation in cell 2 became more marked, its activation became delayed in the fifth beat, conduction block occurred in the sixth beat, and within 1 second following the increase in heart rate the ventricles were fibrillating.[10]

The possibility that the detection of changes in the QT interval, and especially short-term variations, may have predictive value for the occurrence of arrhythmias needs to be further explored. To our knowledge, shortening of the QT interval, indicative of shortening of the refractory period and therefore possibly indicating a shortening of the wavelength, has not been reported as a factor predicting arrhythmogenesis. The association of QT prolongation with subsequent arrhythmias or sudden death[11,12] may indicate that increased inhomogeneity in recovery of excitability "overrules" the increase in refractory period duration which should be expected to prolong wavelength and thus protect against reentrant arrhythmias.

(For the sake of simplicity, we will not consider here a different arrhythmogenic mechanism that may well underly some of the arrhythmias associated with the long QT syndrome, namely, triggered activity based on early afterdepolarization which preferentially occurs in situations when action potential duration is prolonged.)

In the following, we will concentrate on a method using body surface mapping to detect early changes in conduction velocity caused by ischemia.

BODY SURFACE MAPPING DURING BRIEF PERIODS OF ISCHEMIA

There is some controversy regarding the changes in R wave in the conventional electrocardiogram (ECG) during ischemia and about the mechanisms that cause them. Thus, both a decrease and an increase in R wave amplitude have been reported[13,14] and both changes in conduction velocity[13] and changes in intracardiac volume[15] have been considered to underly the changes in R wave amplitude.

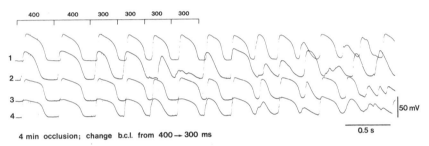

FIGURE 1. An increase in heart rate unmasks inhomogeneity in recovery of excitability in acutely ischemic myocardium. Four transmembrane potentials were simultaneously recorded from the anterior surface of the left ventricle of a porcine heart, 4 minutes after coronary artery occlusion. The atrium was paced at a cycle length of 400 mseconds, and the four cells were more or less synchronously activated. Upon a sudden shortening of the pacing cycle to 300 mseconds, this synchronicity becomes lost: cell 2 is activated with delay (beat 5) and shows conduction block (beat 6). Within seconds the ventricles fibrillate. (Reproduced from Reference 10 with permission.)

Body surface mapping provides more information than standard ECG leads, and this technique has recently been applied during percutaneous transluminal coronary angioplasty.[16,17] We have studied 25 patients, and recorded simultaneously from 62 sites on the thorax, using a specially designed radiotransparent electrode array.[18] Recordings were made before, during, and after balloon inflation during coronary angioplasty. Ten patients had single vessel disease of the left anterior descending coronary artery, five patients of the right coronary artery, and five patients of the circumflex branch. The other patients had multivessel disease. The 62 unipolar electrocardiograms (Wilsons central terminal was used as reference) were sampled with a frequency of 500 Hz and recorded on an Apple IIe computer with an 8 bit A/D converter. The use of high quality monolithic amplifiers and shielding of cables ensured that noise and mains interference was always lower than 1 bit (4 μV). Data were transferred to a PDP 11/73 minicomputer equipped with an electrostatic plotter, and

body surface map

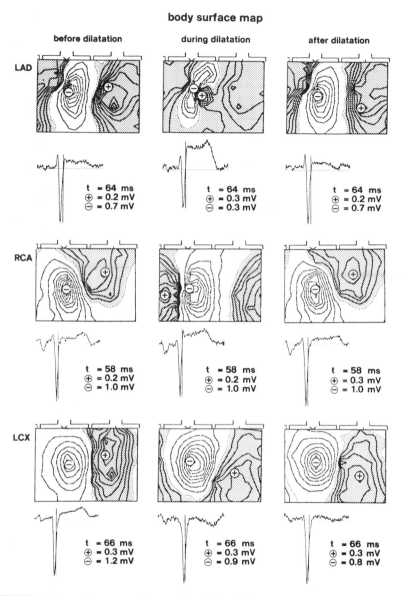

FIGURE 2. Body surface maps of three patients before, during, and after percutaneous translu-minal coronary angioplasty. The recordings during dilatation were made 50 seconds after balloon inflation in respectively the left anterior descending artery (LAD), the right coronary artery (RCA), and the circumflex branch (LCX). Each map represents the unfolded thorax. The right vertical line is the right posterior axillary line and is connected to the left vertical line. Above each map the shoulders, sternum, neck, and spinal column are indicated. Shaded areas are zones of positive potentials, white areas have negative potentials. Isopotential lines are indicated. t = time in QRS complex at which the maps were made; the voltage extremes are indicated below each map. Note characteristic changes in potential distribution during the moment in the QRS complex indicated in the V_1 lead under each map. See text for further discussion.

body surface maps were constructed. Equal positive potentials were connected by solid isopotential lines, negative potentials by dotted isopotential lines. A more detailed description of the methods used can be found elsewhere.[19]

FIGURE 2 shows body surface maps of three patients. All patients had single vessel disease with a normal electrocardiogram at rest. For each of the three patients a similar time interval was selected at the end of the QRS complex, before, during, and after balloon inflation during coronary angioplasty. The time is indicated in the V_1 lead below each map. Isopotential lines were calculated by linear interpolation. Voltages of the extremes are indicated. Each map represents the unfolded thorax in which the right vertical side of the map is connected to the left vertical side. This edge represents the right posterior axillary line. Above each map the shoulders, sternum, neck and spinal column are indicated. In all three patients, the maps before and after dilatation show similar patterns and voltages. During dilatation, 50 seconds after the onset of coronary occlusion, characteristic changes are observed. Thus, during occlusion of the left anterior descending artery (LAD), positivity is found on the left side of the anterior thorax. During occlusion of the right coronary artery (RCA), positivity is on the lower right part of the anterolateral thorax. And during circumflex occlusion (LCX), positivity is on the lower part of the back. Similar patterns were found in the other patients: in all cases the localization of the area of positivity corresponded to the ischemic area. The most likely cause for these changes is a decrease in conduction velocity in the ischemic area. The leads overlying the ischemic area show positive potentials at a time during the activation process where these areas had already become negative before or after ischemia. Our data did not reveal a change in total QRS duration but only a temporal change within the QRS complex. It is surprising that these changes occur so rapidly, i.e., within 40 to 50 seconds after the beginning of balloon inflation. Animal experiments indicate that slowing of conduction within the ischemic zone can be detected only 2 minutes after abrupt coronary occlusion.[20] A possible explanation for the earlier slowing of conduction in these patients may be that the insertion of the guiding wire and of the uninflated balloon in an already narrowed vessel causes a further reduction of the lumen diameter, inducing "low flow ischemia." In animal experiments it was shown that when complete coronary artery occlusion was performed following a period of coronary stenosis, extracellular potassium concentration in the myocardium perfused by the stenotic artery had already risen substantially at the onset of complete occlusion. Since the rate of rise in extracellular K^+ during complete occlusion was similar with or without a previous period of low flow ischemia, the levels of extracellular K^+ where conduction of the impulse would be slowed were reached much earlier during an occlusion preceded by a period of coronary stenosis.[21]

From our results it appears that very early changes in conduction velocity during acute transmural ischemia may be detected by body surface mapping. It remains to be established whether this technique when applied during exercise in patients with coronary artery disease may be more sensitive in detecting early changes in arrhythmia substrate than conventional electrocardiography.

REFERENCES

1. BRUGADA, P. & H. J. J. WELLENS. 1983. The role of triggered activity in clinical arrhythmias. In Frontiers of Electrocardiography. M. Rosenbaum & M. Elizari, Eds.: 195–216. Martinus Nijhoff. The Hague, the Netherlands.
2. BIGGER, J. T. & B. N. GOLDREYER. 1970. The mechanism of supraventricular tachycardia. Circulation 42: 673–688.
3. ALLESSIE, M. A., F. I. M. BONKE & F. SCHOPMAN. 1973. Circus movement in rabbit atrial muscle as a mechanism for tachycardia. Circ. Res. 33: 54–62.

4. JANSE, M. J. 1986. Reentry rhythms. *In* The Heart and Cardiovascular System. H. A. Fozzard, R. B. Jennings, A. M. Katz & H. E. Morgan, Eds.: 1203–1238. Raven Press. New York, N.Y.
5. MINES, G. R. 1913. On dynamic equilibrium in the heart. J. Physiol. 46: 349–383.
6. WIENER, N. & A. ROSENBLUETH. 1946. The mathematical formulation of the problem of conduction of impulses in a network of connected excitable elements, specifically in cardiac muscle. Arch. Inst. Cardiol. Mex. 16: 205–265.
7. RENSMA, P. L., M. A. ALLESSIE, W. J. E. P. LAMMERS, F. I. M. BONKE & M. J. SCHALIJ. 1988. Length of excitation wave and susceptibility to reentrant atrial arrhythmias in normal conscious dogs. Circ. Res. 62: 395–410.
8. SURAWICZ, B. & S. B. KNOEBEL. 1984. Long QT: Good, bad or indifferent? J. Am. Coll. Cardiol. 4: 398–413.
9. VASSALLO, J. A., D. M. CASSIDY, E. KINWALL, F. E. MARCHLINSKI & M. E. JOSEPHSON. 1988. Nonuniform recovery of excitability in the left ventricle. Circulation 78: 1365–1372.
10. JANSE, M. J., A. G. KLEBER, E. DOWNAR & D. DURRER. 1977. Changements electrophysiologiques pendant l'ischemie myocardique et mecanisme possible des troubles du rythme ventriculaire. Ann. Cardiol. Angeiol. Paris 26: 551–554.
11. SCHWARTZ, P. J. & S. WOLF. 1978. QT prolongation as predictor of sudden death in patients with myocardial infarction. Circulation 57: 1074–1077.
12. TAYLOR, G. J., R. S. CROMPTON, R. S. GIBSON, P. T. STEBBINS, M. T. G. WALDMAN & G. A. BELLAR. 1981. Prolonged QT interval at onset of acute myocardial infarction in predicting early phase ventricular tachycardia. Am. Heart J. 102: 16–24.
13. DAVID, D., M. NAITO, E. MICHELSON, Y. WATANABE, C. C. CHEN, J. MORGANROTH, M. SCHAFFENBURG & T. BLENKO. 1982. Intramyocardial conduction: a major determinant of R-wave amplitude during acute myocardial ischemia. Circulation 65: 161–167.
14. BONORIS, P. E., P. S. GREENBERG, M. J. CASTELLANET & M. H. ELLERSTAD. 1978. Significant changes in R wave amplitude during treadmill stress testing: angiographic correlation. Am. J. Cardiol. 41: 846–851.
15. BRODY, D. A. 1956. A theoretical analysis of intracavitary blood mass influence on the heart-lead relationship. Circ. Res. 6: 731–739.
16. HAMEL, D., P. SAVARD, D. DEROME, L. LEGENDRE, R. NADEAU, M. DUBUC & M. SHENASSA. 1988. Detection of localized ischemic changes with body surface potential mapping in patients undergoing coronary angioplasty. (abstr.) Circ. Suppl. 78: II–577.
17. SPEKHORST, H., A. SIPPENSGROENEWEGEN, G. K. DAVID & M. J. JANSE. 1988. Body surface mapping during percutaneous transluminal coronary angioplasty (PTCA): evidence of regional conduction delay. (abstr.) Circ. Suppl. 78: II–577.
18. SPEKHORST, H., A. SIPPENSGROENEWEGEN, G. K. DAVID, C. METTING VAN RIJN & P. BROEKHUIJSEN. 1988. Radiotransparent carbon electrode for ECG recordings in the catheterization laboratory. IEEE Trans. Biomed. BME-35 5: 402.
19. SPEKHORST, H., A. SIPPENSGROENEWEGEN, G. K. DAVID, M. J. JANSE & A. J. DUNNING. 1990. Body surface mapping during percutaneous transluminal coronary angioplasty: QRS changes indicating regional myocardial conduction delay. Circulation 81: 840–849.
20. KLEBER, A. G., M. J. JANSE, F. J. G. WILMS-SCHOPMAN, A. A. M. WILDE & R. CORONEL. 1986. Changes in conduction velocity during acute ischemia in ventricular myocardium of the isolated porcine heart. Circulation 73: 189–198.
21. CORONEL, R., J. W. T. FIOLET, F. J. G. WILMS-SCHOPMAN, T. OPTHOF, A. F. M. SCHAAPHERDER & M. J. JANSE. 1989. Distribution of extracellular potassium and electrophysiologic changes during two-stage coronary ligation in the isolated, perfused canine heart. Circulation 80: 165–177.

Electrocardiography

Past, Present, and Future

HEIN J. J. WELLENS

Department of Cardiology
Academic Hospital
University of Maastricht
Post Office Box 1968
6201 Bx Maastricht, the Netherlands

Ever since Einthoven introduced electrocardiography as a new method to diagnose heart disease in man,[1] its use and importance has expanded. This is not surprising, for as pointed out by Fisch,[2] the electrocardiogram (ECG) is a noninvasive technique which does not harm the patient, is inexpensive, simple, and reproducible, allows serial studies, and is the only practical means to record the cardiac action potential.

Fisch also stressed that the ECG (1) still serves as an independent marker of myocardial infarction; (2) reflects anatomic, metabolic, and hemodynamic alterations; (3) demonstrates a variety of complex electrophysiologic concepts through deductive reasoning; (4) is a stimulus for laboratory confirmation of postulated mechanisms and concepts; (5) is vital for proper diagnosis and therapy; (6) is without peer for the diagnosis of arrhythmias.[2]

It is worrysome therefore that with the increasing use of sophisticated invasive (and noninvasive) techniques, there is a decreasing ability of our younger colleagues to interprete the electrocardiogram correctly. The escalating costs of our health system call for reassessment of the value of the different diagnostic tests in an effort to select those with the best cost/benefit ratio. Electrocardiography is a typical example of a test that, when interpreted correctly, can be extremely cost-effective.

WHY IS OUR KNOWLEDGE OF ELECTROCARDIOGRAPHY STILL EXPANDING?

Essential in the expansion of our knowledge of electrocardiography has been and will be the reexamination of the electrocardiogram in the light of information obtained through invasive and noninvasive techniques. A list (which is far from complete!) of new diagnostic pointers on the electrocardiogram and the techniques that played an essential role in their recognition is given in TABLE 1. It should be stressed, however, that one should not only look for new electrocardiographic signs by using other techniques, but also by critically evaluating the value of accepted ECG criteria against information from new techniques. This philosophy has always been followed in our department and has led to new electrocardiographic findings. Let me illustrate this with a few examples demonstrating that our knowledge of the 12 lead electrocardiogram is still expanding.

TABLE 1. Examples of Recently Described Electrocardiographic Diagnostic Findings and the Techniques that Contributed to Their Recognition

ECG	Technique
Localization of AV and intraventricular conduction disturbances.	Anatomic dissection,[3] electrography of the conduction system and pacing.[4-8]
Significance of site of AV and intraventricular block in myocardial infarction.	Electrography of the conduction system and clinical follow-up.[9,10]
Diagnosis of site of origin of wide and narrow QRS tachycardia.	Intracardiac electrography using mapping and programmed stimulation.[11-16]
Localization of accessory pathways and recognition of multiple accessory pathways.	Programmed stimulation and intracardiac and intraoperative mapping.[17-21]
Localization of ventricular impulse formation.	Intracardiac electrography, surgery, pacing.[11,22,23]
Right ventricular dysplasia.	Intracardiac mapping, surgery, LV angio, echocardiography.[24,25]
Critical high LAD stenosis, left main and severe three vessel disease.	Coronary angiography.[26-28]
Right ventricular infarction.	Autopsy. hemodynamic, echocardiographic, and radionuclide studies.[29-36]
QRS score, infarct size, and LV function after myocardial infarction.	LV angiography.[37,38]
QRS-T findings and LV wall motion.	LV angiography.[39]
Digitalis intoxication.	Pacing.[40-42]
Abnormal depolarization–induced T wave changes.	Pacing, intracardiac electrography.[43-45]

THE ECG IN RISK STRATIFICATION OF PATIENTS WITH UNSTABLE ANGINA

De Zwaan *et al.* described a group of patients who were admitted to hospital with unstable angina and subsequently (in the pain-free period) developed negative T waves in the precordial leads without Q waves and no or minimal enzyme level elevation.[26,27] Coronary angiography in these patients revealed a critical stenosis high in the left anterior descending coronary artery close to the first septal branch. Recognition of these patients is of obvious importance, because of the risk of losing an important portion of left ventricular muscle if occlusion occurs at that site. The same holds for the patient with unstable angina having left main or severe three vessel disease. Gorgels found that ST segment depression in 8 leads together with ST segment elevation in leads AVR and V1 (FIGURE 1) during pain in a patient with unstable angina indicates a very high chance of left main or serious three vessel disease.[28]

THE ECG OF RIGHT VENTRICULAR INFARCTION

Infarct localization studies using 99 m Technetium pyrophosphate scintigraphy showed that right ventricular involvement is present in approximately 45% of patients with an acute inferoposterior infarction.[33] By combining the radionuclide studies with right-sided chest leads, it was found that ST segment elevation of 1 mm or more in lead V_4R has a high sensitivity and specificity to detect right ventricular infarction.[34] This electrocardiographic finding not only indicates a proximal occlusion of the right coronary artery but also identifies a subgroup of patients having a high chance (approximately 50%) of developing high degree AV block.[35] The duration of ST segment elevation in lead V_4R, however, is short lived having disappeared in half of the patients 10 hours after the onset of the pain of myocardial infarction. Recently it was shown that lead V_4R in acute inferoposterior infarction can identify the site of obstruction in the coronary artery. FIGURE 2 demonstrates how the ST-T segment in lead V_4R indicates where and which coronary artery is occluded.[36]

THE ECG OF THE PATIENT SHOWING A WIDE OR
NARROW QRS TACHYCARDIA

The introduction by Durrer[18] and Coumel[46] of programmed stimulation of the heart together with the simultaneous recording of intracardiac and extracardiac electrical activity has been of great help in understanding the ECG of patients showing either a wide or a narrow QRS tachycardia.[13-16] Intracardiac electrograms make it possible to identify the site of origin and the pathway of a tachycardia. By carefully correlating this information with the configurational characteristics of the 12 lead ECG, the site of origin of a wide or narrow QRS tachycardia can correctly be predicted in most patients.[47,48]

THE ECG IN THE PATIENT WITH PREEXCITATION

Several groups have pointed to the value of the 12 lead ECG in predicting the location of the accessory pathway in the patient with preexcitation.[49-52] That knowl-

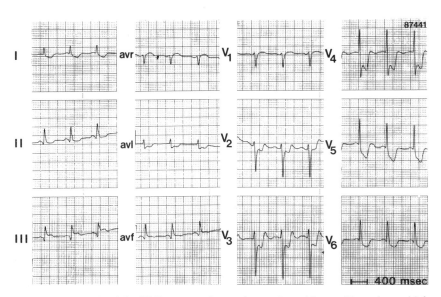

FIGURE 1. Example of the ST-T segment changes in a patient with unstable angina and left main disease. Note the presence of ST segment depression in 9 leads and ST segment elevation in leads AVR and V_1. As described by Gorgels,[28] these findings are typical for left main or severe three vessel disease.

edge was obtained by combining information from intracardiac and perioperative activation mapping studies used to localize the accessory connection with findings on the 12 lead ECG. We have recently shown that the 12 lead ECG during sinus rhythm and tachycardia may show clues indicating the presence of more than one accessory pathway.[21]

THE FUTURE OF ELECTROCARDIOGRAPHY

If we want to continue to expand our knowledge of electrocardiography we have to realize that there are developments that may hamper our efforts.

Although of great importance for screening, epidemiologic studies, and storing, presently used computer programs for ECG interpretation tend to "freeze" our knowledge. New programs should be developed allowing recognition of new specific ECG findings in certain conditions by using both detailed electrocardiographic analy-

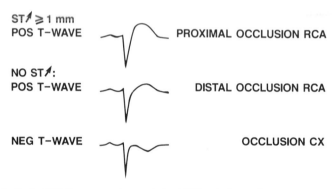

FIGURE 2. Typical ST-T segment changes in lead V_4R pointing to the coronary artery which is occluded in acute inferoposterior myocardial infarction. Note that it is also possible to differentiate between an occlusion proximal or distal in the right coronary artery. See also Braat et al.[36]

sis and diagnostic information from other techniques. This requires the cooperation from cardiologists active and knowledgeable in the different noninvasive and invasive techniques.

Another problem in the advancement of electrocardiography is the increasing use of single lead monitoring in the coronary care unit (CCU). Although useful in alerting the physician to conduction disturbances and ectopic activity, single lead recordings usually do not allow detailed analysis of site and mechanism of abnormal impulse formation and prevent the physician from getting experience in the interpretation and understanding of complex arrhythmias.

A third problem is the growing interest in invasive techniques. They are considered to give more detailed information leading to faster and more reliable decision making. While invasive tests are of great importance, especially when surgical or electrical interventions have to be performed, the correct interpretation of the ECG will indicate that in a number of patients such investigations are not indicated.

CONCLUSION

It has been shown that also in recent years several new contributions have been made in the field of electrocardiography. This stresses the necessity of implementing sufficient electrocardiography in the training program of the cardiologist and internist. It is important to realize that the correct interpretation of the ECG requires all-around knowledge of cardiac anatomy, electrophysiology, and hemodynamics.

In view of the above, electrocardiography should also be a recurrent item in postgraduate teaching. I completely agree with Dr. Charles Fisch when he writes, "He who maintains that new knowledge of electrocardiography is no longer possible or contributive, ignores history."[2]

REFERENCES

1. EINTHOVEN, W. 1906. Le télécardiogramme. Arch. Int. Physiol. **4:** 132–164.
2. FISCH, C. 1980. The clinical electrocardiogram: a classic. Circulation **62**(3): 1–4.
3. ROSENBAUM, M. B., M. V. ELIZARI, & J. O. LAZZARI. 1968. Los Hemibloqueos. Paidos. Buenos Aires, Argentina.
4. SCHERLAG, B. J., S. H. LAU, R. H. HELFANT, W. D. BERKOWITZ, E. STEIN & A. N. DAMATO. 1969. Catheter technique for recording His bundle activity in man. Circulation **39:** 13–22.
5. DAMATO, A. N. & S. H. LAU. 1970. The clinical value of the electrogram of the conducting system. Progr. Cardiovasc. Dis. **13:** 119–140.
6. NARULA, O. S., B. J. SCHERLAG, P. SAMET & R. P. JAVIER. 1971. Atrioventricular block. Localization and classification by His bundle recordings. Am. J. Med. **50:** 146–161.
7. ROSEN, K. M. 1972. Evaluation of cardiac conduction in the catheterization laboratory. Am. J. Cardiol. **30:** 701–703.
8. PEUCH, P. & R. GROLLEAU. 1972. L'Activité du Faisceau de His Normale et Pathologique. Ed Sandoz. Paris, France.
9. LIE, K. I., H. J. J. WELLENS & R. M. SCHUILENBURG. 1974. Factors influencing prognosis of bundle branch block complicating acute myocardial infarction. Circulation **50:** 935–948.
10. TANS, A. C. & K. I. LIE. 1976. AV nodal block in acute myocardial infarction. *In* The Conduction System of the Heart. H. J. J. Wellens, K. I. Lie & M. J. Janse, (Eds).: 655–661. Lea and Febiger. Philadelphia, Pa.
11. JOSEPHSON, M. E., H. L. WAXMAN, F. E. MARCHILINSKI, L. N. HOROWITZ & S. R. SPIELMAN. 1981. Relation between site of origin and QRS configuration in ventricular rhythms. *In* What's New in Electrocardiography. H. J. J. Wellens & H. E. Kulbertus, Eds.: 200–228. Martinus Nijhoff. The Hague, the Netherlands.
12. WELLENS, H. J. J., F. W. H. M. BAR & K. I. LIE. 1978. The value of the electrocardiogram in the differential diagnosis of a tachycardia with a widened QRS complex. Am. J. Med. **64:** 27–33.
13. WU, D., P. DENES, F. AMAT-Y-LEON, R. DHINGRA, C. R. C. WYNDHAM, R. BAUERFEIND, P. LAFIT & K. M. ROSEN. 1978. Clinical, electrocardiographic and electrophysiologic observations in patients with paroxysmal supraventricular tachycardia. Am. J. Cardiol. **41:** 1045–1051.
14. FARSHIDI, A., M. E. JOSEPHSON & L. N. HOROWITZ. 1978. Electrophysiologic characteristics of concealed bypass tracts: clinical and electrocardiographic correlates. Am. J. Cardiol. **41:** 1052–1060.
15. FARRE, J. & H. J. J. WELLENS. 1981. The value of the electrocardiogram in diagnosing site of origin and mechanism of supraventricular tachycardia. *In* What's New in Electrocardiography. H. J. J. Wellens & H. E. Kulbertus, Eds.: 131–171. Martinus Nijhoff. The Hague, the Netherlands.
16. COUMEL, P. 1975. Junctional reciprocating tachycardia. The permanent and paroxysmal forms of AV nodal reciprocating tachycardias. J. Electrocardiol. **8:** 79–90.

17. DURRER, D., L. SCHOO, R. M. SCHUILENBURG & H. J. J. WELLENS. 1967. The role of premature beats in the initiation and termination of supraventricular tachycardia in the Wolff-Parkinson-White syndrome. Circulation 36: 644–655.

18. SLAMA, R., P. COUMEL & Y. BOUVRAIN. 1973. Les syndromes de Wolff-Parkinson-White de type A inapparents ou latents en rhythme sinusal. Arch. Mal. Coeur 66: 639–647.

19. ZIPES, D. P., R. L. DEJOSEPH & D. A. ROTHBAUM. 1974. Unusual properties of accessory pathways. Circulation 49: 1200–1209.

20. GALLAGHER, J. J., E. L. C. PRITCHETT, W. C. SEALY, J. KASELL & A. G. WALLACE. 1978. The pre-excitation syndromes. Progr. Cardiovasc. Dis. 20: 285–327.

21. WELLENS, H. J. J., J. ATIE, J. L. SMEETS, F. E. S. CRUZ, A. P. GORGELS & P. BRUGADA. The electrocardiogram in multiple accessory AV pathways. J. Am. Coll. Cardiol. (In press.)

22. HARKEN, A. H. & M. F. JOSEPHSON. 1984. Surgical management of ventricular tachycardia. In Tachycardias: Mechanisms, Diagnosis, Treatment. M. E. Josephson & H. J. J. Wellens, Eds.: 475. Lea and Febiger. Philadelphia, Pa.

23. JOSEPHSON, M. E., H. L. WAXMAN, M. E. CAIN, M. J. GARDNER & A. E. BUXTON. 1982. Ventricular activation during endocardial pacing. II. Role of pace-mapping to localize origin of ventricular tachycardia. Am. J. Cardiol. 50: 11–22.

24. FONTAINE, G., G. GUIRAUDON & R. FRANK. 1977. Stimulation studies and epicardial mapping in ventricular tachycardia: study of mechanism and selection for surgery. In Re-entrant Arrhythmias. H. E. Kulbertus, Ed.: 334. MTP Press. Lancaster, Pa.

25. MARCUS, F. I., G. FONTAINE, R. FRANK & Y. GROSGOGEAT. 1982. Right ventricular dysplasia: a report of 24 cases. Circulation 69: 384–392.

26. DE ZWAAN, C., F. W. H. M. BÄR & H. J. J. WELLENS. 1982. Characteristic electrocardiographic pattern indicating a critical stenosis high in left anterior descending coronary artery in patients admitted because of impending myocardial infarction. Am. Heart J. 103: 730–735.

27. DE ZWAAN, C., F. W. BÄR, J. H. A. JANSSEN, et al. 1989. Angiographic and clinical characteristic showing an electrocardiographic pattern pointing to a critical narrowing in the left anterior descending coronary artery. Am. Heart J. 117: 657–665.

28. GORGELS, A. P., M. A. VOS, F. W. BÄR & H. J. J. WELLENS. 1988. An electrocardiographic pattern, characteristic for extensive myocardial ischemia. Circulation 78(II): 422.

29. WADE, W. G. 1959. The pathenogenesis of infarction of the right ventricle. Br. Heart J. 21: 545–554.

30. COHN, J. N., N. H. GUIHA, M. I. BRODER & C. J. LIMAS. 1974. Right ventricular infarction. Clinical and hemodynamic features. Am. J. Cardiol. 33: 209–214.

31. CANDELL-RIERA, J., J. FIGUREAS, V. VALLE, A. ALVAREZ, L. GUTIERREZ, J. CORTADELLAS, J. CINCA, A. SALAS & J. RIUS. 1981. Right ventricular infarction. Relationships between ST-segment elevation in V_4R and hemodynamic, scintigraphic and echocardiographic findings in patients with an acute inferior myocardial infarction. Am. Heart J. 101: 281–287.

32. ERHARDT, L. R., A. SJOGREN & J. WAHLBERG. 1976. Single right sided precordial lead in the diagnosis of right ventricular involvement in inferior myocardial infarction. Am. Heart J. 91: 571–576.

33. WACKERS, F. J., K. I. LIE, E. B. SOKOLE, J. RES, J. B. VAN DER SCHOOT & D. DURRER. 1978. Prevalence of right ventricular involvement in inferior wall infarction assessed with myocardial imaging with Thallium 201 and Technetium 99m pyrophosphate. Am. J. Cardiol. 42: 358–362.

34. BRAAT, S. H., P. BRUGADA, C. DE ZWAAN, J. M. COENEGRACHT & H. J. J. WELLENS. 1983. Value of electrocardiogram in diagnosing right ventricular involvement in patients with an acute inferior wall myocardial infarction. Br. Heart J. 49: 368–372.

35. BRAAT, S. H., C. DE ZWAAN, P. BRUGADA, J. M. COENEGRACHT & H. J. J. WELLENS. 1984. Right ventricular involvement with acute inferior wall myocardial infarction identifies high risk of developing atrioventricular nodal conduction disturbances. Am. Heart J. 107: 1183–1186.

36. BRAAT, S. H., A. P. M. GORGELS, F. W. BÄR & H. J. J. WELLENS. 1988. Value of the ST-T

segment in lead V₄R in inferior wall acute myocardial infarction to predict the site of coronary artery occlusion. Am. J. Cardiol. **62:** 140–143.

37. WAGNER, G. S., C. J. FREYE, S. T. PALMERI, S. F. ROARK, N. C. STACK, R. E. IDEKER, R. E. HARRELL, JR. & R. H. SELVESTER. 1982. Evaluation of a QRS scoring system for estimating infarct size 1. Specificity and observer agreement. Circulation **65:** 342–349.

38. PALMERI, S. T., D. G. HARRISON, F. R. COBB, K. O. MORRIS, F. E. HARRELL, R. E. IDEKER, R. H. SELVESTER & G. S. WAGNER. 1982. A QRS scoring system for accessory left ventricular function after myocardial infarction. N. Engl. J. Med. **306:** 4–8.

39. BÄR, F. W., P. BRUGADA, W. R. DASSEN, T. VAN DER WERF & H. J. J. WELLENS. 1984. Prognostic value of Q waves, R/S ratio, loss of R wave voltage, ST-T segment abnormalities, electrical axis, low voltage and notching: correlation of electrocardiogram and left ventriculogram. J. Am. Coll. Cardiol. **4:** 17–27.

40. ROSEN, M. R. & R. F. REDER. 1981. Does triggered activity have a role in the genesis of cardiac arrhythmias? Ann. Intern. Med. **94:** 794–801.

41. GORGELS, A. P. M., H. D. M. BEEKMAN, P. BRUGADA, W. R. M. DASSEN, D. A. B. RICHARDS & H. J. J. WELLENS. 1983. Extrastimulus related shortening of the first postpacing interval in digitalis induced ventricular tachycardia. J. Am. Coll. Cardiol. **1:** 840–857.

42. WELLENS, H. J. J. 1976. The electrocardiogram in digitalis intoxication. *In:* Progress in Cardiology. P. N. Yu & J. F. Goodwin, Eds. **5:** 271–290. Lea and Febiger. Philadelphia, Pa.

43. CHATTERJEE, K., A. HARRIS, G. DAVIES & A. LEATHAM. 1969. Electrocardiographic changes subsequent to artificial ventricular depolarization. Br. Heart J. **31:** 770–779.

44. NICOLAI, P., J. L. MEDVEDOWSKY, R. DELAAGE, P. MARTIN-NOEL, R. FRANK, C. BARNAY, J. C. AGELOW & E. BLANCHE. 1978. Preexcitations ventriculaires. Diagnostic topographique des faisceaux de Kent. *In* Les Troubles du Rhythme Cardiaque. P. Puech & R. Slama, Eds.: 164–178. Roussel. Paris, France.

45. ROSENBAUM, M. B., H. H. BLANCO, M. V. ELIZARI, J. O. LAZZARI & H. M. VETULLI. 1981. Electrotonic modulation of ventricular repolarization and cardiac memory. *In* Frontiers of Cardiac Electrophysiology. M. B. Rosenbaum & M. V. Elizari, Eds.: 67–99. Martinus Nijhoff. The Hague, the Netherlands.

46. COUMEL, P. L., C. CABROL, A. FABIATO, E. GOURGON & R. SLAMA. 1967. Tachycardia permanente par rhythme réciproque. Arch. Mal. Coeur **60:** 1830–1845.

47. WELLENS, H. J. J., F. W. BÄR, E. J. VANAGT, P. BRUGADA & J. FARRE. 1981. The differentiation between ventricular tachycardia and supraventricular tachycardia with aberrant conduction: the value of the 12-lead electrocardiogram. *In* What's New in Electrocardiography. H. J. J. Wellens & H. E. Kulbertus, Eds.: 184–199. Martinus Nijhoff. The Hague, the Netherlands.

48. WELLENS, H. J. J., P. BRUGADA & F. W. BÄR. 1987. When to use intracardiac electrophysiological studies for diagnosing site of origin and mechanism of tachycardias. Circulation **75(III):** 110–115.

49. GALLAGHER, J. J., E. L. C. PRITCHETT, W. C. SEALY, J. KASELL & A. G. WALLACE. 1978. The pre-excitation syndromes. Prog. Cardiovasc. Dis. **20:** 285–327.

50. MILSTEIN, S., A. D. SHARMA, G. M. GUIRAUDON & G. J. KLEIN. 1987. An algorithm for the electrocardiographic localization of accessory pathways in the Wolff-Parkinson-White syndrome. PACE **10:** 555–563.

51. LEMERY, R., S. C. HAMMILL, D. L. WOOD, et al. 1987. Value of the resting 12 lead electrocardiogram and vectorcardiogram for locating the accessory pathway in patients with the Wolff-Parkinson-White syndrome. Br. Heart J. **58:** 324–332.

52. LINDSAY, B. D., K. J. CROSSEN & M. E. CAIN. 1987. Concordance of distinguishing electrocardiographic features during sinus rhythm with the location of accessory pathways in the Wolff-Parkinson-White syndrome. Am. J. Cardiol. **59:** 1093–1102.

Noninvasive Exploration of Cardiac Arrhythmias

PHILIPPE COUMEL

Lariboisière Hospital
2, rue Ambroise-Paré
75010 Paris, France

INTRODUCTION

The noninvasive exploration of arrhythmias essentially refers to long-term ambulatory electrocardiography (ECG), a technique developed by Holter more than 25 years ago.[1] In principle the exercise test also constitutes a noninvasive exploration, but it can be at least qualified as provocative. Holter monitoring is aimed at recording spontaneous, frequently occurring arrhythmias, thus explaining why from the beginning the Holter technique was used as an epidemiological rather than an electrophysiological method, with a statistical rather than a comprehensive approach. Dynamic ECG however should not be confined to documenting paroxysmal arrhythmias or counting trivial extrasystoles. For us this represents the past of this technique. Its future should exploit the advances in data processing and the knowledge of arrhythmias to explore not only the arrhythmia itself but also its context, its environment of cardiac frequency. On the one hand the sinus rate is the marker of the vagosympathetic balance, an important, constantly present determinant of arrhythmias. On the other hand, cycle length variations also directly condition the arrhythmia through the phenomena of rate dependence, and these two aspects are crucial when one tries to understand arrhythmia behavior.

In the 10 years after Holter's discovery, people were somewhat deceived in that, after all, the ambulatory monitoring technique gave nothing more than a 24-hour ECG. Then, during the next decade, dynamic ECG was essentially used to feed counting machines on the basis that quantifying arrhythmic events was sufficient. Actually, the result has been apparently an evaluation of drug efficacy that is much more precise than it was before in the case of spontaneous, nonsustained arrhythmias. The problem is that there are many ways for quantifying arrhythmias, the validity of which in fact depends on whether the different types of arrhythmia disturbances have been correctly weighted. Another problem is to determine what is the correspondence, if any, between spontaneous and provokable arrhythmias that form the domain of invasive electrophysiology. Both are probably also different from what should be after all the ultimate target of our therapeutic efforts, that is, the arrhythmias responsible for serious symptoms or even sudden death. One should not be surprised if in certain circumstances extrapolations from theories to reality are somewhat disappointing.

The context of an arrhythmia consists of nonarrhythmic events, and in practice the prevailing one is the sinus rhythm. The sinus rhythm contains two types of information, the exploration of which should be the basis of any analysis. First, it is a marker of the vagosympathetic balance, and more generally of the interplay between the various parameters implicated in the autonomic nervous system (ANS). Of course, the meaning of this marker is limited to exploring the ANS in the sinoatrial node, and no doubt in the future it should be extended to the ventricular repolarization phase. Even though this limitation is kept in mind, this factor is essential, since there is not a single

312

arrhythmia that is really free of any ANS influence. The second type of information to be drawn from the dominant rhythm is simply the heart rate. Invasive electrophysiology daily shows that the cardiac rate by itself is an important determinant of many arrhythmias, e.g., ventricular extrasystoles. It follows from the two preceding principles that the arrhythmia's behavior or even simply its presence or absence should be studied as a function of the "environment," the aim being to differentiate between the first and the second principle. Using dynamic ECG with this philosophy makes it a technique essentially designed for research on arrhythmia mechanisms.

At least two ingredients are necessary to produce an arrhythmia: an electrophysiological substrate and a triggering factor.[2] In many cases the presence of the substrate can be checked by invasive electrophysiology: inducing a tachyarrhythmia precisely consists in providing artificially the necessary trigger. On the other hand, the simple fact that the tachyarrhythmia is not permanent or incessant implies that its spontaneous trigger is not available at any time or with the adequate characteristics. The triggering factor is usually formed by extrasystoles that are explored through the Holter technique. This opposition between the two techniques however should not be too manichean: exploring the rate dependence of extrasystoles can be carried out in the best conditions of ANS stability by artificial pacing, and the repetitive activity that forms the "complex arrhythmias" in the Holter terminology reflects in fact the activity of the substrate.

THE ARRHYTHMIAS, THE HEART RATE, AND THE ADRENERGIC DRIVE

If the concepts of rate-dependence and adrenergic dependence are clearly different, in the clinical situation the difficulty is to dissociate these two factors which must be evaluated through the same parameter. We naturally tend to take a rapid heart rate as the marker of an increased sympathetic drive. That is generally true but with notable exceptions: at the end of an exercise test for instance a complex situation combines a high level of circulating catecholamines with a vagal rebound that dramatically slows the heart rate, a very unstable and conflicting status that precisely explains why severe tachyarrhythmias tend to occur at this time rather than during the exercise test.[3] In practice, it is our experience that the most convenient way for distinguishing the two determinants is to consider separately the relationships between the arrhythmias and the last few cycles that precede them on the one hand, and the heart rate environment on a larger scale of the order of a few minutes on the other hand. The two arrhythmia components are usually not dependent to the same extent on the rate and on the ANS balance, and we shall now exemplify these theoretical notions with some clinical cases.

Events and Nonevents

FIGURE 1 illustrates rate dependence, a phenomenon initially described in fact by Langendorf as the rule of bigeminy.[4] It can be easily studied by the Holter technique on the condition to develop specific programs of analysis. In a patient with frequent ventricular premature beats, the sequences of bigeminy were frequently separated by a few sinus beats. Determining why extrasystoles did or did not reappear could be achieved by comparing in a three-hour period sequences of cycles following the last extrasystole. In FIGURE 1 the 70 sequences including 7 consecutive sinus beats in between two extrasystoles are compared with the 274 sequences in which the 8th beat after the last extrasystole was of sinus origin. The only difference between the two populations of "events" and "nonevents" was the duration of the 7th sinus cycle

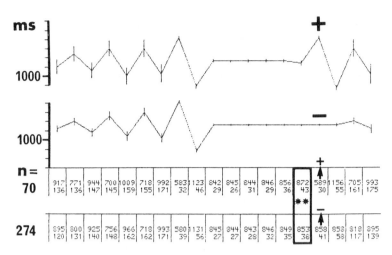

FIGURE 1. Events, nonevents and rate dependence. Two series of sequences have been selected by the computer in a 3-hour Holter recording of a patient with numerous ventricular premature beats. Both sequences are characterized by a ventricular premature beat (isolated or the last of a bigeminy) followed by a compensatory pause and six consecutive cycles of sinus origin, thus totaling seven sinus beats in a row. Then the eighth beat may be a ventricular extrasystole ($n = 70$ events labeled " + ") or a sinus beat ($n = 274$ nonevents labeled " − "). The mean values of all cycles are represented (± standard error of the mean [SEM]) and given in mseconds (± standard deviation [SD]). From the comparison of the two series it appears that the only difference explaining the occurence of a ventricular extrasystole is the longer duration of the seventh cycle (** = $p < 0.01$ by Anova).

following the last premature beat: it was significantly longer in the first population than in the second (872 ± 43 mseconds vs. $853 \pm 38, p < 0.001$). This precisely defines the "upper threshold" of extrasystoles.

FIGURES 2 and 3 are another technical approach to the same problem. One can choose to compare specifically the cycles that are followed by an extrasystole with those that are not in the form of R-R interval histograms.[5] The sinus cycles followed by "nonevents" are much more numerous (open population labeled "N1" = 41,404) than those followed by extrasystoles (solid population labeled "N2" = 1,706). Thus, identification of the heart rate below which ventricular extrasystoles disappear is possible. In the case of FIGURE 2, an upper limit can be identified, above which shorter sinus cycles are not followed by extrasystoles, and its statistical significance is assessed through the analysis of contingency tables by considering proportions. This upper limit is defined as the sinus cycle length below which 5% of sinus cycles generating extrasystoles were distributed. The percentage of sinus cycles not followed by extrasystoles below this limit is compared with these 5%. Such an analysis does not make the likelihood of significant results depend on the number of extrasystoles, as long as this number exceeds 100. In case the limit falls in the middle of a 20 msecond class interval defined by the computerized analysis, the distribution of sinus cycles is deemed regular in the class interval, a method that explains the apparent precision of 596 mseconds for the upper threshold which is significant at p < 0.05. The same mode of calculation can apply to determining the "lower threshold" that represents the symmetrical situation: extrasystoles may tend to disappear when the basic rate becomes too low, and FIGURE 3 is an example of such a situation. The same method permits us to define a significant lower threshold of 746 mseconds. Values of 919 mseconds for the lower threshold in FIGURE 2 and 612 mseconds for the upper threshold in FIGURE 3 were not found significant, and this may correspond to two possibilities: a real absence of such thresholds implying that the extrasystolic phenomenon is not rate dependent, or an observed range of sinus rate not large enough to evidence the phenomenon.

This mode of analysis was used in 10 untreated apparently healthy patients with fixed, coupled, isolated monomorphic ventricular extrasystoles, and the thresholds were looked for during successive one hour periods.[5] Upper and lower limits were observed in 10 and 8 of the patients respectively. An upper and a lower limit were

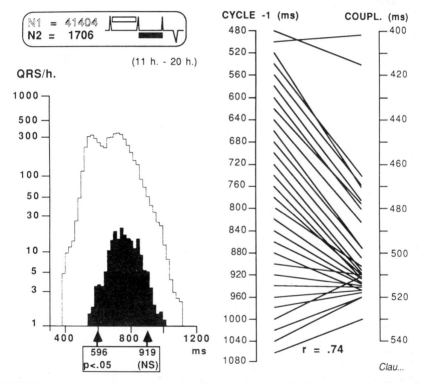

FIGURE 2. Rate dependence and coupling interval of the ventricular extrasystoles. The left upper panel schematizes the sinus cycles followed by another sinus beat (open population $N1 = 41,404$) or by a ventricular extrasystole (solid population $N2 = 1706$) in a 9 hour recording. The lower left diagram represents these two populations, and comparing the number of cycles in each 20 msecond class of cycle duration allows us to determine the value and the significance of an upper and a lower limit of cycle length that conditions the presence or the absence of an extrasystole as the next beat. In the present case an upper (referring to the rate rather than the cycle length) limit of 596 mseconds was found significant ($p < 0.05$) whereas the lower limit was not. The right diagram represents the relationship between the last sinus cycle of the N2 population and the coupling interval of the following extrasystole. The number of events in each 20-msecond class of cycle −1 is not taken into account (sample units) to determine the coefficient of correlation which is positive at 0.74.

identifiable in 9.3 ± 5.1 and 8.4 ± 5.8 hours per recording respectively. Values of both types of limits varied throughout tape recording. A positive significant correlation was found between the values of upper and lower limits and the mean cycle length during the corresponding hour in 9 of the 10 and 8 of the 8 patients respectively. The type of relation observed suggests that heart rate directly alters limits or that heart rate and limits are under the same influence of the ANS.

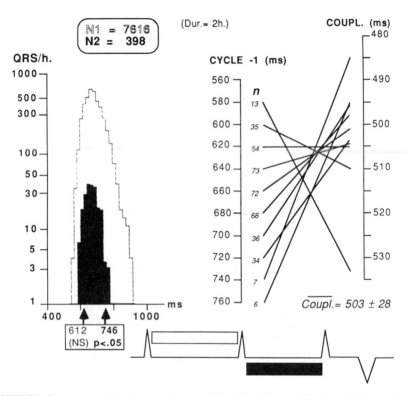

FIGURE 3. Inverse correlation between sinus cycle length and the coupling interval. The mode of presentation is the same as in FIGURE 2, and the example refers to a 2 hour tracing. In this patient there was no evidence of an upper limit of sinus cycle length for the presence of ventricular extrasystoles, but a lower limit was found significant at 746 mseconds. The right part of the diagram shows that the cycle −1 and the coupling interval (mean value 503 ± 28 mseconds) are correlated negatively: the longer the cycle −1, the shorter the coupling interval. The number "*n*" of events in each class of cycle −1 is given.

Among other things, this rate dependence of the extrasystolic phenomenon obviously implies that it should be taken into account when the arrhythmias are studied in terms of spontaneous variability, or changes related to therapy.[6–9] Unfortunately, as the various commercially available systems of analysis are not designed for this purpose, this very important factor is never explored, to the point that the heart rate changes induced by drugs in the therapeutic trials often are not even mentioned.

The Behavior of the Coupling Interval

The right panel of FIGURE 2 specifically studies the relationships between the last sinus cycle (labeled cycle -1) and the coupling interval of the extrasystoles. Two different patterns can be observed, and the most usual one is presented in FIGURE 2, where there is clearly a direct relationship between the sinus cycle duration and the coupling interval. The correlation (r coefficient $= 0.74$) is statistically significant ($n = 30$, $p < 0.001$) even if the different classes are considered as sample units. Had the number of the events been taken into account, the level of significance would have been of course even higher. This pattern is in sharp contrast with FIGURE 3, where the relationships between the cycle -1 and the coupling interval are opposite: the longer the sinus cycle, the shorter the coupling interval ($r = -0.80$, $n = 10$, $p < 0.01$). This opposite behavior must have a significance in terms of electrophysiological mechanism. The case of FIGURE 3 strongly suggests a parasystole. In the case of FIGURE 2 one also has to take into account the role of adrenergic stimulation on the parameters that influence the coupling interval. We observed for instance that the pattern of a direct relationship between the sinus cycle duration and the coupling interval may change in the same patient from day to night or on beta-blocking treatment.

Interaction between the Extrasystolic Phenomenon and the Following Cycles

We have just seen that the sinus rate preceding the extrasystoles could be crucial for their occurrence, and that the duration of the last cycle had an effect on the coupling interval. But the extrasystoles themselves and their coupling interval may have an influence on the sinus rate, as demonstrated in FIGURE 4. During a one-hour period two morphologically different types of extrasystoles were recorded, and they had different coupling intervals: 580 ± 33 mseconds and 627 ± 30 mseconds ($n = 59$ and 22 respectively, $p < 0.001$). The two populations did not differ in terms of preceding sinus cycle duration (869 ± 18 mseconds vs. 864 ± 12). However, the sinus cycles that followed the two types of extrasystoles were indeed different (mean value 847 ± 23 mseconds vs. 870 ± 15, $p < 0.001$), a phenomenon that may be related to the difference in the hemodynamic changes provoked by the extrasystoles. As a matter of fact, it was recently demonstrated that the neural traffic in the sympathetic nerves was immediately influenced by the postextrasystolic compensatory pause,[10] and the changes were proportional to the prematurity of the extrasystole.[11] The present postextrasystolic heart rate acceleration probably is an illustration of this very particular modality of sympathetic stimulation which may actually constitute a negative feedback factor in the case of very stable situations. Indeed, a sequence of bigeminated extrasystoles almost always tends to accelerate the heart rate, probably as a result of its hemodynamic consequences sensed by the carotid sinus, and this acceleration tends to shorten the sequence as a consequence of the upper threshold phenomenon. Hence, one can evaluate how complex may be the interaction of phenomena that govern the simplest arrhythmias.

The Role of Adrenergic Stimulation in the Genesis of Arrhythmias

The ANS modulates to a varying extent all the normal and abnormal electrophysiological phenomena. Delicate changes in the balance condition many critical thresholds responsible for the repetitive activity supposed to characterize the substrate and whatever its mechanism of reentry, triggered activity, abnormal automaticity. Occa-

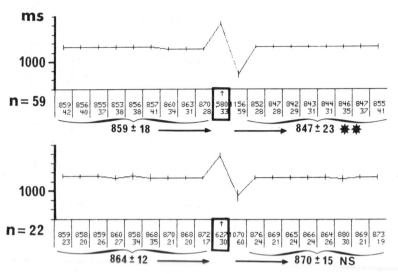

FIGURE 4. Influence of the coupling interval on the following sinus cycles. In the same 1-hour Holter recording with a very stable cardiac frequency two different types of ventricular extrasystoles have been collected according to their shorter (580 ± 33 mseconds, $n = 59$) or longer (627 ± 30, $n = 22$) coupling interval. The average value of the 9 sinus cycles preceding each type of extrasystole do not differ (859 ± 18 and 864 ± 12 mseconds, $p = $ not significant [NS]). However, the mean durations of the postextrasystolic cycles are indeed different (847 ± 23 vs. 870 ± 15 mseconds, $p < 0.01$), thus suggesting that extrasystoles with a shorter coupling interval do have a feedback effect on the sinus rate, possibly due to different hemodynamic consequences.

sionally, isolated extrasystoles (or the first beat of tachyarrhythmias) we are used to designating as the initiating (or triggering) factor also suppose a substrate in which other types of arrhythmogenic mechanisms (parasystole, reflection, afterdepolarization) may also be modulated by the ANS. The easiest method for monitoring the ANS changes is to look at the heart rate, the increase or the decrease of which in principle indicates the predominance of the adrenergic or vagal drive, respectively. The necessary limitations of such a schematic statement are not a sufficient reason not to take into account the background of the heart rate to interpret the mechanism of the arrhythmia onset or the type of this arrhythmia, and the two following examples are by all means not rare. What is rarely carried out indeed, unfortunately, is the type of analysis they suppose.

FIGURE 5 shows in the same tracing the coexistence of isolated premature beats and doublets, without any obvious reason for the latter to occur preferably to the former. FIGURE 6 however shows that the heart rate observed during the 10 preceding cycles is always faster for the doublets than for the isolated extrasystoles, by an average of more than 50 mseconds, so that the role of the adrenergic stimulation is easily evidenced. In this case the great number of events (440 isolated extrasystoles versus 212 doublets) in the 12-hour period makes highly significant the difference between the two populations. But a few events can allow the same important deductions provided some attention is paid to them, and FIGURE 7 is demonstrative in this regard. In a patient with a chronic coronary heart disease, the significance of a short attack of ventricular tachycardia of 2 minutes duration was in fact in close keeping with the very few events observed in the 45 minutes encompassing this tachyarrhythmia: no more than 12 isolated extrasystoles and a salvo of 7 beats were visible in addition to the ventricular tachycardia, but they were all preceded in the 4 to 7 preceding minutes by a short heart rate acceleration indicative of an adrenergic stimulation.

Such findings do not have only an anecdotical meaning, if one considers that they reflect in fact a situation that is common to trivial arrhythmias and sudden death. We have demonstrated that a close positive correlation existed between the shorter or longer duration of the repetitive phenomena (from doublets to salvos) and the heart rate observed in the three minutes preceding these events.[12] This rule applies to benign extrasystoles in undiseased hearts as well as to nonsustained ventricular tachycardias in severe cardiopathies,[13] with the only difference that in the latter the correlation becomes apparently weaker as the impairment of the cardiac function progresses. Rather than suggesting a less marked importance of the ANS in this context, this fact well illustrates the phenomenon of the adrenergic paradox.[2] This paradox implies that the lesser the evidence of a heart rate acceleration before the onset of a tachyarrhythmia, the more dependent on the adrenergic stimulation its substrate must be. The phenomenon may be explained by an increased sensitivity of the substrate if one refers for instance to the denervation of infarcted areas and the denervation supersensitivity that ensues.[14] Another explanation of the adrenergic paradox may be the loss of sensitivity of the marker itself, i.e., the sinus node, if one takes into account the down regulation of the beta-adrenergic receptors, due to heart failure.[15] Whatever the explanation, the fact is that overlooking the importance of the phenomenon leads to misunderstanding the message contained in the consistent results of various trials that demonstrate the efficacy of beta-blocking therapy in sudden death prevention. Not only does this provide indirect evidence of the sudden death mechanism, but invites us to look after the direct evidence of this role in the determination of sudden death.

This evidence can be found in the analysis of the now relatively frequent cases of sudden death recorded at Holter in ambulatory patients.[16] In addition to the expected

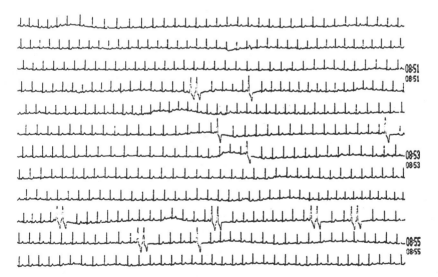

FIGURE 5. Compact tracing of a patient with either isolated ventricular premature beats or doublets throughout the 24-hour period (see also FIGURE 6).

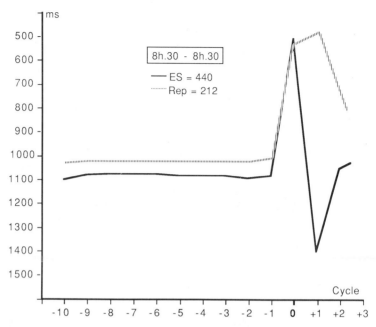

FIGURE 6. Determinism of isolated extrasystoles and doublets. The 440 isolated extrasystoles ("ES") and the 212 doublets ("Rep") of the patient of FIGURE 5 recorded during the 24-hour recording have been collected as well as the 10 cycles that preceded each of these events. The difference that conditions the occurrence of a doublet is obviously formed by a higher heart rate, which reflects a higher sympathetic drive.

but limited role of ischemia, the main factor present was the heart rate acceleration observed just before the arrhythmia onset when compared with the mean heart rate observed one hour before: the difference exceeded 10 beats/minute, a value that was at the same time very important and highly significant in our patients,[17] but that could also be easily missed because it took place over a relatively long period of time. The phenomenon was particularly evident in the absence of any pause just prior to the tachyarrhythmia. The presence of a postextrasystolic pause provoking the arrhythmia onset is also frequent. It is not clear whether the role of this pause should be interpreted as a pure electrophysiological phenomenon that it could be indeed, or as a further, immediate neurogenic sympathetic stimulation as discussed above.

THE AUTONOMIC NERVOUS SYSTEM AND HEART RATE VARIABILITY

Variability of Sinus Rhythm

Heart rate variability (HRV) has been considered for a long time as the possible marker of an impaired heart status conditioning a poor prognosis, but with the remarkable exception of some pioneers[18] it did not provoke a large interest from clinicians. Among many reasons including the difficulty of clearly understanding the complexity of the physiology[19] of the autonomic nervous system, a real obstacle was the

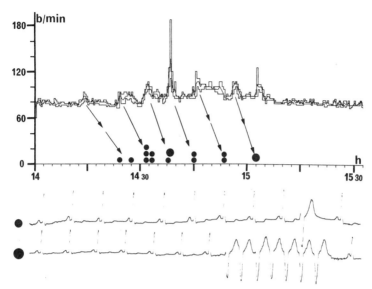

FIGURE 7. Adrenergic stimulation and the occurrence of arrhythmias. A few isolated ventricular premature beats (small solid circles) and two short attacks of ventricular tachycardia (a 7-beat and a 2-minute run, bigger circles) were recorded within one hour in this patient. These events were apparently punctuated by the previous changes of sinus rate acceleration reflecting an adrenergic stimulation 5 to 10 minutes before.

difficulty of standardizing the techniques of evaluation. They require specially oriented laboratory investigations, mainly based on the measurement of the respiration- or blood pressure–related variations of the heart rate on a short-term basis. In essence, monitoring continuously the heart rate on a long-term basis during normal activity rather than on the occasion of somewhat experimental and time-limited conditions was the main obstacle. Curiously however the introduction of the Holter technique did not provoke a renewed attention to this problem. The difficulty of evaluating and quantifying HRV certainly was a technical obstacle, but the fact is that the interest of cardiologists was focused on pathology of arrhythmias rather than on cardiac physiology.

Heart rate variations are dependent upon the ANS and its different components, which not only differ in their function of accelerating or decelerating the heart, but in their neurogenic or humoral origin which conditions the time constant of their influence. When defining the mechanism of the different types of heart rate variations, it is essential not to be manichean because most phenomena depend on a balance rather than on the effect of a single action of a part of the system. Of course, roughly speaking the main function of the vagus is to slow the heart rate whereas the sympathetics accelerate it. However, these functions in fact depend on the starting balance of the system, and the decrease of the sympathetic tone or the increase of the vagal drive may slow the heart without producing the same pattern of HRV. The vagal drive is responsible for short-term heart rate changes,[20] and the respiratory R-R interval variations are easily visible on beat-by-beat tachograms of Holter recordings (FIGURE 8). According to the reference method formed by the power spectral analysis,[21,22] these fluctuations associated with breathing are responsible for the high-frequency peak

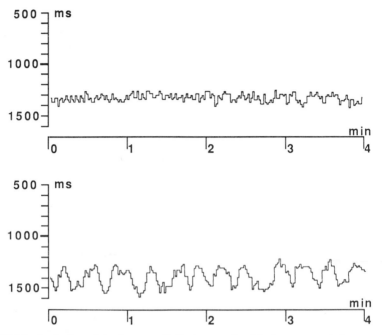

FIGURE 8. Oscillations of the sinus rate. Ordinary example of the heart rate variations recorded at Holter. Every indentation of the tachogram represents a sinus cycle. Accelerations and decelerations are permanently observed and they have different wavelengths. Respiration-related changes classically reflect the vagal influence (upper diagram) whereas longer oscillations involving 10 seconds or more are due to sympathetic activity. Both can be quantified in terms of rate of occurrence, and amplitude.

centered at values of 0.20 to 0.40 Hz. The significance becomes less easy to interpret as the wavelength increases: heart rate oscillations covering 10, 15, 20 seconds, the so-called Mayer waves, certainly have to do with the sympathetic innervation,[22] a fact that does not imply that they only reflect the neurogenic sympathetic activity and that the vagal drive is not concerned. This midfrequency peak centered at 0.08–0.12 Hz was in fact initially related to the frequency effects of the baroceptor reflex. Much longer oscillations covering up to 1 or 2 minutes can also be observed, and they are most probably caused by humoral rather than neurogenic modulations that can involve not only catecholamines but also the renin-angiotensin system.[21]

Without entering into the technical details of the HRV evaluation we are currently using,[23] one can easily conceive that the oscillations visible on FIGURE 8 can be selected according to their wavelength, and quantified in terms of rate per time unit and amplitude (i.e., the difference between the longest and the shortest cycle in each oscillation). Then the physiological meaning of the short and long types of oscillations becomes clear when one considers the pooled hourly values of 23 normal subjects represented in FIGURE 9. In the mean diagram the number of oscillations per hour is closely correlated with the heart rate, positively for the long (sympathetic), negatively for the short (vagal) oscillations. The ratio between the two types is represented in the upper diagram together with the mean heart rate, and the correlation is striking: it is

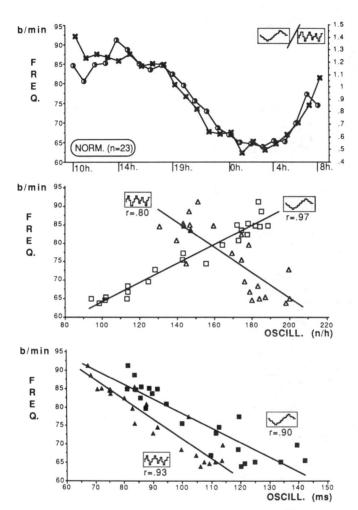

FIGURE 9. Quantification of heart rate variability. The values recorded during a 24-hour period have been pooled in a group of 23 normal subjects. In the upper diagram the hourly values of heart rate (circles) form a curve that closely parallels the ratio (crosses) of the numbers of long (involving 20 cycles or more) over short (respiratory) oscillations. The very close correlation simply reflects the fact that the mean heart rate results from the permanent interplay between the sympathetic and the vagal influences. In the mean diagram the hourly number of either type of long (open squares) and short (open triangles) oscillations are plotted against the mean heart rate in beats per minute, with a close correlation that is positive for the former, negative for the latter. In the lower diagram the amplitude of either type of long (solid squares) and short (solid triangles) oscillations is plotted against the heart rate. The coefficient of correlation r is high and negative in both cases, thus suggesting that the amplitude of the cycle length changes depends on arithmetical rather than physiological rules. Abbreviations: b/min = beats per minute, FREQ = frequency, ms = milliseconds, n/h = number per hour, NORM = normal subjects, OSCILL = oscillations.

important to realize that this figure represents the dependence of the heart rate on the balance between the sympathetic and the vagal drive, rather the reverse cause-to-effect relationship. Finally, the behavior of the oscillation amplitudes in the lower diagram does not relate to their type but to the mean frequency at which they were recorded.

HRV and Clinical Arrhythmias

The following example demonstrates the close relationship between arrhythmias and the autonomic nervous system, not only in terms of heart rate as demonstrated before, but in terms of heart rate oscillations. FIGURE 10 displays the beat-by-beat analysis of the last hour preceding the onset of a paroxysmal atrial fibrillation in a patient with a normal heart. The pattern is quite normal for a sleeping patient during the first 30 minutes after 3:00 AM. After 3:30, progressively larger and ampler oscillations develop, which certainly reflect stronger and stronger adrenergic stimulations of unknown mechanism but most probably of humoral origin as suggested by their long duration over 1 minute or so. Each oscillation is terminated by a dramatic heart rate slowing that probably represents a vagal reflex secondary to the adrenergic

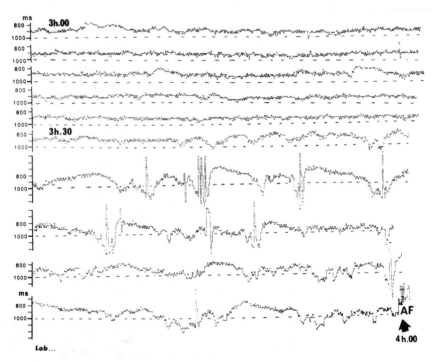

FIGURE 10. Changing pattern of heart rate variability before the onset of paroxysmal idiopathic atrial fibrillation. The beat-by-beat tachogram of a 1 hour recording preceding the onset of an atrial fibrillation (AF) at 4:00 AM is displayed. During the first 30 minutes the pattern is quite usual for a sleeping patient, and the respiration-related changes of the heart rate are only visible. After 3:30 AM progressively greater and greater oscillations are interrupted by dramatic slowings that suggest vagal reactions to adrenergic stimulations. Many of these vagal rebounds provoke atrial premature beats (short cycles figured by peaks), and finally the atrial fibrillation occurs.

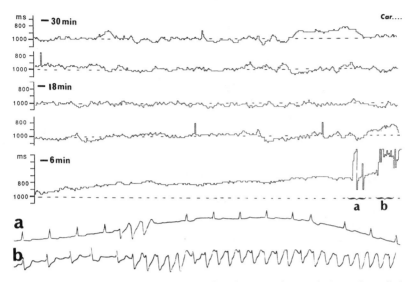

FIGURE 11. Pattern of heart rate variability before the onset of a ventricular tachycardia in a patient with heart failure. Representative samples of beat-by-beat tachograms (each line represents 6 minutes) recorded 30, 18, and 6 minutes before the terminal event are displayed. Bottom tracings a and b correspond to the ventricular extrasystoles and tachycardia occurring in parts a and b of the tachogram. No respiratory oscillations of the heart rate are visible in this severely diseased patient, indicating a predominance of the adrenergic drive that is further suggested by the exclusive presence of long wavelength oscillations. Their amplitude progressively decreases as they are overwhelmed by the heart rate acceleration which finally triggers the ventricular tachyarrhythmia.

stimulation. Almost every heart rate deceleration is heralded by one or several atrial premature beats that finally trigger the attack of atrial fibrillation at 4:00 AM. Such a pattern closely corresponds with the well-known experimental model of acetylcholine-induced atrial fibrillation, which actually has its correspondence in humans.[24]

The pattern of oscillations is quite different in the severely diseased patient of FIGURE 11 who develops a ventricular tachycardia in the setting of a chronic myocardial infarction with heart failure. Basically the HRV is altered in this patient, qualitatively (no respiratory oscillations visible) and quantitatively. Only low-frequency oscillations are present, suggesting that the sympathetic drive is largely predominant. Moreover, as the time progresses towards the attack of ventricular tachycardia (ultimately degenerating into ventricular fibrillation), apparently these oscillations are overwhelmed by the progressive heart rate acceleration certainly resulting from a strong humoral adrenergic stimulation.

HRV and the Prognosis of Cardiopathies

Numerous markers have been proposed to evaluate the prognosis of patients having suffered from a myocardial infarction. They range from parameters as simple as age to complex investigations including hemodynamic studies, coronary angiography, and programmed electrical stimulation. Noninvasive approaches naturally tend to have the clinician's preference, and particularly data derived from Holter recordings, so that an abundant, rather controversial, and frequently revised literature deals with the prognostic value of ventricular arrhythmias. The discussion is still active about the definition of the most sensitive and specific criteria that should be considered. There is some evidence that relying on a limited view of arrhythmic events to assess the long-term prognosis of a disease that by definition concerns many aspects of the cardiac functions would be illusory, and progressively most of the initially proposed criteria have been abandoned or the emphasis on their value has been tempered. The number of ventricular premature beats, their distribution into isolated extrasystoles with or without bigeminy, with or without repetitive activity, the coupling interval have been claimed to constitute valuable markers of low- or high-risk groups of patients. It is now largely admitted that a common primary condition for any prognostic index to be reliable is to be applied in the setting of an impaired cardiac function, the most convenient if not the most reliable image of which being a left ventricular ejection fraction of less than 30 or 40 per 100.

Heart failure diminishes the beta-adrenergic receptor density.[15] On the other hand, the traffic in the sympathetic nerves is increased in patients with cardiopathies.[25] What we are evaluating with HRV is the global result of the very complex interplay of a chain of components forming the ANS. Neural and humoral vectors are permanently interacting behind a sort of curtain formed by the receptors that transmit the balanced influences to the sinus node.[26] The existence of a patent heart failure is otherwise not the common explanation of a decreased HRV: this was not Kleiger's experience,[27] and a decrease in HRV is now widely accepted as a reliable prognostic index, the debate being not closed between the proponents of a decreased parasympathetic drive or the increase of the sympathetic tone.[28,29] Even in the absence of a cardiac insufficiency that by definition indicates the failure of compensatory mechanisms, the intermediate stage of myocardial dysfunction provokes the ANS reactions we are able to evaluate. A decreased flexibility of the ANS indicates that it is stressed for reasons that may not be patent. HRV measures this flexibility, which may be altered at the expense of this or that of its components, thus probably explaining why its features may be different from patient to patient, but with the common result of an impaired adaptative function.

CONCLUSION

Noninvasive investigations of arrhythmias should not be considered less fruitful and less rewarding intellectually than invasive approaches. The term of clinical electrophysiology that was coined more than 20 years ago to qualify the endocavitary studies should no longer be reserved to these techniques but extended to surface long-term ambulatory electrocardiography. We must realize that the vast majority of the fantastic amount of information contained in a 24-hour recording is presently neglected by the type of analysis usually done. The technical limitations are much less responsible for this situation than the lack of curiosity, and making much more sophisticated computerized analyses essentially requires a demand rather than to overcome the difficulties. The next step in the progress of this discipline will be the extension of the Holter technique to more complete information on the surface ECG itself. We are presently using one or at best two channels for interpreting dynamic ECG. There is no technical obstacle for using three-lead recordings, so that continuous, dynamic vectorcardiography can now be thought of, thus adding a new dimension for a global surface electrocardiography.

REFERENCES

1. HOLTER, N. J. 1962. New method for heart studies. Science **134:** 1214–1220.
2. COUMEL, P. 1987. The management of clinical arrhythmias. An overview on invasive versus noninvasive electrophysiology. Eur. Heart J. **8:** 92–99.
3. COUMEL, P., M. ZIMMERMANN & C. FUNCK-BRENTANO. 1987. Exercise test: arrhythmogenic or antiarrhythmic? Rate-dependency vs. adrenergic-dependency of tachyarrhythmias. Eur. Heart J. **8D:** 7–15.
4. LANGENDORF, R., A. PICK & M. I. WINTERNITZ. 1955. Appearance of ectopic beats dependent upon length of the ventricular cycle, the "rule of bigeminy." Circulation **11:** 422–430.
5. FUNCK-BRENTANO, C., P. COUMEL, P. LORENTE, P. MAISON-BLANCHE & R. SLAMA. 1988. Rate-dependence of ventricular extrasystoles. Computer identification and quantitative analysis. Cardiovasc. Res. **22:** 101–107.
6. MORGANROTH, J., E. L. MICHELSON, L. N. HOROWITZ, M. E. JOSEPHSON, A. S. PEARLMAN & W. B. DUNKMAN. 1978. Limitations of routine long-term electrocardiographic monitoring to assess ventricular ectopic frequency. Circulation **58:** 408–414.
7. SCHMIDT, G., K. ULM, P. BARTHEL, L. GOEDEL-MEINEN, G. JAHNS & W. BAEDEKER. 1988. Spontaneous variability of simple and complex ventricular premature contractions during long-term intervals in patients with severe organic heart disease. Circulation **78:** 296–301.
8. ANASTASIOU-NANA, M. I., R. L. MENLOVE, J. N. NANAS & J. L. ANDERSON. 1988. Changes in spontaneous variability of ventricular ectopic activity as a function of time in patients with chronic arrhythmias. Circulation **78:** 286–295.
9. ANDERSON, J. L., A. P. HALLSTROM, L. S. GRIFFITH, R. B. LEDINGHAM, J. A. REIFFEL, S. YUSUF, A. H. BARKER, R. E. FOWLES & J. B. YOUNG. 1989. Relation of baseline characteristics to suppression of ventricular arrhythmias during placebo and active antiarrhythmic therapy in patients after myocardial infarction. Circulation **79:** 610–619.
10. LOMBARDI, F., T. G. RUSCONE & A. MALLIANI. 1989. Ventricular arrhythmias and sympathetic discharge. Cardiovasc. Res. **23:** 205–212.
11. WELCH, W. J., M. L. SMITH, R. F. REA, R. A. BAUERFEIND & D. L. ECKBERG. 1989. Enhancement of sympathetic nerve activity by single premature ventricular beats in humans. J. Am. Coll. Cardiol. **13:** 69–75.
12. ZIMMERMANN, M., P. MAISON-BLANCHE, B. CAUCHEMEZ, J. F. LECLERCQ & P. COUMEL. 1986. Determinants of the spontaneous ectopic activity in repetitive monomorphic idiopathic ventricular tachycardia. J. Am. Coll. Cardiol. **7:** 1219–1227.
13. ZIMMERMANN, M., P. MAISON-BLANCHE, B. CAUCHEMEZ, J. F. LECLERCQ & P. COUMEL. 1986. Déterminants de l'activité répétitive dans les tachycardies ventriculaires en salves. Arch. Mal. Coeur **79:** 1420–1428.
14. BARBER, M. J., T. M. MUELLER, B. G. DAVIES, R. M. GILL & D. P. ZIPES. 1985. Interruption of sympathetic and vagal-mediated afferent responses by transmural myocardial infarction. Circulation **72:** 623–631.
15. BRISTOW, M. R., M. R. GINSBURG, W. MINOBE, R. S. CUBICIOTTI, S. SAGEMAN, K. LUIRE, M. E. BILLINGHAM, D. C. HARRISON & E. B. STINSON. 1982. Decreased catecholamine sensitivity and beta-adrenergic receptor density in failing human hearts. N. Engl. J. Med. **307:** 205–211.
16. BAYES DE LUNA, A., P. COUMEL & J. F. LECLERCQ. 1989. Ambulatory sudden death: mechanisms of production of fatal arrhythmia on the basis of data from 157 cases. Am. Heart J. **117:** 151–159.
17. LECLERCQ, J. F., P. MAISON-BLANCHE, B. CAUCHEMEZ & P. COUMEL. 1988. Respective role of sympathetic tone and of cardiac pauses in the genesis of 62 cases of ventricular fibrillation recorded during Holter monitoring. Eur. Heart J. **9:** 1276–1283.
18. ECKBERG, D. L., M. DRABINSKY & E. BRAUNWALD. 1971. Defective cardiac parasympathetic control in patients with heart disease. N. Engl. J. Med. **285:** 877–883.
19. LEVY, M. N. 1971. Sympathetic-parasympathetic interactions in the heart. Circ. Res. **29:** 437–445.

20. KATONA P. G. & F. JIH. 1975. Respiratory sinus arrhythmia: noninvasive measure of parasympathetic cardiac control. J. Appl. Physiol **39:** 801–805.
21. AKSELROD, S., D. GORDON, F. A. UBEL, D. C. SHANNON, A. C. BARGER & R. J. COHEN. 1981. Power spectrum analysis of heart rate fluctuations: a quantitative probe of beat-to-beat cardiovascular control. Science **213:** 220–222.
22. PAGANI, M., F. LOMBARDI, F. GUZZETTI, O. RIMOLDI, R. FURLAN, P. PIZZINELLI, G. SANDRONE, G. MALFATTO, S. DELL'ORTO, E. PICCALUGA, M. TURIEL, G. BASELLI, S. CERUTTI & A. MALLIANI. 1986. Power spectral analysis of heart rate and arterial pressure variabilities as a marker of sympatho-vagal interaction in man and conscious dog. Circ. Res. **59:** 178–193.
23. COUMEL, M., J. S. HERMIDA, B. WENNERBLÖM, A. LEENHARDT, P. MAISON-BLANCHE & B. CAUCHEMEZ. Heart rate variability in left ventricular hypertrophy and heart failure, and the effects of beta-blockade. Eur. Heart J. (In press.)
24. COUMEL, P., P. ATTUEL, J. P. LAVALLEE, D. FLAMMANG, J. F. LECLERCQ & R. SLAMA. 1978. Syndrome d'arythmie auriculaire d'origine vagale. Arch. Mal. Coeur **71:** 645–656.
25. LEIMBACH, W. N., B. G. WALLIN, R. G. VICTOR, P. E. AYLWARD, G. SUNDLOF & A. L. MARK. 1986. Direct evidence from intraneural recordings for increased central sympathetic outflow in patients with heart failure. Circulation **73:** 913–919.
26. SAUL, J. P., Y. ARAI, R. D. BERGER, L. S. LILLY, W. S. COLUCCI & R. J. COHEN. 1988. Assessment of autonomic regulation in chronic congestive heart failure by heart rate spectral analysis. Am. J. Cardiol. **61:** 1292–1299.
27. KLEIGER, R. E., J. P. MILLER, J. T. BIGGER, A. J. MOSS & THE MULTICENTER POST-INFARCTION RESEARCH GROUP.1987. Decreased heart rate variability and its association with increased mortality after acute myocardial infarction. Am. J. Cardiol. **59:** 256–262.
28. LOMBARDI, F., G. SANDRONE, S. PERNPRUNER, R. SALA, M. GARIMOLDI, S. CERUTTI, G. BASELLI, M. PAGANI & A. MALLIANI. 1987. Heart rate variability as an index of sympathovagal interaction after acute myocardial infarction. Am. J. Cardiol. **60:** 1239–1245.
29. SCHWARTZ, P. J., A. ZAZA, M. PALA, E. LOCATI, G. BERIA & A. ZANCHETTI. 1988. Baroreflex sensitivity and its evolution during the first year after myocardial infarction. J. Am. Coll. Cardiol. **12:** 629–636.

Quantitative Electrocardiography[a]

Standardization and Performance Evaluation

JOS L. WILLEMS

CSE Coordinating Center
University Hospital Gasthuisberg
49, Herestraat
3000 Leuven, Belgium

INTRODUCTION

Although the first attempts to automate electrocardiograph (ECG) analysis by digital computer were made as early as 1957 by H. V. Pipberger and coworkers,[1] it took considerably more time to develop operational computer programs than originally anticipated. However, over the last 15 years computer processing of ECGs has increased rapidly.[2-5] Still, until recently there were no standards in this field. There were no common definitions of waves, no standards for measurement or diagnostic classification, and no uniform terminology for reporting. Even more, data processed by one ECG system can up to today, due to lack of standards, not be transmitted and read by another ECG computer system in routine practice. This has created a situation, whereby large differences in measurement results by different computer programs hamper the exchange of diagnostic criteria and interpretation results.[6,7] More and more microcomputer-based interpretative ECG machines are being put on the market without any prior independent validation.

In order to overcome some of these problems, a concerted action was started in the European Community (EC) in June 1980, striving towards "Common Standards for Quantitative Electrocardiography" (abbreviated CSE).[8,9] In the present paper we will briefly summarize the objectives, present results, and future actions related to this project.

OBJECTIVES AND STAGES OF THE PROJECT

ECG computer processing can basically be reduced to three principal stages:

1. Acquisition, transmission, and storage of digital ECG data.
2. Pattern recognition and measurement.
3. Diagnostic classification.

In each of these stages there are important needs of standardization.
At the start of the CSE project the following objectives were formulated:

1. Standardization of ECG measurement procedures in quantitative terms; comparative studies of measurements performed by different programs; drawing of guidelines, definitions, and standards for measurement.

[a]This research has been supported by the European Commission within the frame of its 2nd, 3rd and 4th Medical and Public Health Research Programs, and by various funding agencies in 10 EC Member States, among which is the Belgian FGWO grant nr. 3.0050.83.

2. Assessment of performance of diagnostic classification computer programs and algorithmic documentation of their operation.
3. Establishment of modest ECG libraries to reach these goals.[8,9]

Over the past nine years a steady course has been followed to achieve these objectives. From the beginning the project was divided into two logically related studies, dealing with measurements first, and next with diagnostic interpretation. The order of these studies has been determined from the inception of the project by the logic that diagnostic criteria can only be exchanged if programs provide the same basic measurement results when analyzing identical ECG recordings. Investigators from 25 institutes in the EC are participating in the project. They constitute the CSE Working Party. Also investigators from six North American and one Japanese center collaborate by processing data or as consultants (see Appendix). As of June 1989 we have started a third project aiming at standards for digital ECG data transmission, encoding, and storage, an essential requirement to interconnect different systems.

STANDARDIZED ECG MEASUREMENT

Main Objectives of the First CSE Study

The main objective of the first CSE study was to reduce the variation of measurement by different ECG computer programs. The aim was to standardize computer-derived ECG measurements, obtaining agreement on definitions of waves and of references for the on- and offsets of P, QRS, and T waves. So that when an ECG of a patient is recorded in Rome with program x, the same measurement results will be printed as when his ECG would have been recorded and analyzed in London with program y. The means and variances of various programs analyzing a common data base should fall within acceptable ranges. Only then can diagnostic criteria for myocardial infarction and other diagnostic categories be exchanged and possibly standardized.

CSE Measurement Reference Libraries

One of the major results of the first CSE study, which has now been completed, was the establishment of such a data bank. In fact two reference data bases have been established in the first CSE study. The first consists of 250 original and 310 so-called artificial ECGs in which 3 leads have been recorded simultaneously, as was current practice until recently.[10] Because different ECG measurement programs apply various principles with respect to analysis (for example some measure single beats, whereas others analyze averaged beats), artificial ECGs have been constructed by selecting one beat from each lead group of the original recordings and making strings of identical beats. The second data base[11] involves 250 original and 250 artificial ECGs in which not 3, but all leads—the 12 standard leads plus the Frank XYZ leads—have been recorded simultaneously, as is being done more and more in microcomputer-based electrocardiographs. The development of these CSE libraries have been described extensively in eight annual CSE Progress Reports and in various publications.[9-16]

The libraries represent a wide variety of ECG configurations; 25% were normal, the remainder abnormal. All ECGs were sampled at 500 Hz, with a resolution of at least 10 bits and a maximal quantization of 5 microvolts. The original and corresponding artificial ECGs were randomly divided into two sets containing nearly equal samples of the various pathologic entities. The results of one set are released; the other is kept secret in the CSE Coordinating Center for independent testing.

Visual ECG Analysis

A group of five cardiologists, each from a different member state, have performed a detailed determination of the on- and offsets of the various ECG waves (P, QRS and T), on very enlarged signals (see example in FIGURE 1).[10] In view of the well-known

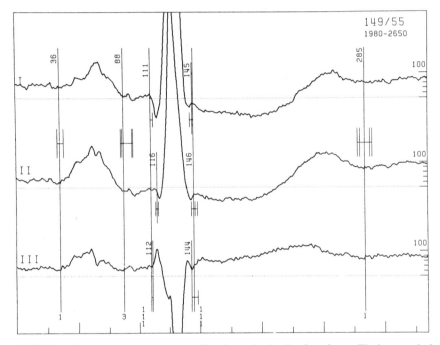

FIGURE 1. Example of wave onset and offset determination by the referees. The long vertical lines denote the median, the short ones the individual estimates of the five referees. (Note that individual referees' estimates may overlap). The adjacent numbers denote time locations (in sample points) with reference of the beat onset. The figures at the bottom of the vertical lines indicate the final reviewing round in which the measurements were obtained.

inter- and intraobserver variability in determining wave recognition points, an elaborate reviewing scheme was derived to establish the CSE three-lead reference library. By using a modified Delphi approach, individual referee "outliers," a point estimate which differs considerably from the median referee result, were eliminated in four successive steps, as illustrated in FIGURE 2. In this way a data bank was established with well-defined wave reference points. Reproducibility tests proved that the final estimates, resulting from the group, proved to be very stable.[10]

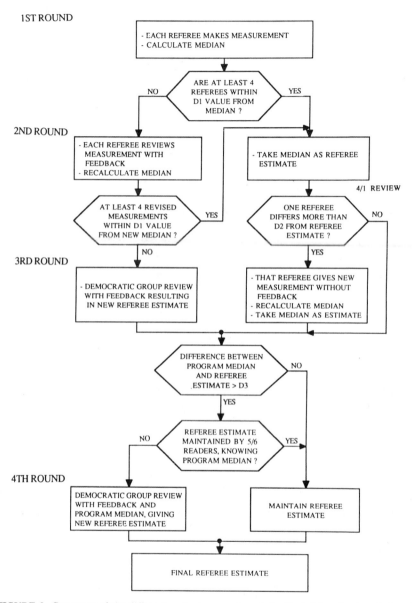

FIGURE 2. Summary of the different reviewing rounds and the final determination of P, and QRS onsets and offsets and for T end by the referees. The limits D1 to D3 used to estimate deviations of individual versus median referee results were respectively as follows: for D1: 10, 10, 6, 10, and 26 mseconds; for D2: 12, 14, 8, 14, and 36 mseconds; and for D3: 12, 12, 6, 10, and 28 mseconds.

Analysis by Different Programs

The same digital ECG recordings have also been measured by in total 9 different VCG and 10 different standard lead ECG programs, from Europe, the United States, Canada, and Japan, including those of major industrial companies.[12] Various graphical and statistical analysis programs have been developed in the Coordinating Center for program to program and referee to program comparison. FIGURE 3 depicts average differences and variances of different individual programs against the final referee results. The reference is indicated by long vertical lines and the variance of the

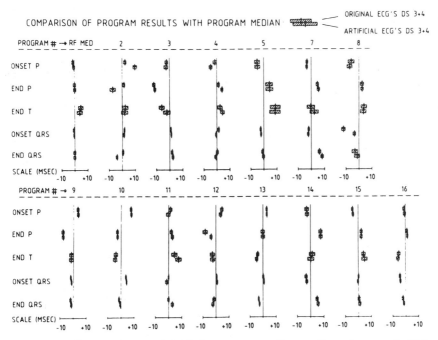

FIGURE 3. Differences between individual program as well as median referee results (RF MED), and the program median in the multilead CSE library.

computer results by horizontal bars. Some programs deviate systematically and some have a significantly higher variance for certain measurements, which means that their algorithms can be improved. However, the median wave recognition results of the 9 VCG and the 10 standard 12-lead ECG analysis programs were almost identical to the final visual estimates obtained by the referees. The program median presented a significantly lower variance than did individual program estimates. This median could therefore be used as a substitute in the determination of the multilead CSE reference library.[11] In general, the measurement performance of XYZ and the so-called 12-simultaneous-lead programs was better than that of conventional 3-lead programs, which nowadays disappear more and more from the market.

Comparison of Derived Interval Measurements

As could be expected from the differences in the basic P, QRS, and T wave onsets and offsets, some programs demonstrated significantly different P and QRS durations as well as PR and QT intervals, compared to others. The duration of the P wave and QT interval derived by the XYZ programs was significantly shorter than that computed by the standard 12-lead programs.[11] In contrast, the QRS duration derived from both lead systems was on the average nearly identical, although some individual results were widely divergent. Among the different standard 12-lead programs, the results were also divergent. Some multilead programs showed statistically shorter and other longer interval measurements. This may be explained by the use of different thresholds or template-matching algorithms, the application of correction procedures or even definition problems. Indeed as demonstrated in TABLE 1 five programs reported Q wave

TABLE 1. Mean Differences and Corresponding Standard Deviations (SD) (in Milliseconds) between Individual Program and Median Q, R, and S Duration Results[a]

CSE Program Number	Q Duration ($n = 2420$)[b]		R Duration ($n = 5619$)[b]		S Duration ($n = 4176$)[b]	
	Mean	SD	Mean	SD	Mean	SD
2	5.7	11.2	2.4	10.1	1.9	9.6
4	−0.1	6.7	−1.3	7.0	1.7	7.1
5	0.5	11.2	1.4	12.4	−2.1	8.7
7	−1.1	12.1	3.9	12.5	9.5	13.4
8	6.8	16.6	2.5	15.2	−3.5	13.3
11	−1.2	7.4	−2.6	7.9	0.3	7.2
12	4.5	13.4	2.3	15.2	6.3	14.0
13	0.8	8.5	−1.7	7.7	0.4	6.9
14	5.8	11.8	2.6	10.4	2.0	8.1
15	−0.1	9.3	0.7	10.4	1.4	10.0
16	5.7	14.9	2.7	12.3	0.4	12.7

[a]The differences (Prog-Median) were only obtained from cases where a result was present for both the respective program and the median. The results are cumulated over all standard leads and all recordings (that is, the original and artificial electrocardiograms) ($n = 492$ ECGs times 12 leads).

[b]n = number of Q, R, or S waves in the median of all 12-lead programs.

durations that were on the average 6 mseconds longer in all leads than the median, because these programs include initial isoelectric segments in the Q or QS wave, when present, whereas others did not. Such differences may lead to significantly different diagnostic results when the same criteria are used in different programs, for example, for myocardial infarction. The inclusion of terminal isoelectric segments in the R wave also at least partially explains the difference in R wave and QRS duration between various programs, and hence also differences in diagnostic statements on ventricular conduction defects.

CSE ECG Measurement Standard

The CSE measurement reference libraries have become an international standard for the evaluation and improvement of ECG measurement programs. The libraries have also been a useful instrument in the establishment of recommendations for more precise measurement rules and definitions.[13] Also noise testing has been performed to study results under degraded operational conditions.[14,15] As a result of CSE, modifications have been made in the wave recognition and measurement programs in several participating institutes. The CSE data bases have also been used by other institutes inside and outside Europe, including Eastern Europe, to improve the accuracy of existing programs or develop new algorithms.

The CSE Working Party does not wish to propose any formal algorithm as the standard for ECG wave recognition. As outlined elsewhere,[2-5,13,16] several mathematical algorithms may lead to similar solutions in pattern recognition. However, the Working Party recommends the CSE reference data bases as standard for 3-lead and 12-SL multilead ECG measurement programs. The meaning of the CSE standard is twofold:

1. A program should approach the reference as close as possible; the mean difference should be close to zero, and
2. The standard deviation of the differences of its results with respect to the reference should not exceed certain limits. These limits have been published in a paper with CSE recommendations.[13]

ASSESSING DIAGNOSTIC PROGRAM PERFORMANCE

Main Objectives of the Second CSE Study

The second CSE study aims at the "assessment of the diagnostic performance of ECG computer programs." The study was started in 1985 and should be finished at the end of 1990.[17-19] The diagnostic CSE study aims at consumer protection of the patient and the medical community. Ultimately a quality label involving minimum performance requirements should be given to ECG computer programs. To this end a library of ECGs is being collected from patients in which the clinical diagnosis is well documented by ECG independent means, such as cardiac catheterization, coronarography, echocardiography, and other techniques. Furthermore statistical methods are being developed to compare various analysis results, provided by both computer and visual ECG interpretation.[20-22]

Material and Methods Used in the Diagnostic CSE Study

Material and Processing Methods

The Working Party agreed on a common protocol for a pilot study, details of which were described previously.[17] This protocol has been used to gather the first 250 validated multilead recordings, comprising seven groups: normal, left, right, and biventricular hypertrophy; anterior, inferior, and combined myocardial infarction.

The so-called normals ($n = 120$) were free of significant cardiopulmonary disease on the basis of a health screening examination ($n = 92$) or invasive cardiac studies ($n = 28$). The diagnosis of LVH ($n = 34$), RVH ($n = 23$), and BVH ($n = 18$) was almost exclusively based on cardiac catheterization findings. Akinesia or dyskinesia in seven different segments of the ventriculogram, coded according to American Heart Association rules, was used as main selection criterion for the infarct classes ($n = 53$).

The ECGs were recorded on digital tape, 15 leads simultaneously, i.e., the standard

TABLE 2. Seven-Group Classification Results (in Percent) Obtained by the Cardiologists

True Group[a]	n	Combined ECG	ECG Results						VCG Results			Combined VCG
			1	2	3	4	5	6	1	2	3	
Normal	120	98.8	89.2	95.4	97.9	97.5	94.2	93.3	74.6	87.5	78.3	85.4
LVH	34	79.9	55.9	88.2	69.1	73.5	80.9	61.8	80.9	64.7	79.4	77.9
RVH	23	45.7	34.8	51.5	39.1	34.8	30.4	47.8	43.5	39.1	56.5	42.8
BVH	18	13.3	20.0	10.0	5.0	0.0	25.0	10.0	5.0	5.0	0.0	2.5
AMI	28	87.5	82.1	78.6	85.7	87.5	85.7	82.1	41.1	78.6	53.6	74.4
IMI	16	80.2	78.1	87.5	81.3	75.0	71.9	56.3	46.9	62.5	46.9	62.5
MIX	9	5.6	11.1	0.0	33.3	22.2	0.0	0.0	55.6	22.2	22.2	22.2
Hyper	75	69.0	59.7	80.3	57.8	58.4	61.7	61.0	75.3	60.4	67.5	68.4
MI	53	85.2	88.7	85.2	84.9	86.8	82.1	73.6	70.8	86.8	68.9	80.8
Total Acc		78.7	69.8	77.8	76.4	75.4	75.2	71.2	60.8	68.4	63.4	68.9
Partial Acc		86.7	78.8	88.3	82.8	82.6	81.4	78.8	72.6	77.4	72.0	77.9

[a]Hyper: any hypertrophy, independent of location; Acc: accuracy.

12 leads plus leads X, Y, and Z with a sampling rate of 500 Hz. The data were collected in two centers. A review board, consisting of three investigators, has verified the clinical information for all cases. ECGs with major ventricular conduction defects (QRS > 120 mseconds) were excluded.

The ECGs have been analyzed by 12 different computer programs and six cardiologists. Three of the referees have also interpreted in an independent way the vector loops and the scalar XYZ leads. Nine of the programs used the standard 12-lead ECG, 3 the VCG. The programs, included in the present study, were respectively: the AVA, Marquette, Louvain, Hannover, HP, IBM, Nagoya, Glasgow, Padova, Modular, and Leuven programs. The AVA results have been derived using clinical prior probabilities, as required by the program developers. Except for age and sex, no prior clinical information was provided to the other processing centers or the referees. A scheme was used to map various diagnostic statements onto a common set of codes. Each statement could be qualified by three degrees of certainty, i.e., definite (A), probable (B), and possible (C). When a program listed minor abnormalities without making reference to any of the seven primary categories listed above, the case was classified in the "so-called normal" group.

Statistical Analysis

The individual program and referee results have been compared with the true case disease category. Different misclassification matrices have been calculated, firstly in a bigroup analysis, i.e., normal vs. abnormal, LVH vs. non-LVH, etc.; next in a three-by-three matrix, i.e., normal vs. infarct vs. hypertrophy; then in a five-by-five and finally in a full seven-by-seven misclassification matrix. Only the diagnostic statement with the highest probability level A, B, or C was taken into consideration. If a program provided two statements with equal probability, of which one was correct and the other incorrect, the corresponding cells of the classification matrix were incremented by one-half. Similarly when three statements appeared on the highest level with equal probability, the cells were incremented by one-third. In this way a normalization was made for the fact that different programs print out various number of statements.

Based on these results, sensitivity, specificity, predictive values of a positive and negative test, total and partial accuracy figures have been determined for each program and each reader, as well as for the combined program and referee results. For the calculation of the partial accuracy figures, BVH was counted as partially correct when the case was classified as LVH or RVH. Similarly, for MIX infarction the output was considered partially correct if AMI or IMI was provided and vice versa. The information content and other measures of performance such as ROC curves, plots of predictive values versus incremental prevalence figures and McNemar statistics[20-22] were calculated, for each diagnostic category and each program individually.

The combined program and also the combined referee results have been derived by means of a point-scoring method. For every statement, each occurence with probability A was allocated three points, probability B two points, and C one point. This was first performed for the results of each processing center. The total sum was subsequently calculated over all centers for each recording and divided by the number of centers, so as to obtain a final combined result between one and three.

Preliminary Results of the CSE Diagnostic Study

Different tables have been prepared comparing program and referee results to the clinical truth. The diagonal elements of the full seven-by-seven misclassification matrices are presented in TABLES 2 and 3, both for the programs and the referees.

Referee Results

The specificity of the visual interpretation varied between 89% and 98%; for the VCG interpretation the range was 75% and 88%. This difference was statistically significant ($p < 0.01$). The sensitivity for AMI and IMI was also significantly higher in the ECG than the VCG interpretation results (see TABLE 2). The referees had a higher accuracy than the majority of the computer programs, at least when using the standard ECG. Their VCG interpretations, however, proved to be less accurate. Interestingly, the combined referee data demonstrated the highest accuracy, higher than that of any individual reader.[19] The accuracy for the six ECG readings combined was 78.7%, against 77.8% for the best and 69.8% for the least accurate reader (median 75.3%).

TABLE 3. Seven-Group Classification Results (in Percent) Obtained by the Various Programs

True Group	Combined Programs	A	B	C	D	E	F	G	H	I	J	K	L
Normal	97.9	72.4	88.3	75.4	94.9	97.5	93.3	95.8	89.6	99.2	83.3	90.8	91.7
LVH	88.2	66.2	94.1	86.8	67.6	72.1	85.3	67.6	76.5	88.2	48.5	87.9	72.1
RVH	42.8	39.1	26.1	26.1	35.7	30.4	34.8	4.3	54.3	34.8	30.4	26.1	47.1
BVH	1.7	10.0	0.0	0.0	0.0	0.0	0.0	0.0	7.5	15.0	0.0	0.0	45.0
AMI	75.0	53.6	64.3	53.6	69.6	67.9	75.0	67.9	66.1	66.1	50.0	82.1	64.3
IMI	68.8	81.3	62.5	53.1	53.3	46.7	56.3	75.0	81.3	68.8	40.6	62.5	81.3
MIX	5.6	0.0	22.2	11.1	0.0	0.0	0.0	0.0	22.2	0.0	0.0	0.0	27.8
Hyper	73.2	65.6	69.5	73.4	64.2	56.5	61.0	42.9	87.7	68.8	55.2	65.1	83.3
MI	72.6	73.6	76.4	66.0	70.2	64.4	67.0	69.8	82.1	68.9	46.2	73.6	88.7
Total Acc	76.1	59.3	69.6	60.2	69.7	70.1	71.6	68.0	72.4	75.8	57.6	71.1	75.1
Partial Acc	84.6	70.1	79.2	69.8	79.1	77.1	77.8	73.6	86.2	82.2	64.8	78.9	87.3

Program Results

As can be seen from TABLE 3, specificity values for the different programs varied between 72.4% and 99.2%. Eight programs had a specificity of 90% or more, two were close to 85%, and two were at the level of 75%. The sensitivity for RVH was as could be expected low for all programs and varied between 4.3% and 54.3%. This is probably due to the fact that most RVH cases were rather mild to moderate. The sensitivity for LVH, in contrast, was rather high for most programs. This may indicate that the enclosed LVH pathology was rather severe. The sensitivity for myocardial infarction (MI), irrespective of the location ($n = 53$), amounted to a low of 46.2% and a high of 88.7%.

Similarly as for the referee results the combined program results also proved to have a higher total accuracy, i.e., 76.1% higher than that of any individual program, the median accuracy of the individual programs being 69.8% and that of the best program 75.8%. After deleting the two extremes, the total accuracy of the remaining nine programs ranged between 59% and 75%. The difference between these values amounts to 30%, as opposed to a difference in range of 10% for the ECG readers.[19]

Discussion of Results of CSE Diagnostic Study

The aims of the CSE diagnostic study are to evaluate and eventually improve diagnostic ECG systems, to compare different diagnostic strategies, and to establish an ECG independent and clinically validated library to carry out these objectives. The development of such a data base cannot be performed by a single center, but needs a joint international effort. The CSE Working Party and foreign consultants agreed that there was an urgent need for such a study, since industry has nowadays to a large extent overtaken academic centers and is placing "cheap" computerized ECG machines on the market. In many cases these lack adequate validation and could potentially pose a real health hazard in the hands of inexperienced users (general practitioners).

According to a predefined protocol, a set of cases was gathered from 15-lead recordings with type A anomalies,[23] which can be validated by ECG independent clinical information. From the results obtained so far, it is obvious that the referees as a whole perform definitely better than a large majority of the computer programs, at least when interpreting the standard 12-lead ECG. The VCG results of the referees were surprisingly less accurate. Similarly, if one excludes the results of the AVA program, which uses clinical prior information, also the VCG programs proved to be less accurate. The reasons for these differences still need to be established. Indeed, it has recently been demonstrated that the ECG and the VCG perform equally well in the differential diagnosis of seven main entities, provided identical procedures are used in the design of the classifiers.[24]

An interesting finding of the diagnostic pilot study was the higher total accuracy of the combined ECG results (78.7%) over all individual referee results (range 69.8% to 77.8%; median 75.3%). The total accuracy for the combined VCG results (68.5%) was also higher than that obtained by any referee individually (range 60.8% to 68.4%; median 63.4%). Although less clear-cut, this was also the case for the program results.[19] The combined program accuracy was 76.1%, as opposed to a range of 57.6% to 75.8% (median 69.8%) for the individual program results, enclosed in the present study. Seven of these 11 programs showed a total accuracy of <71%, four <69%. These findings support the superiority of group opinions over individual interpretations. On the other hand, it may also be noted that the best programs performed almost as well as the best of six cardiologists.

Further Prospects

It should be underlined that these results are preliminary, since they are only based on 250 recordings. Several performance indices of diagnostic accuracy depend heavily on the composition of the test groups and the fraction of test cases in each group. For some diagnostic categories only few cases were available. In the coming months we will continue the collection of cases for an expanded validated data base in three centers. In parallel to the data collection some methodological problems need to be solved further. In December 88 we reached a total of 500 cases. They have been mailed to the processing centers and the referees for intermediate analysis at the beginning of 1989. We hope to reach 1000 cases by the end of 1989.

A standardization and performance testing task, such as undertaken by CSE, is difficult and can only be done by means of the international collaboration of clinicians, engineers, and computer specialists. By including contributions and expertise from different centers with international reputation, results will not be restricted to a "special ECG School," but will be accepted by the medical community as a whole, and also by industry.

STANDARDS FOR TRANSMISSION, ENCODING, AND STORAGE OF DIGITAL ECG DATA

Standardization Needs

In addition to the needs and objectives listed above, there is a growing need to harmonize and standardize the technical and telecommunication areas of acquisition, transmission, encoding, and storage of computer-processed ECG data.[18,25] Until recently, transmission of ECGs was mainly done with analog techniques. Almost all newer electrocardiographs offer features of digital recording and interpretation. These stand-alone microcomputer-based machines can be connected to larger minicomputer-based management systems for long-term storage and serial comparison of ECGs. There is now even the possibility of storing ECG data on personal microchip cards. However, standards are also lacking in this information technology area (IT).

Indeed, various manufacturers use different techniques not only for measurement and interpretation, but also for transmission and storage of data. As a result, equipment cannot be linked and monopoly situations loom in and over hospital and regional authorities buying equipment and trying to link these electrocardiographs with larger ECG management systems. It is in the general public interest if users are not restricted in their options by incompatible technical features and services of different systems and manufacturers. Digital acquisition and transmission of data offers the possibility of increased fidelity and flexibility, but at the same time requires the development of efficient encoding, compression, and even also encryption schemes.

Proposed Actions

To meet these objectives we have worked out a proposal for the "Conformance Testing Services" (CTS) and the "Advanced Medical Informatics" (AIM) Programs of Directorate General XIII of the European Community. The aims are to establish standards and to set up testing services in at least two laboratories in two different EC member states. These centers should be capable to implement, execute, and if necessary further refine IEC specifications with regard to performance and safety of computer-based electrocardiographs, along various technical steps from signal acquisition up to the measurement part. This is an area in the IT field, which is in line with other activities supported by CTS and the European Standardization Bodies CEN/CENELEC.[25]

In the CTS and the complementary AIM project, which started June 1 1989, an investigation will be made of the complete chain of acquisition of signals, of transmission and communication of data to determine at each step:

- The standards and specifications that can be applied.
- The tests that have to be executed according to existing IEC recommendations and eventually supplementary tests.
- The work to be done to move from this stage to an operational testing service

IEC recommendations with respect to electrocardiographic devices date from 1977 and definitely need to be updated. ISO or CEN/CENELEC standards will be followed with respect to the IT specific issues. Specifications will be drafted on the basis of consensus with participation of all interested parties, i.e., academia, industry, professional standardization bodies, and user-cardiologists.

CONCLUSION

Medical technology is developing at an increasingly greater speed. Progress in medical informatics and computing will in the future depend more and more on the adoption of standards for interpreting and communicating medical data, signals, and images. The basic aim of the standards already developed in CSE and still planned for the future is to increase the availability and compatibility of objective decision support by means of quantitative electrocardiography throughout the European Community and the world at large. The importance of the development of quantitative test procedures and reference libraries for assessing the precision and accuracy of ECG computer programs has been emphasized on several occasions, as early as 1971.[2,23] However, before CSE, no one had been able to proceed with some action in this direction. Performance evaluation tests are needed for consumer protection, both for the patient and the medical community. Ultimately, a quality label or conformity certificate of minimum performance requirements should be given to computer programs, before they are put on the market. In CSE, groundwork has been performed for this to happen in the future.

ACKNOWLEDGMENT

We are grateful to Ms. I. Tassens for secretarial assistance and to Mr. I. Schoolmeesters for computer programming help.

REFERENCES

1. PIPBERGER, H. V., R. J. ARMS & F. W. STALLMAN. 1961. Automatic screening of normal and abnormal electrocardiograms by means of a digital electronic computer. Proc. Soc. Exp. Biol. Med. **106:** 130.

2. ZYWIETZ, C. & B. SCHNEIDER. 1973. Computer Application in ECG and VCG Analysis. North Holland. Amsterdam, the Netherlands.
3. VAN BEMMEL, J. H. & J. L. WILLEMS, Eds. 1977. Trends in Computer Processed Electrocardiograms. North Holland. Amsterdam, the Netherlands.
4. WOLF, H. K. & P. W. MACFARLANE, Eds. 1980. Optimization of Computer ECG Processing. North Holland. Amsterdam, the Netherlands.
5. WILLEMS, J. L., J. H. VAN BEMMEL & C. ZYWIETZ, Eds. 1985. Computer ECG Analysis: Towards Standardization. North Holland. Amsterdam, the Netherlands.
6. WILLEMS, J. L. 1980. A plea for common standards in computer aided ECG analysis. Comp. Biomed. Res. **13:** 120–131.
7. WILLEMS, J. L. & J. PARDAENS. 1977. Differences in measurement results obtained by four different ECG computer programs. In Proceedings of Computers in Cardiology 1977. H. G. Ostrow & K. L. Ripley, Eds: 115–121. IEEE Computer Society. Long Beach, Calif.
8. 1980. Official Journal of the European Communities. L78: 24–28.
9. WILLEMS, J. L., P. ARNAUD, R. DEGANI, P. W. MACFARLANE, J. H. VAN BEMMEL, & C. ZYWIETZ. 1980. Protocol for the concerted action project "Common Standards for Quantitative Electrocardiography" 2nd R & D programme in the field of Medical and Public Health Research of the EEC (80/344/EEC), CSE Ref. 80-06-00. Acco Publ. Leuven, 1-152, Belgium.
10. WILLEMS, J. L., P. ARNAUD, J. H. VAN BEMMEL, et al. 1985. Establishment of a reference library for evaluating computer ECG measurement programs. Comp. Biomed. Res. **18:** 439–457.
11. WILLEMS, J. L., P. ARNAUD, J. H. VAN BEMMEL, et al. 1987. A reference data base for multilead electrocardiographic computer measurement programs. J. Am. Coll. Cardiol. **6:** 1313–1321.
12. WILLEMS, J. L., P. ARNAUD, J. H. VAN BEMMEL, et al. 1985. Assessment of the performance of electrocardiographic computer programs with the use of a reference data base. Circulation **71:** 523–534.
13. The CSE Working Party. 1985. Recommendations for measurement standards in quantitative electrocardiography. Eur. Heart J. **6:**815–825.
14. WILLEMS, J. L., C. ZYWIETZ, P. ARNAUD, J. H. VAN BEMMEL, R. DEGANI & P. W. MACFARLANE. 1987. Influence of noise on wave boundary recognition by ECG measurement programs. Comp. Biomed. Res. **20:** 543–562.
15. ZYWIETZ, C., J. L. WILLEMS, P. ARNAUD, J. H. VAN BEMMEL, R. DEGANI & P. W. MACFARLANE. 1990. Stability of computer ECG measurements in the presence of noise. Comp. Biomed. Res. **23:** 10–31.
16. WILLEMS, J. L. (CSE Project Leader). 1981–1989. Annual CSE Progress Reports. Acco Publ. Leuven, Belgium.
17. WILLEMS, J. L., C. ABREU-LIMA, P. ARNAUD, J. H. VAN BEMMEL, C. BROHET, R. DEGANI, B. DENIS, I. GRAHAM, G. VAN HERPEN, P. W. MACFARLANE, J. MICHAELIS, S. MOULOPOULOS, S. POPPL & C. ZYWIETZ. 1987. Testing the performance of ECG computer programs. The CSE diagnostic pilot study. J. Electrocardiol. **20:** S298–S301.
18. WILLEMS, J. L. 1988. 8th CSE Progress Report, Common Standards for Quantitative Electrocardiography. ACCO Publ. Leuven, Belgium.
19. WILLEMS, J. L., C. ABREU-LIMA, P. ARNAUD, et al. (for the CSE Working Party). 1988. Effect of combining electrocardiographic interpretation results on diagnostic accuracy. Eur. Heart J. **10:** 1348–1355.
20. BAILEY, J. J., G. CAMPBELL, M. R. HORTON, R. I. SHRAGER & J. L. WILLEMS. 1988. Determination of statistically significant differences in the performance of ECG diagnostic algorithm: an improved method. J. Electrocardiol. **21:** S188–S192.
21. MICHAELIS, J. & J. L. WILLEMS. 1988. Performance evaluation of diagnostic ECG programs. In Computers in Cardiology 1987 K. L. Ripley, Ed.: 25–30. IEEE Computer Society. Long Beach, Calif.
22. WILLEMS, J. L., G. CAMPBELL & J. J. BAILEY. 1989. Progress on the CSE diagnostic study. Application of McNemar's test revisited. J. Electrocardiol. **22:** S135–S140.
23. RAUTAHARJU, P. M., M. ARIET, T. A. PRYOR, R. C. ARZBAECHER, J. J. BAILEY, R.

BONNER, et al. 1978. Task Force III: computers in diagnostic electrocardiology. Am. J. Cardiol. **41**: 158–170.
24. WILLEMS, J. L., E. LESAFFRE & J. PARDAENS. 1987. Comparison of the classification ability of the ECG and VCG. Am. J. Cardiol. **59**: 119–124.
25. WILLEMS, J. L. 1988. An example of standardization need: common standards for quantitative electrocardiography. Abstract Book of CEN/CENELEC Workshop on European Standardization of Medical Devices, Brussels, Belgium, 12–14 December 1988.

APPENDIX
CSE Organizational Structure

CSE European Working Party

Belgium: C. Brohet (University of Louvain), J. L. Willems (University of Leuven)
West Germany: J. Meyer and J. Michaelis (University of Mainz), S. J. Pöppl (Institute of Medical Data Processing, München), C. Zywietz (University of Hannover)
Denmark: J. Damgaard Andersen (University of Copenhagen)
France: P. Arnaud (INSERM U121 Lyon), B. Denis (University of Grenoble), P. Rubel (INSA, Lyon)
Great Britain: P. J. Bourdillon (University of London), P. W. Macfarlane (University of Glasgow)
Greece: S. Moulopoulos (University of Athens), E. Skordalakis (Technical University of Athens)
Ireland: I. Graham (University of Dublin)
Italy: S. Dalla Volta (University of Padova), R. Degani (Ladseb CNR, Padova), G. Mazzocca (University of Pisa)
The Netherlands: J. H. van Bemmel and J. Kors (Erasmus University, Rotterdam), H. J. Ritsema van Eck (Rotterdam), G. van Herpen (University of Leiden)
Portugal: C. Abreu-Lima (University of Porto), H. B. Machado (University Hospital, Lisbon)

Consultants

J. J. Bailey (National Institutes of Health) and H. V. Pipberger (George Washington University, United States), P. M. Rautaharju (University of Dalhousie, Canada), E. O. Robles de Medina (University of Utrecht, NL)

Non-European Participants

United States: C. Monroe, S. Charlesworth (Hewlett-Packard), K. Michler (Telemed), I. Rowlandson (Marquette), D. W. Mortara (Mortara Instruments)
Canada: P. M. Rautaharju, P. Macinnis (University of Dalhousie)
Japan: M. Okajima, N. Okamoto, M. Yokoi (University of Nagoya), N. Ohsawa (Fukuda Denshi)

Representing BME-COMAC

J. Marques-Montes (University of Madrid, Spain) and U. Faust (University of Stuttgart, FRG)

CSE Coordinating Center

Division of Medical Informatics, University of Leuven, Leuven, Belgium

Computerized Electrocardiography

A Historical Perspective

IAN ROWLANDSON

Marquette Electronics Inc.
8200 West Tower Avenue
Milwaukee, Wisconsin 53223

INTRODUCTION

Periodically it is beneficial to review the advancement of a technology. This exercise can often lead to insights about the future.

Beginning with the first recorded electrocardiogram (ECG), the topic of computerized electrocardiography will be presented via a historical perspective. Particular attention will be paid to those aspects that have affected automated analysis. Based on this perspective, future trends are predicted.

BEFORE THE COMPUTER

Many of us who use the ECG on a daily basis recognize the name Einthoven and are aware that he was one of the great men of electrocardiography. What is typically not appreciated is the fact that the science is over a century old and that many of the diagnostic patterns we see today were first documented before 1930.

The first human ECG was taken in 1887, by Waller.[1] He used a glass capillary electrometer which was based on the principle that the surface tension at the junction of mercury and dilute sulfuric acid changes when the electric potential between them is altered. The movements of the meniscus were magnified and recorded on moving photographic paper.

In 1895, Einthoven introduced the terms P, Q, R, S, and T from his work with the capillary electrometer. Frustrated with the frequency resolution of the electrometer, Einthoven developed the string galvanometer and published his first results in 1903.

The string galvanometer used a quartz fiber, coated with silver, suspended between the poles of a magnet. Small currents from the heart were conducted through the quartz string. The varying magnetic field generated by the current resulted in a deflection of the string at right angles to the field of the magnet. A strong beam of light was used to cast a shadow of the string on a moving photographic plate. This method resulted in a high resolution photographic record of the string's movement.

Even though the instrument was not a portable, direct writing electrocardiograph, many of the abnormalities that we recognize today were observed and documented in the early use of the string galvanometer. Consider:[1]

- Repolarization changes due to digitalis (Nicolai, 1909).
- Bundle branch block (Eppinger, 1910).
- Ventricular fibrillation and recovery (Hoffman, 1912).
- Delta waves, WPW syndrome (Wilson, 1915).

- Repolarization changes due to infarction (Pardee, 1920).
- ST/T change before, during, and after angina (Feil, 1928).

By the 1950s, advancements in amplifier technology led to the advent of a portable, direct writing ECG cart and, as a result, the widespread popularity of these instruments. Although the number of leads and format of the ECG had changed (Wilson terminal, 1932—precordial lead standardization, 1938), the resolution and quality of the ECG signal had not advanced.[1] In addition to amplifier technology, another advancement—the cathode-ray oscilloscope—brought the manifestation (1936) of Einthoven's early theories regarding the cardiac vector.

By 1959, the first analog to digital (A/D) conversion system was specifically designed for ECGs.[2] Within a few years, several labs were converting the analog ECG signal into digital form. The motivation of these investigators was threefold. They felt:

1. there was information being missed by the naked eye;
2. the intuitive "reading" of the ECG could be quantified; and
3. the efficiency of ECG recording could be increased.

The realization of the first two goals is still subject to debate. However, there is no question that the recording, storing, processing, and retrieval of digital ECGs has led to a dramatic increase in efficiency.

A/D CONVERSION

It is critical that the "front end"—that is, everything that comes before a digital sample—removes noise and faithfully captures the analog signal. Once the signal enters the digital domain, filtering out these distortions is very difficult.

One source of noise that must be rejected by the front end comes from electrical fields outside the body. The ability of the cart to reject that signal, so that it does not appear on the ECG tracing, is called common mode rejection.

Recall that every lead of the ECG results from the subtraction of two inputs. Therefore, if the input terminals are electrically matched, the noise generated by the external fields will be subtracted when the ECG leads are generated. Advances in high quality, differential amplifiers have made this possible.

Another method of removing the influence of the external fields is to have the front end generate a signal that is in direct opposition to them. This is the purpose of a "right leg driver."[3] The front end sums the signals from the limb electrodes, inverts the result, and drives it out through the right leg electrode, thus nullifying the effect of the signals generated by the external fields.

A relatively recent advancement in eliminating noise from the ECG has come from the use of a patient cable that performs digitization at the patient.[4] Since the digitization occurs at the body, the entire cable length is not subject to artifact. This is especially germane to stress testing, where the patient cables are typically over 15 feet in length and subject to a great deal of movement.

The manifestation of these three concepts (balanced input terminals, right leg driver, and intelligent patient cable) has resulted in front ends with a common mode rejection of greater than 130 dB.

Besides rejecting the common mode signal, there is another step that must be done before digitization: frequencies above half the sampling rate must be removed from the signal. If the sampling rate is less than twice the highest frequency in the signal, the resultant digitized values generate an artifactual low frequency signal (see FIGURE 1).

Filters that are used to eliminate these high frequency signals are known as antialiasing filters.

A/D converters were, at one time, an expensive, special item. Cost reduction has led to their use in household appliances and automobiles. Two parameters that are often used to describe an A/D converter are its sampling rate and bit length.

The sampling rate of most resting ECG carts is 250 samples per second (sps). This is quickly being replaced by 500 sps as memory, transmission speeds, and processing power enable this to be a practical standard for clinical use. Other applications—like late potential analysis—require sampling rates on the order of 1000 sps. Other applications—like ambulatory and bedside monitoring—require less sampling (120 sps) since their intent is to analyze rhythm and the ST/T.

Bit length refers to the number of bits that the A/D converter generates per sample. This determines the number of gradations that are possible with the converter. For example, a 12 bit converter divides the input range by 4096 (2^{12}). In order to determine the resolution of the sampled data, one must also know the range of values to be digitized. For example, an input range of ± 20 mV with an A/D converter of 12 bits results in a resolution of 10 μV per bit (i.e., 40 mV divided by 4096).

In order for a 12 bit converter to attain a resolution of 10 μV, and yet digitize ECGs that can be floating on a DC offset as large as 300 mV some additional technology must be applied to the problem.

One approach is to remove the DC offset with a high pass filter; this is often

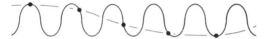

FIGURE 1. Antialiasing filters.

referred to as an A/C-coupled front end. Most analog high pass filters add phase distortion to the waveform, which can result in artifactual ST segment deviations[5] (see Signal Conditioning).

A second approach is to allow the front end to sample and hold the DC offset. This value is then subtracted from the incoming signal. First implemented in 1968 by Marquette Electronics, the DC-coupled front end preserved low frequency response, leaving the ST segments intact.

Recent advancements in the music industry (optical disk players) have generated A/D converters of much longer bit lengths, higher accuracy, and lower cost. This will be the ultimate answer to the dynamic range versus resolution dilemma.

In the mid-1960s there were several labs that were directly digitizing the analog signal from the patient's body.[2] However, most computerized ECGs that were taken during this era were done in two steps: that is, the ECG was first put onto analog tape, or transmitted via voice grade lines, before it was digitized at a central system.

In 1979, the first commercially available digital cart was introduced (Marquette Electronics—MAC I). Direct digitization resulted in several key breakthroughs:

1. All the ECG leads could be acquired simultaneously. Previously the bandwidth of the phone lines had restricted the transmission of analog data to three channels at a time.
2. The ECG was transmitted digitally, using a communication protocol which

supported error checking. Artifacts generated by phone line noise etc. were eliminated from the ECG.
3. Digital filters could be applied at the bedside, resulting in cleaner, artifact-free tracings.

SIGNAL CONDITIONING

The purpose of signal-conditioning algorithms is to eliminate artifacts from the ECG, without contaminating the physiological signal. This is difficult since the ECG and the artifact often overlap.

Note that the ECG has a broad spectrum. ST/T waves start at about 0.5 Hz. QRSs begin in the frequencies of the T wave and extend all the way up to 100–125 Hz. Baseline sway is in the low frequency domain; this often overlaps with the ST/T. Power line interference is in the frequency range of the QRS, but it has other characteristics that make it a prime candidate for filtering. Muscle artifact covers a wide spectrum, beginning at 30 Hz and encompassing the upper limits of the QRS.

Of the three artifacts, power line interference is the easiest to characterize and remove. Since it comprises a discrete frequency, the computer can model it using a sine wave that has a period equal to that of 50/60 Hz. The computer can constantly

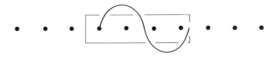

FIGURE 2. Low pass filter/boxcar filter.

compare its model against the actual artifact, because power line interference is, typically, a continuous signal. If the comparison results in a discrepancy, the computer can adapt the model so that it is equal to the power line interference. Changes to this model must take place slowly, otherwise the adaptive filter would make erroneous changes during a QRS, etc. As the model is generated it is subtracted from the original signal. This results in the elimination of the 50/60 Hz noise.

Muscle artifact, as opposed to power line noise, is neither periodic nor continuous. There is no technique available for filtering out the artifact without also disturbing valuable information in the QRS. Nevertheless, a low pass filter, with a cutoff frequency of 40 Hz, is typically applied to this problem. FIGURE 2 is an example of a simple low pass filter. The output of the filter is equal to the sum of the data points within the box. The box is then moved down by one sample, and another output is generated in the same manner. Not surprisingly, this filter is often referred to as a "boxcar filter." Note that a sinusoidal waveform—equal in length to the boxcar— would result in zero. Similarly, higher frequencies would be attenuated by the filter, regardless of whether or not they came from the QRS or the muscle artifact.

Now that muscle artifact and power line noise have been discussed, there is one remaining artifact that must be dealt with: baseline sway. Recently there have been some important advances in removing this artifact, resulting in more accurate detections of ischemic heart disease, etc. Baseline sway begins at DC and rarely extends

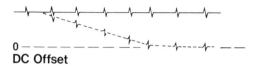

DC Offset

FIGURE 3. High pass filter. Use of estimate for baseline sway correction.

beyond 0.5 Hz. On the other hand, the signal generated by the heart has been shown to start at no lower than 0.5 Hz.[6] Theoretically there should be a filter that could eliminate baseline sway without harming the information in the ST/T.

One method that has been used for removing baseline sway is the use of a baseline estimate that is constantly subtracted from the raw, incoming data. This concept is portrayed in FIGURE 3. Note that the baseline of the raw data has a DC offset. Initially, the computer assumes the baseline is zero. It subtracts this estimate from the raw data. A fraction of this difference is then added to the next estimate. After each successive sample, the estimate grows and the DC offset is gradually removed.

One of the problems with this technique, however, is that it can generate an artifactual ST segment deviation. Note that as the filter enters a QRS (see FIGURE 4) it has no way of discriminating it from baseline sway. As a result, it begins to build up its estimate of the baseline. When the QRS is complete, the charged up estimate continues to be subtracted from the baseline, resulting in an artifactual ST segment deviation.

This scenario reveals an important aspect about filters: they have a phase as well as an amplitude response. The amplitude response is what is most often quoted when characterizing a filter and it refers to how much a filter will attenuate the amplitude of a given frequency. The phase response, however, describes how much the filter will delay a signal of a particular frequency. This simple, aforementioned filter has poor phase response (a nonlinear phase response) because it selectively delays certain frequencies more than others.

This phenomenon was recognized by the American Heart Association (AHA) when they published their recommendations for the resting ECG in 1975.[7] They asked that the amplitude response of this filter be limited to 0.05 Hz, and made no mention of phase response. At the time, there were no baseline filters available that could avoid the creation of this ST artifact. Therefore, they limited the aggressiveness of this filter so that the artifact would be inconsequentially small. However, it also limited the ability of the filter to remove baseline sway.

In 1975, ECG carts were only equipped with analog filters that could not uncouple their phase and amplitude response. The filter that was portrayed in FIGURE 3 is the

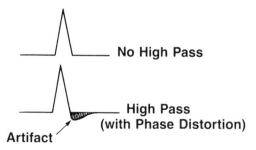

No High Pass

High Pass
(with Phase Distortion)

Artifact

FIGURE 4. Artifactual ST segment deviation via high pass filter.

digital equivalent to the filter most often implemented in analog carts (and in A/C-coupled front ends). When it is used aggressively and not counteracted—as it is in some commercial equipment—it can result in artifact and an improper diagnosis.[6]

In contrast, digital filters can uncouple their phase and amplitude response. With the advent of digital carts, there are now filters that will not generate this artifact. This is an important advancement. Digital filters can now more aggressively remove baseline sway, up to 0.5 Hz, without corrupting the ST segment.[6]

Ironically, the phase distortion of the filter portrayed in FIGURE 3 can be removed if, after a forward pass through the data, the filter is executed backwards.[6] Low frequency components that had suffered delays in the forward pass are similarly delayed in the opposite direction. This bidirectional approach was first made commercially available in 1982 (Marquette Electronics—MAC II).

Other more sophisticated linear phase response filters (finite impulse response, cubic spline,[8,9] etc.) have also been implemented in applications like Holter or stress testing, where running the data backwards through a filter is impractical.

QRS DETECTION

The first computer program used for the detection of QRSs was reported in 1961.[2] The hardware used to execute the program filled a small room. By the mid-1980s, computerized ECG carts, which contain more computer power than these early mainframes, were reduced to the size of book (Marquette Electronics, MAC PC, 1985). Although the hardware has dramatically changed, the algorithms used for QRS detection have remained almost the same.

The first step includes band-pass filtering the data: that is, removing frequencies below 5 Hz and above 30 Hz. The point of this step is to remove those frequencies that are not the major components of the QRS.

In modern programs, this process is performed on quasi-orthogonal leads, with the reason being that the cardiac vector will be apparent in at least one of three orthogonal leads. Previous to the advancement of simultaneous acquisition, programs that operated on 12 lead ECGs could not take advantage of this concept.

The next step of QRS detection requires adding up the absolute values of each of the filter outputs and comparing them against a threshold. When they exceed the threshold, a QRS is "detected" by the program.

The threshold that is most often used by programs has a contour similar to that in FIGURE 5. The first 200 mseconds of the threshold serves as a refractory period: that is, once the threshold is exceeded, the program continues to look for a maximum output of the band-pass filter. This is so that the program will avoid detecting two portions of the same QRS. This is followed by another 200 mseconds, with a threshold equal to one-half the detected QRS. The purpose of this is to avoid detecting the T wave and yet still provide the program a good chance of detecting heart rates on the order of 300 beats per minute (bpm). Finally, the threshold drops to one quarter of the detection value. In this way, the program uses a threshold that is based on the QRS that will allow it to "float" over artifacts and not detect them as QRSs.

The threshold contour can be made increasingly more complicated by the program designer by taking into account the last eight detected beats, etc. Although this approach will be accurate over 90% of the time, it will ultimately fail on a complicated rhythm or on an ECG with a challenging artifact. Other clues must be used by state-of-the-art algorithms—with the important one being the knowledge of what shapes it is detecting (i.e., correlation).

QRS CORRELATION

Before the advent of simultaneous lead acquisition, the computer had to pick a "favorite beat" in order to measure the QRS waveform. Although the computer tried to find a beat with the best signal to noise ratio, it was often left with a QRS surrounded with so much artifact that accurate measurement became impossible.

The concept of a favorite beat was the state-of-the-art approach until the mid-1970s. At that time, computers were being confronted by the challenge of stress test data that were so noisy that the use of a favorite beat was impossible. A new solution was required. It was evident that the computer should take advantage of the repetitive nature of the ECG and average the QRSs together so that the artifact could be minimized.[10] In order for the computer to do this, it had to first recognize which were the normally conducted beats. This is the purpose of correlation.

Computers correlate (that is, compare a template with the raw data) by comparing one, or a combination of, the following: actual sample values, certain features from each waveform, or frequencies from each waveform.

It is important that the comparison be done at the same place on the waveforms, otherwise a mismatch will result, even when the QRSs are identical. Most programs try

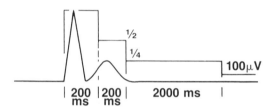

FIGURE 5. QRS detection—threshold profile.

several points around the QRS trigger (i.e., where the program detected a beat). However, the trigger is often very unstable: one time it will trigger on the R wave, the next time the S wave.

A better idea is to continuously perform correlation, looking for an optimal match between the templates and raw data. This approach also has the significant advantage of allowing the program to continuously look for shapes that are familiar to it. These clues can markedly improve the accuracy of the QRS detector, allowing it to throw out detections that are obviously artifact—given the context of the other beats.

Continuous correlation is not used by most programs since it is computationally expensive, especially for real-time analysis. Marquette Electronics first used a continuous correlator in the 12SL program. Recently it has been applied to Holter analysis via a real time recorder (SEER, Marquette Electronics).

SIGNAL AVERAGING

After the QRSs have been detected, grouped by shape, and aligned in time, the computer can average the QRSs and markedly reduce the amount of noise.

Some computer algorithms form a median[4,10] instead of an average. A median is formed by taking, at each sample time, the middle voltage of the aligned beats. This process is computationally more expensive since a sort is required. However, the method generates a cleaner complex since it disregards outliers.

A median would be an exceptional advantage during stress testing, where there is so much noise.[8] However, since the data stream is continuous during stress testing, the formation of a median complex is impractical. Another technique—called incremental updating—also has the advantage of eliminating the influence of outliers but it is computationally less expensive and it provides a continuous, artifact-free image of the incoming data.[11] It does this by adjusting the template by small increments. If there is a consistent discrepancy between the raw data and template, the incremental updating process will track it. However, artifacts will only influence it by an inconsequential amount.

MEASUREMENTS

Programs that employ simultaneous lead acquisition have a large advantage over programs that do not. This is because they do not have to resolve the differences resulting from the measurement of a different beat from each lead group. The onsets and offsets are determined by analyzing the noise level and the simultaneous slopes in all 12 leads.

After the P, QRS, and T complexes have been demarcated, the waves for each complex are identified. The measurement matrix contains the amplitudes (with respect to QRS onset) and durations of all these individual waves.

CRITERIA IMPLEMENTATION

After the computer has made its measurements, it executes a criteria package in order to generate diagnostic statements. These packages vary in complexity from program to program. Most commercially available programs use decision-tree type logic in order to generate statements. They have the great advantage that the diagnostic criteria are usually familiar to the cardiologist. Other packages are based on multivariate analysis and/or "fuzzy logic." In contrast, these methods are not easy to explain or understand. Regardless of which method is used, a large data base for developing and testing the programs is required.

DATA COMPRESSION/CLINICAL DATA BASES

Digital carts must compress the ECG data in order to minimize transmission time and conserve computer storage space. Some compression algorithms irreversibly change the acquired data, while other methods preserve the original data.

In 1980 Marquette Electronics introduced the use of Huffman encoding[12] for the storage and transmission of ECGs. Huffman encoding simply converts the data from a fixed length binary code into a variable length binary code (see TABLE 1). In order to compress the data, those values that occur frequently in the ECG are assigned shorter bit length codes. This form of compression allows any ECG (regardless of its origin) to be used for criteria development and reanalysis. This feature expedites the growth of clinically correlated data bases, which are necessary for the development and validation of the program.

FUTURE TRENDS

Although computerized electrocardiography is now a mature technology, continued evolution is expected.

Recently, extensive and sophisticated calculations that are almost impossible to do by hand (like ST/HR index,[8] RR variability, late potential analysis, etc.) are being performed on the computer with promising results. This trend will continue, opening up a new era for computerized electrocardiography.

As has been demonstrated since 1960, the hardware will continue to advance. Smaller, cost-effective devices that do more will bring the computerized ECG into new environments (like the home, ambulance, etc.). In addition, advances in networks and storage systems will result in expedient information management; ECGs associated with other data will be routed anywhere the cardiologist cares to practice.

Advances in software will also occur, but the challenge is now different. In the last 25 years a lot of progress has been made in signal-processing techniques that remove

TABLE 1. Huffman Truth Table

Value	Binary	Huffman
0	00	0
1	01	10
2	10	110
3	11	111

artifact and accentuate the physiological signal for detection. These techniques have begun to reach their limit in pushing forward the accuracy of automated analysis. Programs must now become more "expert" and take into account the other clues that the human reader uses when analyzing the ECG. This further development of artificial intelligence will require access to appropriate data bases and statistical tools in order to insure that changes to the program are in the correct direction.

REFERENCES

1. BURCH, G. E. & N. P. DEPASQUALE. 1964. A history of electrocardiography. Year Book Medical Publishers. Chicago, Ill.
2. PIPBERGER, H. V., et al. 1975. Computer methods in electrocardiography. Annu. Rev. Biophys. Bioeng. 4: 15–42.
3. WINTER, B. B. & J. G. WEBSTER. 1982. Reduction of interference due to common mode voltage in biopotential amplifiers. IEEE Trans. Biomed. Eng. 30: 58–62.
4. Marquette Electronics Inc. 1988. Physician's Guide for Resting Analysis. Milwaukee, Wis.
5. BERSON, A. S. & H. V. PIPBERGER. 1966. The low frequency response of electrocardiographs, a frequent source of recording errors. Am. Heart J. 71: 779.
6. TAYLER, D. I. & R. VINCENT. 1985. Artefactual ST segment abnormalities due to electrocardiographic design. Br. Heart J. 54: 121–128.

7. PIPBERGER, H. V. *et al.* 1975. Recommendations for standardization of leads and of specifications for instruments in electrocardiography and vectorcardiography. Circulation **52:** 11.
8. FROELICHER, V. F. 1987. Exercise and the heart. 2nd edit. Year Book Medical Publishers. Chicago, Ill.
9. MEYER, C. R. & H. N. KEISER. 1977. Electrocardiogram baseline noise estimation and removal using cubic spline and state space computation techniques. Biomed Res. **10:** 83–92.
10. MERTENS, J. & D. MORTARA. 1984. A new algorithm for QRS averaging. *In* Computers in Cardiology: 367–369. IEEE Computer Society. Los Angeles, Calif.
11. SIMOONS, M. L. & P. G. HUGENHOLTZ. 1981. Quantitation of exercise electrocardiography. Circulation **63:** 471–475.
12. HUFFMAN, D. A. 1952. A method for the construction of minimum redundancy codes. Proc. Inst. Radio Eng.: 1098–1101.

Computer-Assisted Analysis of Holter Recordings

PAUL KLIGFIELD, KENNETH M. STEIN, AND
EDMUND M. HERROLD

Division of Cardiology
Department of Medicine
Cornell Medical Center
525 East 68th Street
New York, New York 10021

INTRODUCTION

Early work in radiotelemetry and signal processing by Holter[1] made it possible to detect changes in heart rate and cardiac rhythm in ambulatory subjects. Heart rhythm was identified by cycle-length-dependent superimposition of electrocardiographic complexes, with a 60-fold ratio of playback to recording speed to allow data analysis in compressed time. By 1964, Gilson *et al.* were able to report that simple arrhythmias, brief changes in electrocardiographic morphology, and a wide range of artifacts could be detected by these methods in apparently normal subjects.[2] Useful association of transient arrhythmias with symptoms was observed by Corday *et al.* in patients studied with 10-hour continuous recordings,[3] and limitations and advantages of early ambulatory recording methods were reviewed by Hinkle *et al.* in 1967.[4]

Advancing technology soon made it practical to acquire longer samples of analog electrocardiographic data on a lightweight, portable, battery-powered recorder, using reel-to-reel tape as the storage medium. The advantage of extending continuous electrocardiographic monitoring to 24 hours to fully characterize highly sporadic and variable ambulatory rhythms was demonstrated by Lopes *et al.*[5] While more prolonged recording periods may further increase the detection of sporadic arrhythmias,[6] which may demonstrate striking spontaneous and activity-related variability,[7,8] 24-hour continuous recordings have evolved as the most widely used compromise between technology and convenience in ambulatory populations.

CLINICAL EVOLUTION OF AMBULATORY MONITORING

Computer analysis of ambulatory recordings requires acquisition, processing, storage, retrieval, and interpretation of data. Most current ambulatory electrocardiographic recording and analysis systems are later-generation computer-assisted descendants of the original Holter method,[1,2] which focus on the quantitative analysis of recorded analog data during playback. These use simultaneous visual complex superimposition, visual cycle-length display, audio transformation of cycle length, and computer sorting and storage of interval and configuration data to identify arrhythmias and changes in morphology.[9] As "full disclosure" systems, these allow all electrocardiographic data to be printed on paper for visual inspection, validation, and interpretation as needed.

Advances in computer-based signal analysis have led to increasing use of "real-

353

time" devices[10] that generate summaries of heart rate, rhythm, and repolarization variability with time, but generally without "full disclosure." Compression of data by devices that continuously analyze rhythm and configuration, but only store detected abnormalities, can lead to false-negative conclusions even when a selection of sampled rhythm strips can be retrieved for review. On the other hand, solid state recorders, made possible by advances in computer-based memory technology, offer advantages of real-time analysis combined with full disclosure capability for review and reanalysis of the acquired data.

Current clinical applications of ambulatory electrocardiographic monitoring are summarized in TABLE 1. During the past 25 years, ambulatory monitoring has evolved from a tool used *to correlate* arryhthmias with symptoms in individuals, to a method that can be applied *to profile* patient populations with disease and *to predict* risk within these populations.[11] Newer, computer-intensive applications of ambulatory recording should expand its future role as a method *to derive pathophysiologic insight* into disease mechanism.

The recent derivation of heart rate variability indices that can be related to autonomic tone[12-15] has led to potentially useful applications of ambulatory monitoring to the study of neurophysiologic influences in health and disease.[16-22] New algorithms for the analysis and interpretation of arrhythmias as random or clustered events, based on fractal geometry and chaos theory,[23-28] may provide additional insight into mechanisms surrounding sudden death in various forms of heart disease. Recently developed

TABLE 1. Evolution of Clinical Applications of Ambulatory Electrocardiography

To correlate symptoms with transient electrocardiographic findings
To profile normal and diseased populations
To predict cardiovascular risk
To probe for pathophysiologic insights into the mechanism of disease

methods for heart rate correction of exercise-related ST segment depression[29-32] may find application in the assessment of dynamic changes in coronary tone in patients with ischemic heart disease, and expanded multilead capability of recording devices also should lead to improved detection and localization of ischemia.[33] Advances in signal processing may also allow derivation of late potentials and other information in the high resolution electrocardiogram from ambulatory recordings.[34]

EVALUATION OF THE RELATIONSHIP OF SYMPTOMS TO ARRHYTHMIAS

Since dizziness, syncope, palpitation, and chest pain are commonly sporadic in occurrence and brief in duration, ambulatory electrocardiography has long been used to evaluate the association of symptoms with transient disorders of rhythm and repolarization. However, data bearing on the causal relationship of arrhythmias to symptoms, and to transient alterations of consciousness most specifically, have been conflicting. Several studies have suggested good correlation between arrhythmias and sporadic alteration of consciousness,[35,36] but a causal relationship between other presenting complaints and asymptomatic arrhythmias detected by ambulatory monitoring can be difficult to establish with certainty.[37,38] The often striking discrepancy between patient symptoms and arrhythmias detected by ambulatory electrocardiography was well illustrated by Zeldis *et al.*[39]

The value of ST segment depression recorded during ambulatory monitoring as a marker for coronary artery disease has been controversial,[40] but several principles have emerged. Despite the high specificity of prolonged horizontal and downsloping ST segment depression found by Deanfield *et al.*,[41] most studies of ambulatory repolarization findings have focused on patient populations with a high prevalence of known and generally highly symptomatic ischemic disease.[42-44] Detection of asymptomatic episodes of "silent ischemia" in these groups has provided important pathophysiologic insights into the relationship of myocardial blood supply and demand factors in coronary disease. These observations have highlighted the common role of neurohumoral influences on coronary artery tone and blood flow, rather than augmentation of demand, in the provocation of myocardial ischemia in some patients, but the highly symptomatic status of these patients requires emphasis.

PROFILING OF CARDIAC RHYTHM IN NORMAL AND DISEASED POPULATIONS

Ambulatory electrocardiography has been widely used to study the prevalence of disorders of impulse formation and impulse conduction in specific populations. Of course, the interpretation of arrhythmias in individuals and in groups of patients with specific types of heart disease depends on an understanding of the prevalence of rhythm findings in clinically normal populations.[11]

Data bearing on cardiac rhythm in apparently normal populations are available for newborn infants,[45] healthy children,[46] male medical students,[47] young women,[48] working adults,[49-51] and active elderly people.[52-54] Several important trends and observations emerge from these studies. Most obvious is the extraordinarily high prevalence of potentially significant arrhythmias present in ambulatory subjects of all ages. Also apparent is a shift in the type of prevalent arrhythmia that accompanies aging. A high prevalence of episodic sinus pauses is common in normal children but uncommon in normal adults. Atrial and ventricular arrhythmias are quite unusual in children, but common in young adults and rather expected in the elderly, in whom complex ventricular forms such as ventricular couplets and brief bursts of nonsustained ventricular tachycardia may occur in the absence of disease.

Ambulatory electrocardiography can profile the arrhythmias found in populations with recognized cardiac abnormalities, and mitral valve prolapse serves as a useful model of the value and limitations of this process.[55] During prolonged recording, which has varied in duration among studies, atrial premature complexes have been recorded in 35%–90%, atrial tachycardia in 3%–32%, and ventricular premature complexes in 58%–89% of prolapse populations.[56] Complex ventricular arrhythmias have been reported in 43%–56% of adult patients. However, patient selection has varied widely for these study populations, and this can introduce significant bias in the interpretation of data when highly symptomatic patients are concentrated in a study group.[57] When ambulatory populations of adult patients with mitral prolapse are compared with comparably aged symptomatic, or comparably aged asymptomatic, control subjects, it is difficult to demonstrate a higher prevalence of complex arrhythmias other than paroxysmal atrial tachycardia in patients with mitral prolapse who do not have mitral regurgitation.[50,58]

In contrast, mitral prolapse patients with important mitral regurgitation are more likely to have frequent and complex atrial and ventricular arrhythmias than patients without regurgitation, and similar prevalences of complex arrhythmias have been demonstrated in patients with comparable mitral regurgitation, whether or not the regurgitation is related to underlying mitral prolapse.[55,59] Therefore, these arrhythmias appear to be more strongly related to the physiologic effects of mitral regurgitation than to direct structural or functional consequences of mitral prolapse itself.

PROGNOSTIC VALUE OF VENTRICULAR ARRHYTHMIAS IN PATIENTS WITH HEART DISEASE

Ambulatory electrocardiography has been widely applied to evaluation of the prognostic value of ventricular arrhythmias, most commonly in populations with ischemic heart disease.[11] Observations in these populations support the early findings of the Lahey Clinic study that excess mortality among cardiac patients with ventricular arrhythmias is largely found in the postinfarction subset.[60]

The independent risk conferred by variably complex ventricular ectopy above and beyond the effect of ventricular dysfunction after myocardial infarction has been controversial.[11,61–66] All sudden death reported in the early experience of Schulze et al.[61] occurred in the subset of patients who had both complex ventricular arrhythmias on 24-hour ambulatory electrocardiography and poor left ventricular function by radionuclide evaluation of ejection fraction. While multivariate analysis by Ruberman et al. has suggested that the presence of complex arrhythmias is the strongest independent risk factor for sudden death after infarction,[63] other studies have questioned the independent predictive value of arrhythmias alone.[64–66] Sudden death occurring during ambulatory electrocardiography has been reported by several groups,[67,68] with potentially fatal arrhythmias often, but not invariably, associated with complex or early-cycle ventricular ectopy in patients with ischemic or myopathic hearts.[68,69]

Sudden death can also be related to complex ventricular arrhythmias detected by ambulatory monitoring in some populations with valvular heart disease.[11,70,71] In contrast to the low mortality in patients with uncomplicated mitral valve prolapse, sudden death appears to be strongly concentrated in prolapse patients who have developed hemodynamically important mitral regurgitation,[55,70] and complex ventricular arrhythmias are common in this group.[59] With mitral regurgitation of varied etiology as a model, sudden death can be shown to be highly concentrated in patients who have developed systolic ventricular dysfunction,[70] and repetitive forms of ventricular arrhythmias can be found prior to death in this subgroup.[71] At the same time, similarly complex arrhythmias are not strongly predictive of sudden death in patients with mitral regurgitation when ventricular function remains normal.

Data supporting a primary predictive role for repetitive ventricular arrhythmias in sudden death, independent of significantly depressed ventricular function alone, can be found in the dilated cardiomyopathy population.[72] In these patients, mortality appears to be significantly increased when either ventricular couplets or nonsustained ventricular tachycardia is detected by ambulatory monitoring than when complex arrhythmias are absent in patients with similar ventricular dysfunction.

Taken together, these data are consistent with an interaction of ventricular dysfunction and repetitive ventricular arrhythmias in the precipitation of sudden death in some forms of heart disease. This has been characterized by Keefe et al. as the interaction of "substrate" and "trigger,"[73] but their prognostic value in general populations has been limited by poor specificity and by poor predictive value when event rates are low. Fatal arrhythmias might also result from a temporally unique cluster of pathophysiologic conditions that might or might not be detectable by ambulatory monitoring. As has been suggested by Coumel et al.,[74] additional insight into both the mechanism and the prediction of fatal arrhythmogenesis may be available from consideration of potential "third factors" that can be related to neurohumoral interactions with the heart.[75] Evaluation of these factors, which influence heart rate variability and arrhythmia clustering among many others, has been facilitated by advances in computer-based analysis of ambulatory electrocardiographic recordings.

HEART RATE VARIABILITY

Heart rate varies in response to complex interactions of the sympathetic and parasympathetic branches of the nervous system,[75] and ambulatory electrocardiography can provide a set of data for studying these interactions by analysis of beat-to-beat variation of cycle length. Precision of measurement within ambulatory recording and playback equipment can markedly affect the accuracy of such time-dependent data. Several computer-based methods of data analysis have been used to assess heart rate variability.

One approach to the evaluation of heart rate variability involves the use of power spectrum analysis, which represents a complex dynamic function as a unique sum of a series of sine waves of varying amplitude and frequency, with each frequency having a corresponding amplitude.[76] Heart rate variability examined in this way has been found to be a marker for heart transplant rejection[17,18] and has been examined following myocardial infarction and in patients with dilated cardiomypathy.[19,20]

Another approach to the evaluation of heart rate variability is to calculate the standard deviation, or a related measure, of observed cycle lengths during prolonged recording or during discrete time intervals.[21,22,77] Decreased variability measured in this way has been found to predict mortality in patients with ischemic disease.[21,22] While cycle-length variability appears to be greater during periods of increased parasympathetic tone,[78,79,81] heart rate itself can be related to the magnitude of sympathetic and parasympathetic activity,[79,80] and the interdependence of rate and variability requires further exploration. Accordingly, more detailed insights into the physiologic correlates of heart rate variability might emerge from computer-assisted analyses of ambulatory data that look beyond the standard deviation of cycle length alone.

Mitral valve prolapse has been associated with variable autonomic changes,[81–84] and both greater mean daily cycle length[58] and absence of an age-related decrease in simple estimates of heart rate variability[81,83] have been reported in these patients. We examined relationships among cycle length, standard deviation of overall cycle length, and beat-to-beat variation of cycle length derived from ambulatory recordings of 15 normal subjects and 8 patients with mitral valve prolapse without hemodynamically important mitral regurgitation.

In this small population, a trend toward higher mean daily standard deviation of cycle length (SD of RR) was apparent when patients with prolapse were compared with normal subjects (141 vs. 114 mseconds, $p = 0.06$). SD of RR in our normal subjects was inversely related to age (FIGURE 1), as has been reported previously,[12,15,22] but this relationship was not present in the prolapse patients, a finding consistent with observations on respiratory effects on cycle-length variation by Weissman *et al.*[83] In addition, patients with prolapse also had longer mean cycle lengths, or slower average daily heart rates, than did the normal subjects (745 vs. 680 mseconds, $p = 0.06$).

However, when SD of RR was compared with mean daily cycle length in these groups, it was apparent that SD of RR was positively correlated with mean RR itself

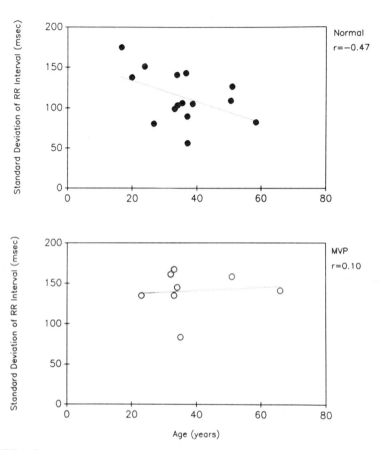

FIGURE 1. Standard deviation of daily cycle lengths (SD of RR) in relation to age in 15 normal subjects (top panel) and in 8 patients with uncomplicated mitral valve prolapse (MVP, bottom panel).

(FIGURE 2), as also noted by Kleiger *et al.* in patients after myocardial infarction.[22] It is therefore unclear whether the higher SD of RR in the prolapse patients is a function of greater intrinsic variability, or merely the consequence of slower heart rate. Derivation of a coefficient of variability for cycle length by dividing SD of RR by mean RR in each subject eliminated group differences between normal subjects and prolapse patients (FIGURE 3, 17% vs. 15% respectively), and this coefficient effectively normalized SD of RR for cycle length in the combined population. At the same time, the age-related changes remained different in prolapse patients and normal subjects (FIGURE 4). These findings suggest that after adjustment for underlying cycle length, heart rate variability in groups of patients with mitral valve prolapse is similar to that in normal subjects. Even so, the change in heart rate variability with respect to age may differ between these groups.

The relationship between heart rate variability and heart rate itself was explored further in this population by examining the magnitude and variance of beat-to-beat changes in cycle length throughout the period of ambulatory recording as a function of absolute RR intervals themselves. Because heart rate variability might have different characteristics with respect to decreasing and increasing RR intervals, negative and positive changes in serially paired RR intervals were evaluated separately. Each measured change in the RR interval between current and preceding cycle length (the delta RR interval) was stored as data relating to the current RR interval, as either a positive or negative value. Estimated accuracy of time measurement was ±5–10 mseconds, and the range of cycle lengths observed during ambulatory activity were grouped in 20 msecond increments. In order to confer a degree of statistical stability to the pattern of changing RR intervals, only cycle-length interval ranges that had at least 100 occurrences during the 24-hour period were included.

In effect, this algorithm allows all increasing and decreasing cycle-length increments between successive electrocardiographic complexes to be stored in relation to a continuum of small ranges of cycle-length intervals that occur throughout a prolonged period of recording. Within any specified range of underlying cycle lengths, all positive and negative increments from the previous cycle (the delta RR interval) can be examined. These increments can be represented as the mean positive and negative values occurring at any cycle length (the mean delta RR), and an estimate of the variability of these increments, at any cycle length, can be represented as the standard deviation of the delta RR (SD of delta RR).

Findings in a normal subject are shown in FIGURE 5. For each panel, the horizontal axis represents the measured cycle lengths found during approximately 20 hours of ambulatory monitoring, according to increasing RR intervals in 20 msecond groups. In FIGURE 5a, the number of intervals within each cycle-length group is shown as a histogram. In FIGURE 5b, the mean positive delta RR associated with each cycle-length group interval is plotted above, and the mean negative delta RR is plotted below, the horizontal axis. FIGURE 5c shows the SD of delta RR for both positive and negative delta RR values along the same cycle-length axis.

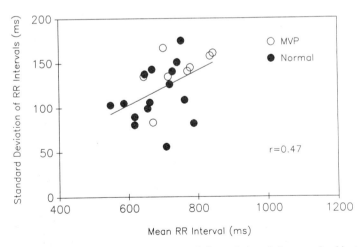

FIGURE 2. Relationship of SD of RR to mean daily cycle length in normal subjects and in patients with MVP.

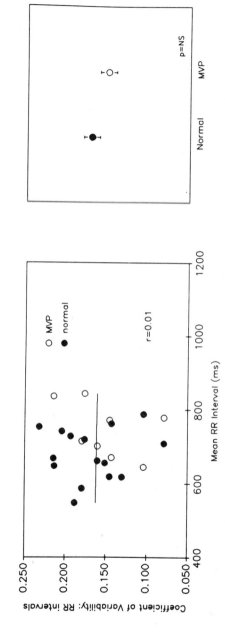

FIGURE 3. Derivation of a coefficient of variability (SD of **RR**/mean **RR**), which is not related to mean cycle length (left panel) and is similar in normal subjects and patients with MVP (right panel).

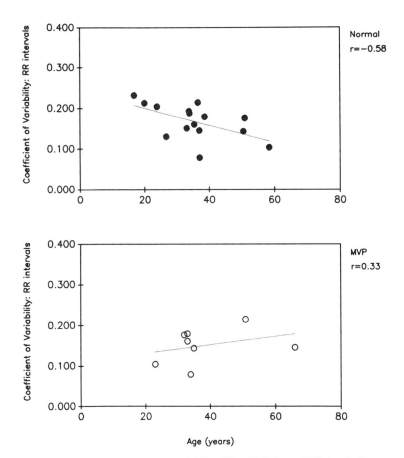

FIGURE 4. Coefficient of cycle length variability (SD of RR/mean RR) in relation to age in normal subjects (top panel) and in patients with MVP (bottom panel).

Examination of these data reveals several interesting findings. Most striking is the extremely strong dependence of both the delta RR interval and the SD of the delta RR on underlying cycle length. Both estimates of beat-to-beat variability are greatest at longer RR intervals, the region of presumed strongest parasympathetic activity, and least at the faster rates that might coincide with periods of sympathetic tone. Indeed, the data appear to be composed of two linear components, separated at approximately 900–1000 msecond cycle lengths. Most of the corresponding patterns in our subjects were similar in form, and these observations raise the intriguing possibility that separate quantification of these components might provide insight into autonomic tone. This, of course, requires specific testing.

Several approaches to analysis of these data are being explored for derivation of descriptive variables that are independent of heart rate itself. The slopes of the mean delta RR and the SD of delta RR relationship to cycle length, derived separately over their linear portions at both shorter and longer RR intervals, appear logical and promising as markers of neurohumoral tone. Alternatively, the apparent exponential

Frequency

Mean Delta R-R

SD of Delta R-R

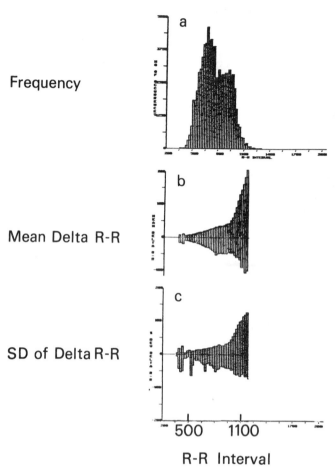

500   1100

R-R Interval

FIGURE 5. Heart rate variability from beat-to-beat evaluation of a normal subject, with cycle-length histogram for 20 msecond increments of RR interval in the top panel (a). Mean positive and negative delta RR intervals from the immediately preceding cycle during 24 hours of recording are shown in relation to resulting cycle length in the middle panel (b). The corresponding standard deviations of mean delta RR intervals are shown in the bottom panel (c).

envelope of the data suggests that a single slope of logarithmically transformed values over the entire range of observed cycle lengths can be derived. Finally, it is possible that one of the cycle-length-dependent variables taken at a fixed RR interval might provide rate-independent information of physiologic value.

FRACTAL DISTRIBUTION OF VENTRICULAR PREMATURE COMPLEXES

Fractals are a class of irregularly irregular geometric objects, first described by Mandelbrot[23,24] and recently reviewed by Peitgen and Saupe.[25] The timing of ventricular premature complexes can be shown to be represented by a particular kind of fractal—the fractal dust. This makes it possible to measure a quantity that describes the tendency of ventricular ectopy to be clustered, which may provide insight into the correlates and prognostic value of arrhythmias.

If an object can be subdivided into n similar constituent parts, each part represents $(1/r)$ of the whole. Where n is related to r by the equation:

$$n = (1/r)^D \qquad (1)$$

then the object's similarity dimension (also known as fractal dimension) is defined by Mandelbrot as:

$$D = \log(n)/\log(1/r) \qquad (2)$$

A cube of edge length x, for example, can be divided into 8 cubes of edge length

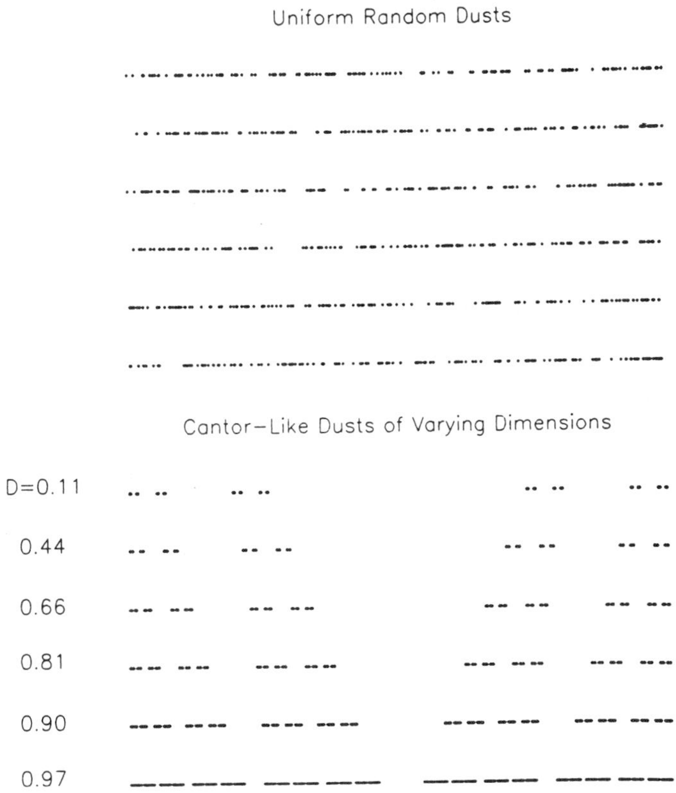

FIGURE 6. Examples of random data generated by computer and clustered data derived from "Cantor dusts." The fractal dimension (D) is close to 1.0 for the uniform distribution of the random data, but decreases with the extent of clustering.

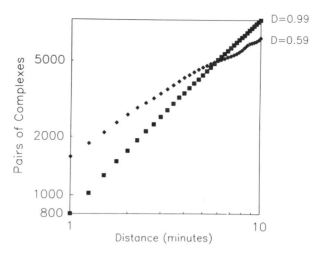

FIGURE 7. Correlation functions relating the log of the number of ventricular premature complexes that can be paired within increasing time scales (vertical axis) to the log of the time scale (horizontal axis) in two patients with dilated cardiomyopathy. The slope of each regression line is the correlation dimension (D) for the patient.

$x/2$, 27 cubes of edge length $x/3$, 64 cubes of edge length $x/4$, and so on, and therefore the dimension of a cube is three. The similarity dimension of any standard Euclidean shape is equal to the shape's topologic dimension, so that a point has a dimension of zero, a line one, a circle two, and a sphere three. However, there are many shapes that have a similarity dimension greater than their topologic dimension, and Mandelbrot names all such shapes "fractals."

One class of objects of particular interest is the set of shapes composed entirely of unconnected points. Such an object is termed a "dust" and if the points are defined by a single coordinate (perhaps a temporal coordinate or a spatial coordinate), it can be called a linear dust. Any such dust, being composed of single points, has a topologic dimension of zero. Therefore, any dust with similarity dimension greater than zero must be a fractal dust.

The "correlation function" is a means of estimating the similarity dimension of a dust from experimentally acquired data. This technique was initially proposed by Procaccia and Grassberger in 1983.[26,27] A review of some of the properties of this function is provided in Schaffer et al.[28] For data that can be represented on a linear scale, the function is created as follows: (1) take an object that is described by a defined number of points; (2) identify all of the possible pairs of these points; (3) make a list of these pairs and for each note the distance separating the two points that make up the pair; (4) take a given distance and count the number of pairs separated by this distance or less; (5) repeat this for different distances to result in a function that relates the number of pairs of points separated by less than any given distance to that distance.

For a wide variety of naturally occurring shapes the correlation function, if plotted on log-log axes, results in a straight line. The "correlation dimension" is defined as the slope of this line, and gives a lower limit for the similarity dimension of the object. In practice this is determined by a least-squares regression of $\log(n)$ against $\log(\text{distance})$ over a range of distances that are relevant to the data. This range of distances can be considered the time scale for the dimension. For our purposes we will use the terms "correlation dimension," "dimension," and "D" interchangeably.

In the case of a linear fractal dust, the correlation dimension is a measure of the clustering of the points that make up the dust. If a set of points is densely clustered in space then, beyond a critical distance, the number of pairs of points counted will no longer increase and for these time scales the slope of the correlation curve (and hence the dimension) will be zero. On the other hand, for a uniformly random set of points the number of pairs continues to increase with increasing distance and, in the limiting case, the slope approaches 1.0. Representative linear arrays of random data point distribution are contrasted with mathematically clustered data that have been adapted from "Cantor dusts"[24] in FIGURE 6.

Fractal geometry can be applied to the study of ventricular premature complexes, where ectopic beats can be considered as points lying along a time line. A correlation function can be constructed by counting the number of pairs of ventricular premature complexes that occur within a given number of minutes (or hours or seconds) of one another. We have done this for 18 patients with dilated cardiomyopathy, looking at the correlation function in the range of one to 10 minutes. Two representative correlation functions are shown in FIGURE 7. Calculated D values in this population ranged from 0.59 to 0.99, with a median value of 0.92. Repetitive ventricular arrhythmias occurred during the period of analysis in nearly all of these patients, and D values indicative of clustering are not explained by episodes of ventricular tachycardia limited to some patients of this group.

Preliminary survival data are available for this patient population, separated according to uniform and clustered ranges of D (FIGURE 8). These retrospective findings suggest that there is a strong association between clustering of ventricular ectopy, independent of the frequency and traditionally defined complexity of these arrhythmias, and mortality in patients with dilated cardiomyopathy ($p < 0.005$). Thus, ventricular premature complexes may be clustered in time, and the degree of this clustering can be quantitated using mathematical methods derived from fractal geometry.

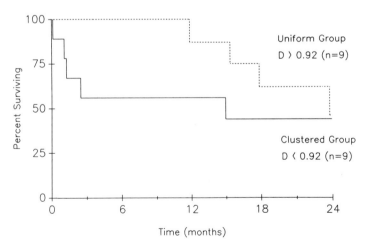

FIGURE 8. Survival in 18 patients with dilated cardiomyopathy separated into uniform and clustered arrhythmia groups defined by a median correlation dimension (D) value of 0.92.

REFERENCES

1. HOLTER, N. J. 1961. New method for heart studies. Science **134:** 1214–1220.
2. GILSON, J. S., N. J. HOLTER & W. R. GLASSCOCK. 1964. Clinical observations using the electrocardiocorder-AVSEP continuous electrocardiographic system: tentative standards and typical patterns. Am. J. Cardiol. **14:** 204–217.
3. CORDAY, E., V. BAZIKA, T-W. LANG, S. PAPPELBAUM, H. GOLD & H. BERNSTEIN. 1965. Detection of phantom arrhythmias and evanescent electrocardiographic abnormalities. J. Am. Med. Assoc. **193:** 417–421.
4. HINKLE, L. E., J. MEYER, M. STEVENS & S. T. CARVER. 1967. Tape recordings of the ECG of active men: limitations and advantages of the Holter-Avionics instruments. Circulation **36:** 752–765.
5. LOPES, M. G., P. RUNGE, D. C. HARRISON & J. S. SCHROEDER. 1975. Comparison of 24 versus 12 hours of ambulatory ECG monitoring. Chest **67:** 269–273.
6. KENNEDY, H. L., V. CHANDRA, K. L. SAYTHER & D. G. CARASIS. 1978. Effectiveness of increasing hours of continuous ambulatory electrocardiography in detecting maximal ventricular ectopy: continuous 48 hour study of patients with coronary heart disease and normal subjects. Am. J. Cardiol. **42:** 925–930.
7. WINKLE, R. A. 1978. Antiarrhythmic drug effect mimicked by spontaneous variability of ventricular ectopy. Circulation **57:** 1116–1121.
8. MORGANROTH, J., E. L. MICHELSON, L. N. HOROWITZ, M. E. JOSEPHSON, A. S. PEARLMAN & W. B. DUNKMAN. 1978. Limitations of routine long-term electrocardiographic monitoring to assess ventricular ectopic frequency. Circulation **58:** 408–414.
9. KENNEDY, H. L. 1981. Ambulatory Electrocardiography, Including Holter Recording Technology. Lea & Febiger. Philadelphia, Pa.
10. MARK, R. G. & K. L. RIPLEY. 1985. Ambulatory ECG monitoring: real-time analysis versus tape scanning systems. MD Comput. **2:** 38–50.
11. KLIGFIELD, P. 1984. Clinical applications of ambulatory electrocardiography. Cardiology **71:** 69–99.
12. O'BRIEN, I. A. D., P. O'HARE & R. J. M. CORRALL. 1986. Heart rate variability in healthy subjects: effect of age and the derivation of normal ranges for tests of autonomic function. Br. Heart J. **55:** 348–354.
13. BERGER, R. D., S. AKSELROD, D. GORDON, & R. J. COHEN. 1986. An efficient algorithm for spectral analysis of heart rate variability. IEEE Trans. Biomed. Eng. BME-**33:** 900–904.
14. COKER, R., A. KOZIELL, C. OLIVER & S. E. SMITH. 1984. Does the sympathetic nervous system influence sinus arrhythmia in man? Evidence from combined autonomic blockade. J. Physiol. **356:** 459–464.
15. WADDINGTON, J. L., M. J. MACCULLOCH & J. E. SAMBROOKS. 1979. Resting heart rate variability in man declines with age. Experientia **35:** 1197–1198.
16. SMITH, S. E. & S. A. SMITH. 1981. Heart rate variability in healthy subjects measured with a bedside computer-based technique. Clin. Sci. **61:** 379–383.
17. SANDS, K. E. F., M. L. APPEL, L. S. LILLY, F. J. SCHOEN, G. H. MUDGE & R. J. COHEN. 1989. Studies after cardiac transplantation: power spectrum analysis of heart rate variability in human cardiac transplant recipients. Circulation **79:** 76–82.
18. ALEXOPOULOS, D., S. YUSUF, J. A. JOHNSTON, J. BOSTOCK, P. SLEIGHT & M. H. YACOUB. 1988. The 24-hour heart rate behavior in long-term survivors of cardiac transplantation. Am. J. Cardiol. **61:** 880–884.
19. LOMBARDI, F., G. SANDRONE, S. PERNPRUNER, R. SALA, M. GARIMOLDI, S. CERUTTI, G. BASELLI, M. PAGANI & A. MALLIANI. 1987. Heart rate variability as an index of sympathovagal interaction after acute myocarcial infarction. Am. J. Cardiol. **60:** 1239–1245.
20. SAUL, J. P., Y. ARAI, R. D. BERGER, L. S. LILLY, W. S. COLUCCI & R. J. COHEN. 1988. Assessment of autonomic regulation in chronic congestive heart failure by heart rate spectral analysis. Am. J. Cardiol. **61:** 1292–1299.
21. MARTIN, G. J., N. M. MAGID, G. MYERS, P. S. BARNETT, J. W. SCHAAD, J. S. WEISS, M. LESCH & D. H. SINGER. 1987. Heart rate variability and sudden death secondary to

coronary artery disease during ambulatory electrocardiographic monitoring. Am. J. Cardiol. **60**: 86–89.

22. KLIEGER, R. E., J. P. MILLER, J. T. BIGGER, A. J. MOSS & the Multicenter Post-Infarct Research Group. 1987. Decreased heart rate variability and its association with increased mortality after acute myocardial infarction. Am. J. Cardiol. **59**: 256–263.

23. MANDELBROT, B. B. 1977. Fractals: Form, Chance, and Dimension. Freeman. New York, N.Y.

24. MANDELBROT, B. B. 1982. The Fractal Geometry of Nature. Freeman. New York, N.Y.

25. PEITGEN, H. O. & D. SAUPE, Eds. 1988. The Science of Fractal Images. Springer-Verlag. New York, N.Y.

26. GRASSBERGER, P. & I. PROCACCIA. 1983. Characterization of strange attractors. Phys. Rev. Lett. **50**: 346–349.

27. GRASSBERGER, P. & I. PROCACCIA. 1983. Measuring the strangeness of strange attractors. Physica **9D**: 189–208.

28. SCHAFFER, W. M., S. ELLNER & M. KOT. 1986. Effects of noise on some dynamical models in ecology. J. Math. Biol. **24**: 479–523.

29. ELAMIN, M. S., R. BOYLE, M. M. KARDASH, D. R. SMITH, J. B. STOKER, W. WHITAKER, D. A. S. G. MARY & R. J. LINDEN. 1982. Accurate detection of coronary heart disease by new exercise test. Br. Heart J. **48**: 311–320.

30. DETRANO, R., E. SALCEDO, M. PASSALAQUA & R. FRIIS. 1986. Exercise electrocardiographic variables: a critical appraisal. J. Am. Coll. Cardiol. **8**: 836–847.

31. OKIN, P. M., P. KLIGFIELD, O. AMEISEN, H. GOLDBERG & J. S. BORER. 1988. Identification of anatomically extensive coronary artery disease by the exercise electrocardiographic ST segment/heart rate slope. Am. Heart J. **115**: 1002–1013.

32. KLIGFIELD, P., O. AMEISEN & P. M. OKIN. 1989. Heart rate adjustment of ST segment depression for improved detection of coronary artery disease. Circulation **79**: 245–255.

33. KRUCOFF, M. 1988. Poor performance of lead V5 in single- and dual-channel ST-segment monitoring during coronary occlusion. J. Electrocardiol. **21**: S30–S34.

34. LANDER, P., J. S. STEINBERG, J. T. BIGGER, JR. & E. J. BERBARI. 1989. Signal averaging of ventricular late potentials using Holter recordings. *In* IEEE Computers in Cardiology: 377–380. IEEE Computer Society Press. Washington, D.C.

35. LIPSKI, J., L. COHEN, J. ESPINOZA, M. MOTRO, S. DACK & E. DONOSO. 1976. Value of Holter monitoring in assessing cardiac arrhythmias in symptomatic patients. Am. J. Cardiol. **37**: 102–107.

36. BOUDOULAS, H., S. F. SCHAAL, R. P. LEWIS & J. L. ROBINSON. 1979. Superiority of 24-hour outpatient monitoring over multi-stage exercise testing for the evaluation of syncope. J. Electrocardiol. **12**: 103–108.

37. VAN DURME J. P. 1975. Tachyarrhythmias and transient cerebral ischemic attacks. Annotations **89**: 538–540.

38. CLARK, P. I., S. P. GLASSER & E. SPOTO. 1980. Arrhythmias detected by ambulatory monitoring: lack of correlation with symptoms of dizziness and syncope. Chest **77**: 722–725.

39. ZELDIS, S. M., B. J. LEVINE, E. L. MICHELSON & J. MORGANROTH. 1980. Cardiovascular complaints: correlation with cardiac arrhythmias on 24-hour electrocardiographic monitoring. Chest **78**: 456–462.

40. KENNEDY, H. L. & R. D. WIENS. 1989. Ambulatory (Holter) electrocardiography and myocardial ischemia. Am. Heart J. **117**: 164–174.

41. DEANFIELD J. E., P. RIBIERO, K. OAKLEY, S. KRIKLER & A. P. SELWYN. 1984. Analysis of ST-segment changes in normal subjects: implications for ambulatory monitoring in angina pectoris. Am. J. Cardiol. **54**: 1321–1325.

42. CECCHI, A. C., E. V. DOVELLINI, F. MARCHI, P. PUCCI, G. M. SANTORO & P. F. FAZZINI. 1983. Silent myocardial ischemia during ambulatory electrocardiographic monitoring in patients with effort angina. J. Am. Coll. Cardiol. **1**: 934–939.

43. BIAGINI, A., M. G. MAZZEI, C. CARPEGGIANI, R. TESTA, R. ANTONELLI, C. MICHELASSI, A. L'ABBATE & A. MASERI. 1982. Vasospastic ischemic mechanism of frequent asymptomatic transient ST-T changes during continuous electrocardiographic monitoring in selected unstable angina patients. Am. Heart J. **103**: 13–20.

44. GOTTLIEB, S. O., M. L. WEISFELDT, P. OUYANG, E. D. MELLITS & G. GERSTENBLITH. 1986. Silent ischemia as a marker for early unfavorable outcomes in patients with unstable angina. N. Engl. J. Med. **314:** 1214–1219.
45. SOUTHALL, D. P., J. RICHARDS, P. MITCHELL, D. J. BROWN, P. G. B. HOHNSTON & E. A. SHINEBOURNE. 1980. Study of cardiac rhythm in healthy newborn infants. Br. Heart J. **43:** 14–20.
46. SOUTHALL, D. P., F. JOHNSTON, E. A. SHINEBOURNE & P. G. B. JOHNSTON. 1981. 24-hour electrocardiographic study of heart rate and rhythm patterns in population of healthy children. Br. Heart J. **45:** 281–291.
47. BRODSKY, M., D. WU, P. DENES, C. KANAKIS & K. M. ROSEN. 1977. Arrhythmias documented by 24 hour continuous electrocardiographic monitoring in 50 male medical students without apparent heart disease. Am. J. Cardiol. **39:** 390–395.
48. SOBOTKA, P. A., J. H. MAYER, R. A. BAUERNFEIND, C. KANAKIS & K. M. ROSEN. 1981. Arrhythmias documented by 24-hour continuous ambulatory electrocardiographic monitoring in young women without apparent heart disease. Am. Heart J. **101:** 753–758.
49. HINKLE, L. E., S. T. CARVER & M. STEVENS. 1969. The frequency of asymptomatic disturbances of cardiac rhythm and conduction in middle-aged men. Am. J. Cardiol. **24:** 629–650.
50. SAVAGE, D. D., D. L. LEVY, R. J. GARRISON, W. P. CASTELLI, P. KLIGFIELD, R. B. DEVEREUX, S. J. ANDERSON, W. B. KANNEL & M. FEINLEIB. 1983. Mitral valve prolapse in the general population, part 3: dysrhythmias. The Framingham Study. Am. Heart J. **106:** 582–586.
51. CLARKE, J. M., J. R. SHELTON, J. HAMER, S. TAYLER & G. R. VENNING. 1976. The rhythm of the normal human heart. Lancet: 508–512.
52. GLASSER, S. P., P. I. CLARK & H. J. APPLEBAUM. 1979. Occurrence of frequent complex arrhythmias detected by ambulatory monitoring: findings in an apparently healthy asymptomatic elderly population. Chest **75:** 565–568.
53. CAMM, A. J., K. E. EVANS, E. D. WARD & A. MARTIN. 1980. The rhythm of the heart in active elderly subjects. Am. Heart J. **99:** 598–603.
54. KANTELIP, J-P., E. SAGE & P. DUCHENE-MARULLAZ. 1986. Findings on ambulatory electrocardiographic monitoring in subjects older than 80 years. Am. J. Cardiol. **57:** 398–401.
55. KLIGFIELD, P., D. LEVY, R. B. DEVEREUX & D. D. SAVAGE. 1987. Arrhythmias and sudden death in mitral valve prolapse. Am. Heart J. **113:** 1298–1307.
56. KLIGFIELD, P. & R. B. DEVEREUX. 1985. Arrhythmias in mitral valve prolapse. Clin. Prog. Electrophysiol. Pacing **3:** 403–418.
57. MOTULSKY, A. G. 1978. Biased ascertainment and the natural history of diseases. N. Engl. J. Med. **298:** 1196–1197.
58. KRAMER, H. M., P. KLIGFIELD, R. B. DEVEREUX, D. D. SAVAGE & R. KRAMER-FOX. 1984. Arrhythmias in mitral valve prolapse: effect of selection bias. Arch. Intern. Med. **144:** 2360–2364.
59. KLIGFIELD, P., C. HOCHREITER, & H. KRAMER, et al. 1973. Complex arrhythmias in MR with and without mitral valve prolapse: contrast to arrhythmias in mitral valve prolapse without MR. Am. J. Cardiol. **55:** 1545–1549.
60. DESAI, D. C., P. L. HERSHBERG & S. ALEXANDER. 1973. Clinical significance of ventricular premature beats in an outpatient population. Chest **64:** 564–569.
61. SCHULZE, R. A., H. W. STRAUSS & B. PITT. 1977. Sudden death in the year following myocardial infarction: relation to ventricular premature contractions in the late hospital phase and left ventricular ejection fraction. Am. J. Med. **62:** 192–199.
62. BIGGER, J. T., C. A. HELLER, T. L. WENGER & F. M. WELD. 1978. Risk stratification after acute myocardial infarction. Am. J. Cardiol. **42:** 202–210.
63. RUBERMAN, W., E. WEINBLATT, J. D. GOLDBERG, C. W. FRANK, B. S. CHAUDHARY & S. SHAPIRO. 1981. Ventricular premature complexes and sudden death after myocardial infarction. Circulation **64:** 297–305.
64. BORER, J. S., D. R. ROSING, R. H. MILLER, R. M. STARK, K. M. KENT, S. L. BACHARACH, M. V. GREEN, C. R. LAKE, H. COHEN, D. HOLMES, D. DONOHUE, W. BAKER & S. E. EPSTEIN. 1980. Natural history of left ventricular function during 1 year after acute

myocardial infarction: comparison with clinical, electrocardiographic and biochemical determinations. Am. J. Cardiol. **46:** 1–12.

65. LURIA, M. H., J. D. KNOKE, J. S. WACHS & M. A. LURIA. 1979. Survival after recovery from acute myocardial infarction: two and five year prognostic indices. Am. J. Med. **67:** 7–14.

66. TAYLOR, G. J., J. O. HUMPHRIES, E. D. MELLITS, B. PITT, R. A. SCHULZE, L. S. C. GRIFFITH & S. C. ACHUFF. 1980. Predictors of clinical course, coronary anatomy and left ventricular function after recovery from acute myocardial infarction. Circulation **62:** 960–970.

67. NIKOLIC, G., R. L. BISHOP & J. B. SINGH. 1982. Sudden death recorded during Holter monitoring. Circulation **66:** 218–225.

68. BAYES DE LUNA, A., P. COUMEL, & J. F. LECLERCQ. 1989. Ambulatory sudden cardiac death: mechanisms of production of fatal arrhythmia on the basis of data from 157 cases. Am. Heart J. **117:** 151–159.

69. MEYERBURG, R. J., C. A. CONDE, R. J. SUNG, A. MAYORGA-CORTES, S. M. MALLON, D. S. SHEPS, R. A. APPEL & A. CASTELLANOS. 1980. Clinical, electrophysiologic and hemodynamic profile of patients resuscitated from prehospital cardiac arrest. Am. J. Med. **68:** 568–576.

70. HOCHREITER, C., N. NILES, R. B. DEVEREUX, P. KLIGFIELD & J. S. BORER. 1986. Mitral regurgitation: relationship of non-invasive right and left ventricular performance descriptors to clinical and hemodynamic findings and to prognosis in medically and surgically treated patients. Circulation **73:** 900–912.

71. KLIGFIELD, P., C. HOCHREITER, N. NILES, R. B. DEVEREUX & J. S. BORER. 1987. Relation of sudden death in pure mitral regurgitation, with and without mitral valve prolapse, to repetitive ventricular arrhythmias and right and left ventricular ejection fractions. Am. J. Cardiol. **60:** 397–399.

72. HOLMES, J. R., S. H. KUBO, R. J. CODY & P. KLIGFIELD. 1985. Arrhythmias in ischemic and nonischemic dilated cardiomyopathy: prediction of mortality by ambulatory electrocardiography. Am. J. Cardiol. **55:** 146–151.

73. KEEFE, D. L., J. SCHWARTZ & J. C. SOMBERG. 1987. The substrate and the trigger: the role of myocardial vulnerability in sudden cardiac death. Am. Heart J. **113:** 218–225.

74. COUMEL, P., J-F. LECLERCQ & A. LEENHARDT. 1987. Arrhythmias as predictors of sudden death. Am. Heart J. **114:** 929–937.

75. LEVY, M. N. 1971. Sympathetic-parasympathetic interactions in the heart. Circ. Res. **29:** 437–445.

76. COOLEY, J. W. & J. W. TUKEY. 1965. An algorithm for the machine calculation of complex Fourier series. Math. Comp. **19:** 297–301.

77. WOLF, M. W., G. VARIGOS, D. HUNT & J. G. SLOMAN. 1978. Sinus arrhythmia in acute myocardial infarction. Med. J. Australia **2:** 52–53.

78. DIBNER-DUNLAP, M. E., D. L. ECKBERG, N. M. MAGID & N. M. CINTRON-TREVINO. 1985. The long-term increase of baseline and reflexly augmented levels of human vagal-cardiac nervous activity induced by scopolamine. Circulation **71:** 797–804.

79. SCHER, A. M. & A. C. YOUNG. 1970. Reflex control of heart rate in the unanesthetized dog. Am. J. Physiol. **218:** 780–789.

80. HERROLD, E. M. 1979. The interactive effects of angiotensin-II infusion into the vertebral artery and the carotid sinus baroreceptor reflex on the heart period and systemic pressure in dogs. Ph.D. Thesis. Case Western Reserve University. Cleveland, Ohio.

81. COGHLAN, H. C., P. PHARES, M. COWLEY, D. COPLEY & T. N. JAMES. 1979. Dysautonomia in mitral valve prolapse. Am. J. Med. **67:** 236–244.

82. GAFFNEY, F. A., B. C. BASTION & L. B. LANE, *et al.* 1983. Abnormal cardiovascular regulation in the mitral valve prolapse syndrome. Am. J. Cardiol. **52:** 316–320.

83. WEISSMAN, N. J., M. K. SHEAR, R. KRAMER-FOX & R. B. DEVEREUX. 1987. Contrasting patterns of autonomic dysfunction in patients with mitral valve prolapse and panic attacks. Am. J. Med. **82:** 880–888.

84. TAYLOR, A. A., A. O. DAVIES, A. MARES, J. RASCHKO, J. L. POOL, E. B. NELSON & J. R. MITCHELL. 1989. Spectrum of dysautonomia in mitral valvular prolapse. Am. J. Med. **86:** 267–274.

The Promise of Electrocardiography in the 21st Century

OSCAR B. GARFEIN

Division of Cardiology
St. Luke's-Roosevelt Hospital Center
Columbia University College of Physicians & Surgeons
428 West 59th Street
New York, New York 10019

The original concept behind this conference was based on the belief that an analysis of the electrical activity of the heart with multiple electrocardiographic techniques could contribute a great deal to the diagnosis of its various physiologic, pathologic, and anatomic abnormalities. Obviously, this had already been wonderfully accomplished by the originators of various isolated electrocardiographic (ECG) techniques. Nonetheless our firm belief was that much more clinically usable information would be available if two conditions were met. First, many of the various electrocardiographic techniques that have been discussed at this conference, such as signal averaging, power spectrum analysis, body surface mapping, and quantitative electrocardiography, would have to be applied to a large clinical population. Second, a data base consisting of a combination of invasive and noninvasive diagnostic tests would have to be developed to correlate these electrocardiographic changes with certain normal and abnormal states so that one could understand the significance of these various ECG-derived waveforms in living patients rather than relying on postmortem materials for correlations that, naturally, have limited applicability. The creation of these two conditions would necessitate the creation of new technologies and organizations. These would consist of new ways of obtaining and recording electrocardiographic data, new ways of analyzing these data, and new ways of presenting them to the clinician. This paper will review the application of various electrocardiographic techniques to the diagnosis of morphologic and physiologic changes in the heart, how they have been correlated with pathologic entities, present a view of a hypothetical electrocardiographic system of the future, and suggest an organizational mechanism by which electrocardiographic interpretation may be furthered.

The electrocardiograph is capable of supplying much more information than has been extracted by it in the past. Information about infarction, hypertrophy, conduction disturbances, and arrhythmias has been available since the late 1940s and early 1950s. But now we have the capacity to use the electrocardiograph more fully and quite differently from ever before. The physiology of the entire organism, the quantitative and qualitative assessment of the activity of the autonomic nervous system, and indirect assessment of ventricular function are all potentially analyzable through detailed study of the power spectrum analysis of the heartbeat variation, analysis of the circadian variability of the heart rate, and a detailed analysis of the ambient heart rate surrounding cardiac arrhythmias.[1-4]

The status of the heart with regard to its potential for arrhythmogenesis can be defined by application of techniques of signal averaging.[5] In the future this technique may be useful in predicting the response, both positive and negative, to various therapeutic interventions and conceivably might be used to assess the probability of atrial arrhythmias as well as ventricular events. Fourier analysis of the various component waveforms of the electrocardiogram, when applied to standardized, orthogonal, quantitative electrocardiography, may offer previously unsuspected insights into changes in the heart that currently defy analysis or even observation. A computer-performed analysis of variations in size, shape, and slope of the ST-T wave that are invisible to the eye may expose conditions that currently cannot even be suspected by the most learned analysis of the scalar electrocardiogram.[6] Various techniques discussed in this program have the ability to refine the diagnosis of different forms of heart disease as well as varying degrees of cardiac dysfunction. Zaret has discussed the potential that the isonitriles will give us to measure the size of an infarct precisely.[7] Weiss has shown us dazzling images of cardiac motion never before seen using magnetic resonance imaging (MRI), and tissue tagging and these images may allow us to make very subtle observations on early cardiac pump malfunction.[8] Grover-McKay presented a cogent statement of positron emission tomography (PET) scanning's ability to define very fundamental metabolic changes in myocardium in states of ischemia and infarction.[9]

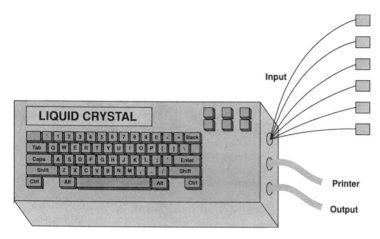

FIGURE 1

We have had an extensive discussion of circadian variability of heart rate,[3] and have learned how certain deductions concerning the role of the autonomic nervous system can be made based on electrocardiographic observations.

Let us now think about combining this information—the new information about the electrocardiograph and the new information derived from noninvasive and invasive testing—and see where it takes us. How will the electrocardiogram look in the future and how will it be used? What will its characteristics be? And what will the report look like, and how we will achieve this?

The reader will now be exposed to a bit of fancy and read a scenario that 20 years ago would have been pure science fiction but is now quite reasonable to consider.

The electrocardiograph will be a rather small, perhaps palm-sized, solid state device without moving parts, the major purpose of which will be to record, store, amplify, and filter the electrocardiographic waveform (FIGURE 1). In addition it would have the capacity to transmit this material telephonically. Certain devices might also possess the capacity to perform certain analytic functions as well and to store information from previous recordings and compare a patient's electrocardiogram at one point in time with a later ECG from the same patient. FIGURE 2 shows some of the characteristics of the recording device and some of its potential outputs. The device will measure approximately 15 × 10 × 5 cm and weigh ½ kg. The electrodes will be shielded at their most distal extremity to prevent electromagnetic interference and consist of an electrode and a transducer converting the electrical input into an optical signal which will then travel to the body of the device by optical fibers or, as Rowlandson has described, digitization of the signal in the patient cable can be used to the same end.[9] Once received in the ECG device, the signal will be amplified and filtered and templates made. The cyclical variation in the size, shape, and frequency content and slope of various individual waveforms will be determined then stored. Individual complexes as well as mean data will be stored so that variability and rate can be analyzed.

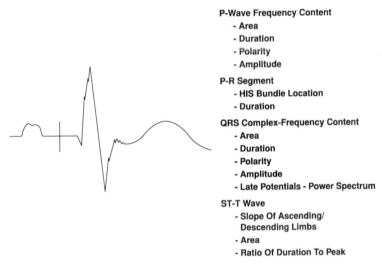

P-Wave Frequency Content
 - Area
 - Duration
 - Polarity
 - Amplitude

P-R Segment
 - HIS Bundle Location
 - Duration

QRS Complex-Frequency Content
 - Area
 - Duration
 - Polarity
 - Amplitude
 - Late Potentials - Power Spectrum

ST-T Wave
 - Slope Of Ascending/
   Descending Limbs
 - Area
 - Ratio Of Duration To Peak

FIGURE 2

Data from the patient such as identification, age, sex, selected bits of clinical history, and ancillary diagnostic criteria could be entered via the alphanumeric keyboard. Long-term storage might be available for individual practitioners who have high volumes of cardiac patients so that prior ECGs can be compared immediately in a single patient. A simple analytic algorithm of limited capabilities might be incorporated in this device although for maximal interpretive power analysis would be performed at a distance (see below).

Under many circumstances when the physician does not need to have an immediate analysis of the electrocardiograph signal the recording device would simply store the signal as raw, unprocessed information able to transfer the data at a later time into a much larger and more sophisticated processing and analyzing unit into which other diagnostic material could be inserted such as echocardiographic, scintigraphic, angio-

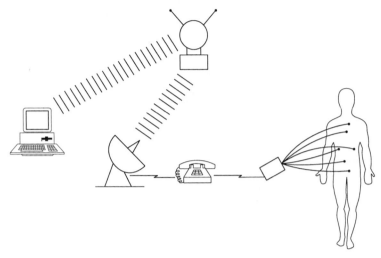

FIGURE 3

graphic, and magnetic resonance imaging data along with selected clinical descriptors to help in analyzing the signal.

The information would be transmitted telephonically to a central processing unit which has access to a data bank, be analyzed, and a report from this could be immediately retrieved by the practitioner (FIGURE 3). A hypothetical report is described in FIGURE 4A. Noteworthy in this report is the absence of a hard copy of the

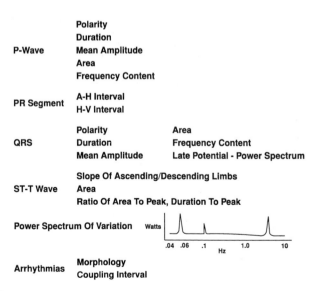

FIGURE 4A

Interpretation	Odds Ratio	Specifity	Sensitivity
Morphology - Left Ventricular Hypertrophy: 1.3 - 1.5 cm Left Atrial Hypertrophy: 4 - 7 mm			
Anatomy - Anteroseptal Myocardial Infarction			
Physiology - Lateral Myocardial Ischemia Low Arrhythmogenic Potential Ejection Fraction - 45% (±5) Left Atrial Hypertension Early Cardiac Decompensation			
Conditioning Factors			

Echocardiographic Data
    Clinical History
    Coronary Arteriography
    Thallium Scintigraphy
    PET Scan			

FIGURE 4B

electrocardiogram. Since so many of the data being analyzed and reported on are not visible to the human eye and not measurable by the brain (e.g., late potentials, His Bundle, ST-T wave slope, areas, ratio of peak to area and time, and power spectrum of the rate variation), the necessity for having hard copies is dramatically diminished and may even be obviated totally. The report resembles a standard ECG report insofar as data are collected and reported and an interpretation rendered. The difference, of course, in addition to the absence of hard copy, resides in the number of different measurements made and the quantity and quality of the interpretations made. Not only will many more functional anatomic parameters be described but the limits of the accuracy of the diagnostic interpretation will be given (FIGURE 4B).

What has been missing from routine electrocardiographic diagnosis up to the present is a consideration of gender-, age-, and race-related variables and how these change the specificity and sensitivity of the established diagnostic criteria. The same is obviously more pertinent when two or more functional or pathologic cardiac conditions exist in the same patient, a condition not at all uncommon. Under circumstances such as these (ischemia, old infarction, hypertrophy, chamber enlargement), standard criteria for the diagnosis of those conditions are certainly not as accurate as they might be and this format allows the clinician to appreciate the likelihood of the diagnosis derived by the computer algorithm.

For example, if the isolated electrocardiographic data were combined with simple, relatively widespread diagnostic techniques such as plain chest x-ray or echocardiography, enhanced diagnostic accuracy could result. For example, a partial interpretation of a transmitted ECG might state "There is a 68% likelihood that this pattern represents an anterior myocardial infarction. If echocardiography shows no evidence of left ventricular hypertrophy (by such and such criteria) then this likelihood increases to 93%" (FIGURE 4B).

Thus far we have discussed technology that could be devised rather easily even if it does not exist. We have also discussed technologies that are not widely applied but do exist and could achieve broad clinical application. These technologies are not the limiting factor in widening the application of the ECG as a sophisticated clinical tool. The limitation is due primarily to the lack of correlative data. Not enough information has been cross-correlated with ECGs that come from living beings. These correlative data would be derived from all the noninvasive tests that are in clinical use as well as some of the more sophisticated techniques that we have heard discussed at this conference. In addition to the analyses of these data, extensive and systematic cross-correlation of electrocardiography with biopsies, body surface mapping, and Holter recordings will be very useful.

To obtain this cross-correlation is a mammoth operation. It is best achieved by a multinational consortium the activities of which are outlined in TABLE 1. This organization will collect data derived from the various invasive and noninvasive techniques and tests we now have at our disposal along with demographic, historical, and clinical data and collect quantitative electrocardiographic information as well. It would then analyze the data, and perform cross-correlation studies.

The data coming into this data base will probably be derived from university medical centers at which the more sophisticated diagnostic techniques are currently performed. These will include but not be limited to those techniques mentioned above. It would also include postmortem examination of the heart. The electrocardiographic data to be recorded would include the standard 12-lead ECG, the quantitative ECG, signal-averaged ECG for late potentials and His Bundle intervals, and computer-analyzed frequency content and morphology of the P-wave, QRS complex, and ST-T wave. In addition, frequency content and power spectrum analysis of the heart rate variability would also be recorded. The quality controls would be performed in a standard manner with core laboratories responsible for validation of the various test data sent into the center. Finally, a working center would be established with access made available to nonparticipants so that practitioners around the world could avail themselves of this powerful tool.

Some of the diagnoses that would come from this enhanced diagnostic capacity are obvious and are mere extensions of the capabilities that now exist. The value of ready availability of His bundle recordings and late potentials is obvious. Variations in the ECG dependent on age, gender, ethnic background, even geography, should become apparent and identified as such rather than being considered manifestations of disease.

TABLE 1. Multinational Electrocardiographic Data Interpretation/Acquisition (Media)

1. Acquire quantitative electrocardiographic data	
2. Acquire simultaneous data	
a. Clinical history	h. Coronary arteriography
b. Demographics	i. Electrophysiologic studies
c. Chest x-ray	j. Body surface mapping
d. Echocardiography	k. Endocardial biopsy
e. Thallium scintigraphy	l. Stress testing
f. PET scanning	m. Postmortem examination
g. Signal averaged ECG	
3. Establish quality controls for data	
4. Correlative studies	
5. Interpretation	
6. Ready access to all input	

Diagnoses of ischemia at rest, especially when it would ordinarily be confused by the administration of certain drugs, ventricular hypertrophy in the presence of conduction disturbances or myocardial infarction, early cardiomyopathy, specific etiologic diagnoses of cardiomyopathy, and functional assessment of the overall status of the cardiovascular system are all possible results from this type of analysis.

The nonspecific ST-T wave changes we know so well and understand so little may yield new diagnostic information when subject to cross-correlation with other techniques and independent analysis of the slope and volume of its various components. Intraventricular conduction defects, with and without other morphologic QRS abnormalities, may be shown to correlate with anatomic or pathologic conditions we cannot possibly recognize at present.

The consortium will consist of clinical cardiologists, epidemiologists, statisticians, computer and communication scientists, and technology-based scientists and engineers. Although it would be a free-standing, independent organization it would function in close association with regional or national cardiologic organizations. The funding would be derived from many sources but primarily from government and from industry. The industries that might find it valuable to contribute would be those heavily involved in medical technology, telecommunications, and computers. Governments could be induced to support the venture for two reasons. First, they are concerned with improving the level of health care of their citizens, and second, they are especially concerned with reducing the costs of these services. It is quite conceivable that electrocardiography as described would eventually supplant many technologically more sophisticated and more extensive technologies in the routine evaluation and follow-up of patients with real or suspected cardiovascular disease.

During discussion of this presentation several months ago with one of my colleagues I was told an anecdote that is hopefully not apposite. A leading scientist was invited to give the keynote lecture at the annual meeting of a major medical society many years ago and his topic was to be "The Future of————." When my colleague mentioned this to me I interrupted and said "and I bet almost everything he had to say came true." "Quite the contrary," he answered. "Within a few years everything he had predicted turned out to be absolutely wrong."

I hope that this is not the case with the above. As has been learned from these proceedings, electrocardiography has much to offer as a safe, simple, inexpensive technique in the diagnosis of cardiac disease and pathophysiology. It will be up to some of those who have been at this meeting to ensure that this potential is fulfilled.

REFERENCES

1. MALLIANI, A., F. LOMBARDI, M. PAGANI & S. CERUTTI. 1990. Clinical exploration of the autonomic nervous system by means of electrocardiography. Ann. N.Y. Acad. Sci. (This volume.)
2. BERBARI, E. J., D. E. ALBERT & P. LANDER. 1990. Spectral estimation of the electrocardiogram. Ann. N.Y. Acad. Sci. (This volume.)
3. CINCA, J., A. MOYA, A. BARDAJI, J. RIUS & J. SOLER-SOLER. 1990. Circadian variations of electrical properties of the heart. Ann. N.Y. Acad. Sci. (This volume.)
4. COUMEL, P. 1990. Noninvasive exploration of cardiac arrhythmias. Ann. N.Y. Acad. Sci. (This volume.)
5. BREITHARDT, G., M. BORGGREFE & A. MARTINEZ-RUBIO. 1990. Signal averaging. Ann. N.Y. Acad. Sci. (This volume.)
6. MOSS, A. J., M. MERRI, J. BENHORIN, M. ALBERTI & E. LOCATI. 1990. Multidimensional quantitation of ventricular repolarization. Ann. N.Y. Acad. Sci. (This volume.)
7. ZARET, B. L. & F. J. WACKERS. 1990. Myocardial perfusion scintigraphy as an aid in

understanding electrocardiographic changes of ischemia and infarction. Ann. N.Y. Acad. Sci. (This volume.)

8. WEISS, J. L., E. P. SHAPIRO, M. BUCHALTER & R. BEYAR. 1990. Magnetic resonance imaging as a noninvasive standard for the quantitative evaluation of left ventricular mass, ischemia, and infarction. Ann. N.Y. Acad. Sci. (This volume.)

9. GROVER-MCKAY, M. 1990. Positron emission tomography as an aid in understanding electrocardiographic changes in ischemia, infarction, and cardiomyopathy. Ann. N.Y. Acad. Sci. (This volume.)

The Reflex Effects of Tachycardias on Autonomic Tone[a]

MENASHE B. WAXMAN AND DOUGLAS A. CAMERON

Department of Medicine
University of Toronto
and
Division of Cardiology
Toronto General Hospital
200 Elizabeth Street
EN 12-215
Toronto, Ontario, M5G 2C4, Canada

CHANGES IN AUTONOMIC TONE RESULTING FROM TACHYCARDIA—INTRODUCTION

Tachycardias, irrespective of their origin, mechanism, or cause, alter cardiovascular function because they affect cardiac filling and stroke volume.[1-3] Blood pressure and pulse pressure decline in direct relationship to the rate, atrioventricular synchrony, and cardiac function.[3,4] This reduces stretch on the pressure-sensitive baroreceptors which are located mainly in the carotid sinuses.[5,6] The reduced pressure decreases the afferent nerve traffic from the baroreceptors to the vasomotor centers. This in turn augments sympathetic efferent tone and withdraws vagal efferent tone. These changes affect the ongoing tachycardia rate, the blood pressure recovery, as well as the overshoot of the blood pressure following termination of the tachycardia.[7] The overshoot of the blood pressure activates vagal tone which in turn slows the heart rate for a period of time after the tachycardia ends.[8]

Tachycardias generally cause a maximum blood pressure fall at their onset,[2,3] and thus the peak stimulus for sympathetic compensation and vagal withdrawal occurs at this time.[8] While autonomic tone may not play a significant role in the initiation of a given tachycardia, once the arrhythmia is established, changes in neural tone can exert significant effects on the arrhythmia depending on its location, innervation, and responsiveness to autonomic tone.[9,10] As well, changes in autonomic tone are vital in restoring cardiac output and blood pressure during the tachycardia.

While the fall in blood pressure leads to a reflex increase in sympathetic tone through extracardiac baroreceptors,[5,6] signals from ventricular and atrial mechanoreceptors may result in an opposite effect.[11,12] During supraventricular and ventricular tachycardias, atrial pressure and ventricular diastolic pressure rise dramatically[2,3,7,13] (FIGURE 1). The increased filling pressure can activate cardiac mechanoreceptors leading to a reflex withdrawal of sympathetic tone and an enhancement of vagal tone.[11,12] Thus, during paroxysmal tachycardia, the cardiac[11,12] and extracardiac baroreceptors[5,6] may result in opposite types of reflex changes in sympathetic tone. It is also pertinent to point out that stretch receptors in the atrium and possibly in the ventricles cause release of atrial natriuretic factor (ANF) which not only promotes a

[a]These studies were supported in part by a grant-in-aid from the Heart and Stroke Foundation of Ontario.

378

diuresis,[14] but this hormone relaxes vascular smooth muscle.[15] Thus, released ANF can impede the recovery of blood pressure during a tachycardia.

The reflex changes accompanying a tachycardia can be readily examined by pacing the atria or the ventricles at various rates for various dura ns of time. This is illustrated in FIGURE 2, in a patient with Wolff-Parkinson-White (WPW) syndrome, in whom right atrial pacing was undertaken at a rate of 200 beats per minute for seven periods as indicated at the bottom (number of beats). Each sequence caused a dramatic fall in blood pressure, following which there was a brisk overshoot of the blood pressure, and its extent is described (as delta BP) at the bottom of the figure.

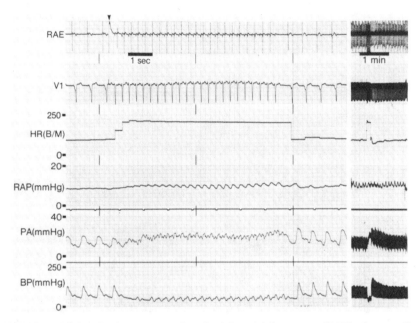

FIGURE 1. This is a simultaneous recording of a right atrial electrogram (RAE), electrocardiograph (ECG) lead V1, beat-to-beat heart rate (HR), right atrial pressure (RAP), pulmonary artery pressure (PA), and systemic arterial blood pressure (BP) from a patient with WPW syndrome. At the arrowhead, a premature atrial beat initiated a run of nonsustained supraventricular tachycardia at a rate of 225 beats per minute. There was considerable hypotension, a small rise in right atrial filling pressure, and a dramatic rise in pulmonary artery pressure, especially the pulmonary artery diastolic pressure. The panel on the right is a compressed record of the same event. (Unpublished observations, M. B. Waxman.)

Coincident with the overshoot in blood pressure, there was a period of reflex sinus bradycardia. During more prolonged pacing, one sees significant improvement in the initial hypotension. Thus, two responses indicate that sympathetic tone was activated by rapid pacing: (a) there was a significant blood pressure recovery during pacing; and (b) there was a brisk overshoot of the blood pressure following termination of the pacing. Assuming that the overshoot of the blood pressure is proportional to the intensity of sympathetic tone, the largest overshoot was seen in the third panel after the heart was paced for 40 beats. This suggests that the extent of sympathetic activation may be greatest during tachycardias of short duration, or in the early part of a tachycardia.

RELATIONSHIP BETWEEN HEART DISEASE AND THE REFLEX RESPONSE TO A TACHYCARDIA

In general there is an inverse relationship between the rate of a tachycardia and the cardiac output or blood pressure. Thus, the higher the tachycardia, the lower the cardiac output and blood pressure are.[16,17] In the presence of ventricular dysfunction, even a modest tachycardia may cause a major reduction in cardiac output and blood pressure.[3] In diseases where coronary perfusion is limited, tachycardias reduce ventricular compliance causing further reductions in cardiac output and blood pressure.[18-20]

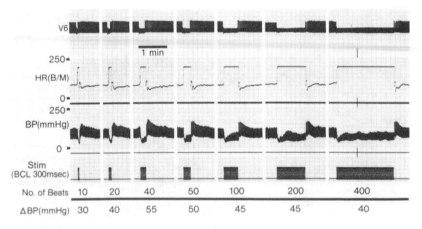

FIGURE 2. This is a simultaneous recording of ECG lead V6, beat-to-beat heart rate, blood pressure, and stimulus code from a patient with WPW syndrome. In each panel the right atrium was paced for the number of beats indicated at the bottom. The blood pressure overshoot following termination of pacing is indicated at the bottom of each panel. (Unpublished observations, M. B. Waxman.)

Thus in the case of heart disease associated with limited coronary reserve, one expects that tachycardias will result in greater hemodynamic compromise and therefore larger increases in sympathetic tone.

Sympathetic tone may cause minimal hemodynamic improvement of the diseased heart because of the combination of cardiac denervation[21,22] and reduced cardiac responsiveness to autonomic tone.[23] Thus, a mechanism for perpetuating enhanced sympathetic tone can develop. The tachycardia drops cardiac output and blood pressure, thereby enhancing sympathetic tone, but the lack of adequate compensation will maintain high sympathetic tone indefinitely. This may be responsible for acceleration of the tachycardia, or its transformation, i.e., ventricular tachycardia to ventricular fibrillation.[24]

Various drugs may be critical in the reflex adjustment to a tachycardia. Beta-adrenergic receptor blocking drugs blunt the heart's contractile response to increased sympathetic tone and hence reduce the blood pressure recovery following the onset of a tachycardia.[25] While beta-adrenergic receptor blocking drugs reduce sudden cardiac death mortality following a myocardial infarction,[26] they can impair the hemodynamic tolerance to an episode of tachycardia. On the other hand, adrenergic receptor blockade may inhibit the transformation of ventricular tachycardia to ventricular fibrillation that results from enhanced sympathetic tone.[24] It should be appreciated that if a beta-adrenergic receptor blocking drug reduces the tachycardia rate, this benefit might offset the blunted cardiac response to sympathetic tone.[8,25] In the case of supraventricular tachycardia, beta-adrenergic receptor blockade significantly slows the tachycardia and hence may reduce the hypotension.[8] Therefore, although cardiac responsiveness to sympathetic tone is blunted by beta-adrenergic receptor blocking drugs, there may be far less need for sympathetic compensation provided the tachycardia is slower to start with.

BRIEF DISTURBANCES IN AUTONOMIC TONE MAY CAUSE LONG-LASTING EFFECTS ON A TACHYCARDIA

Various heart rates induce hemodynamic changes which in turn alter autonomic tone so as to maintain or change the rate. For example, at slow rates the cardiac output and blood pressure may be optimal, thereby maintaining low sympathetic tone and high vagal tone. This could perpetuate a slow rate long after the original slowing. By contrast, a rapid rate reduces cardiac output and blood pressure, and this can maintain high sympathetic tone beyond the original sympathetic stimulus. Therefore transient changes in vagal or sympathetic tone alter the rate of a tachycardia, and the resultant rate can in turn cause long-lasting changes in autonomic tone.

A Transient Increase in Vagal Tone Can Permanently Change the Rate of a Tachycardia without Interrupting It

A transient increase in vagal tone may slow an arrhythmia such as paroxysmal supraventricular tachycardia without causing termination.[27] The slowing may improve cardiac output and blood pressure sufficiently so as to create a self-perpetuating increase in vagal tone and reduction in sympathetic tone. This is illustrated in a patient with paroxysmal supraventricular tachycardia (FIGURE 3). Supraventricular tachycardia was initiated by a premature atrial beat and the heart rate jumped to 200 beats per minute, and there was marked hypotension (systolic BP 30 mmHg). The hypotension undoubtedly activated sympathetic tone as the tachycardia accelerated to 260 beats per minute and the blood pressure recovered modestly. The very high tachycardia rate prevented the systolic blood pressure from rising above 75 mmHg and the persistent hypotension maintained high sympathetic tone. Thus the high rate and low blood pressure were linked in a positive feedback loop. Carotid sinus massage (CSM) slowed the tachycardia rate to 200 beats per minute normalizing rate-related right bundle branch block. The slowing persisted indefinitely despite the transient nature of carotid sinus massage. Once the rate slowed by about 60–70 beats per minute, the blood pressure rose and this reduced sympathetic tone further.As a consequence, the tachycardia rate did not reaccelerate and in turn, this maintained the higher blood pressure.

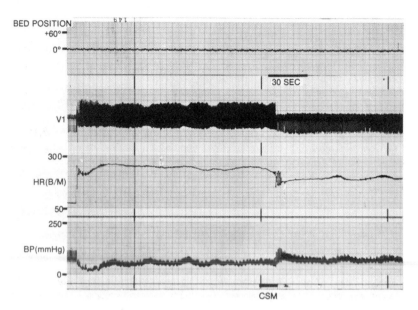

FIGURE 3. This is a simultaneous recording of surface ECG lead V1, beat-to-beat heart rate, and blood pressure from a patient with recurrent paroxysmal supraventricular tachycardia. A single premature atrial beat started the tachycardia and its initial rate was 200 beats per minute. There was considerable hypotension and the rate rose to 260 beats per minute while the blood pressure recovered modestly. Carotid sinus massage (CSM) caused a dramatic reduction in heart rate, and this was accompanied by a considerable augmentation in blood pressure. The fall in heart rate and the increase in blood pressure persisted indefinitely. (Unpublished observations, M. B. Waxman.)

Transient Increases in Sympathetic Tone Can Permanently Affect the Rate of the Tachycardia

A transient increase in sympathetic tone may increase the rate of a tachycardia and cause a self-sustaining mechanism to keep sympathetic tone elevated. This is illustrated in a patient with atrial flutter who conducted with a 2:1 ratio at rest (FIGURE 4). The patient was passively tilted to +60° (first arrow), and this raised sympathetic tone, withdrew vagal tone, and caused a 1:1 ventricular response, thus doubling the heart rate.[16,17] The patient was returned to 0° (second arrow), but 1:1 conduction persisted for 40 minutes as the dependent body position did not raise vagal tone sufficiently to overcome the high level of sympathetic tone which was perpetuated by the hemodynamic effects of the fast rate. Additional vagal tone and sympathetic withdrawal created by carotid sinus massage were necessary to slow and permanently stop the 1:1 conduction ratio. It is also interesting that carotid sinus massage, a maneuver that enhances vagal tone for only a few seconds, caused a permanent reduction in heart rate. The rise in cardiac output and blood pressure following the rate slowing provided feedback to maintain increased vagal tone and reduced sympathetic tone long after the original effects of carotid sinus massage had elapsed. This maintained the rate permanently slowed.

SPONTANEOUS TERMINATION OF SUPRAVENTRICULAR TACHYCARDIA

The reflex neural effects following the onset of a tachycardia are responsible for spontaneous early termination of paroxysmal supraventricular tachycardia.[8] We examined the reflex neural effects of spontaneous early termination of paroxysmal supraventricular tachycardia in 20 patients and found 9 individuals in whom the tachycardia consistently terminated spontaneously within a mean of 28 ± 5 seconds after its onset. The mechanism was due to reflex changes in autonomic tone. The onset of the tachycardia caused hypotension which activated powerful sympathetic reflexes which restored the blood pressure to control or even above control values. The blood pressure elevation then stimulated baroreceptors which in turn increased efferent vagal tone, and the latter depressed conduction in the AV node and terminated the tachycardia.[27] This is illustrated in FIGURE 5. At the arrow, an artificial premature atrial beat initiated paroxysmal supraventricular tachycardia. The initial rate was 175 beats per

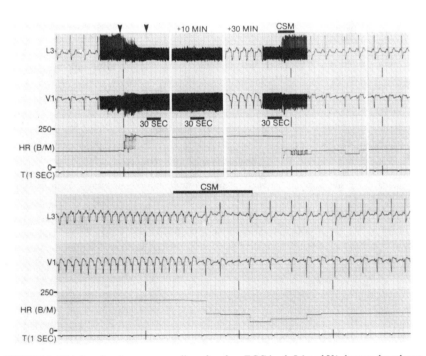

FIGURE 4. This is a simultaneous recording of surface ECG leads L3 and V1, beat-to-beat heart rate and time code marker from a patient with atrial flutter. Initially there was a 2:1 ventricular response, producing a heart rate of 105 beats per minute. At the first arrowhead, the patient was turned to +60° and, within several seconds, the ventricular response doubled to 210 beats per minute as 1:1 conduction ensued. At the second arrowhead, the patient was returned to 0°, but despite this, 1:1 conduction persisted for the next 40 minutes. Carotid sinus massage (CSM) was then performed and it abruptly slowed the rate permanently. The bottom panel is a blow-up of the transformation from 1:1 conduction (with rate-related left anterior hemiblock) to a higher degree of block in response to CSM. (Reproduced with permission from Reference 17.)

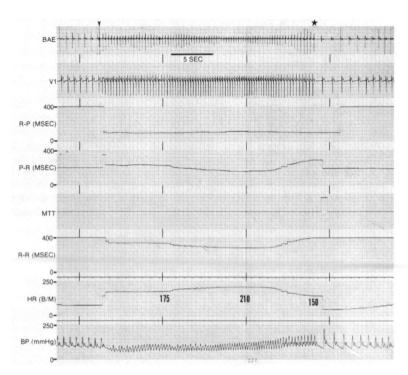

FIGURE 5. This is a simultaneous recording of a bipolar atrial electrogram (BAE), surface ECG lead V1, R-P interval, P-R interval, mode of tachycardia termination (MTT), R-R interval, beat-to-beat heart rate, and blood pressure from a patient with paroxysmal supraventricular tachycardia. At the arrow, a premature atrial beat initiated paroxysmal supraventricular tachycardia at a rate of 175 beats per minute. This was accompanied by considerable hypotension. As the hypotension recovered, there was acceleration of the tachycardia rate to 210 beats per minute and this was traceable to a shortening of the P-R interval while the R-P interval remained constant. As the blood pressure reached control levels and then exceeded these values, the tachycardia rate slowed to 150 beats per minute and then terminated back to sinus rhythm. The tachycardia rate slowing was traceable to prolongation of the P-R interval. The positive pip on the MTT tracing indicates that the tachycardia ended with a retrograde P wave. (Reproduced with permission from Reference 8.)

minute and there was considerable hypotension. In response to the hypotension, sympathetic tone increased, and this was manifest by a rise in blood pressure above the pretachycardia level, and a parallel increase in the rate to 210 beats per minute. As the blood pressure approached the pretachycardia levels, vagal tone was activated, and the tachycardia slowed to 150 beats per minute and terminated spontaneously. A continuous display of the P-R interval revealed that the tachycardia accelerated and slowed as a consequence of P-R interval shortening and lengthening respectively. These are the typical effects of sympathetic and vagal tone respectively on AV nodal conduction velocity.[28,29] The tachycardia broke because of anterograde block within the AV node. Consequently the tachycardia ended with a retrograde P wave (star), and this is denoted by the positive pip on the MTT tracing. Activation of vagal tone was the essential final mechanism responsible for spontaneous termination of the tachycardias.

Pretreatment with atropine (FIGURE 6) prevented the spontaneous termination of tachycardia, without interfering with the blood pressure recovery.

Cardiac adrenergic responsiveness to the tachycardia was another essential component of spontaneous termination of paroxysmal supraventricular tachycardia. Beta-adrenergic receptor blocking drugs inhibited spontaneous termination by two mechanisms. In some, propranolol greatly slowed the rate of the induced tachycardia. Therefore the initial hypotension at the onset of tachycardia was blunted, and as a consequence, there was minimal rise of sympathetic tone, and hence the tachycardia did not undergo spontaneous termination. This is illustrated in FIGURE 7. In this example, the first three episodes of induced supraventricular tachycardia were associated with hypotension at the onset which was followed by recovery and spontaneous termination within 30 seconds or less. The recovery of blood pressure was accompanied by a rise in the rate of the tachycardia. After the patient was placed in a head dependent position of −20° (panels 3 and 4), background sympathetic tone was reduced. The two episodes of induced tachycardia manifested a greatly reduced rate, and this attenuated the initial hypotension. As a consequence, there was minimal need for blood pressure recovery and the tachycardia did not exhibit spontaneous termination. In the last two panels, the patient was returned to 0° and pretreated with 10 mg of propranolol. Again episodes of induced tachycardia were greatly slowed, and this resulted in a small initial blood pressure fall and there was no tendency for spontaneous

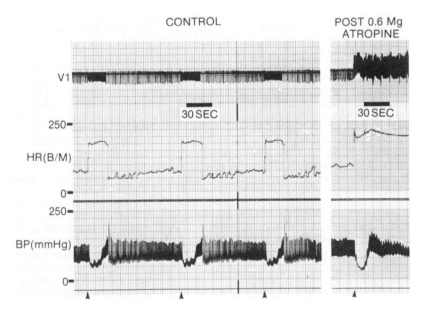

FIGURE 6. This is a simultaneous recording of surface ECG lead V1, beat-to-beat heart rate, and blood pressure from a patient with paroxysmal supraventricular tachycardia. During control conditions, three episodes of tachycardia were started by premature atrial beats delivered at the arrowheads. Each episode caused considerable hypotension which resolved spontaneously, and when the blood pressure exceeded the control levels the tachycardias terminated. Following pre-treatment with atropine (right-hand panel), another episode of supraventricular tachycardia was started by a premature atrial beat. The rate was higher and the hypotension was greater. Despite this, the blood pressure was restored above the control levels, but the tachycardia did not end. (Reproduced with permission from Reference 8.)

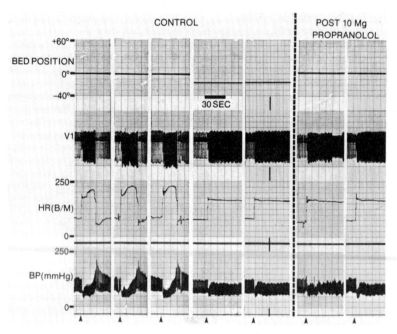

FIGURE 7. This is a simultaneous recording of bed position, surface ECG lead V1, beat-to-beat heart rate, and blood pressure from a patient with paroxysmal supraventricular tachycardia. During control conditions (first three panels), three episodes of tachycardia were initiated at 0°. Each episode caused considerable hypotension, but the blood pressure recovered sufficiently to cause reflex termination of the tachycardia in each case, within 30 seconds or less. In the fourth and fifth panels, two episodes of tachycardia were induced after the patient was placed in a head dependent position of −20° and the rate of the tachycardia was considerably reduced to 170 beats per minute. The hypotension was considerably less, and the tachycardias did not terminate spontaneously. In the sixth and seventh panels supraventricular tachycardia was initiated following 10 mg of propranolol and the rate of the tachycardia slowed to 170 beats per minute. The hypotension was less compared to the control record, and the tachycardias did not terminate spontaneously. (Reproduced with permission from Reference 8.)

termination of the tachycardia. It is noteworthy that the result following propranolol is almost identical to the result seen in the preceding two panels when the patient was at −20°. Thus, one of the mechanisms by which propranolol blocks spontaneous termination of supraventricular tachycardia is by reducing the tachycardia rate, thereby decreasing the initial hypotensive stimulus that is necessary for the augmentation of sympathetic tone.

Beta-adrenergic receptor blockade inhibited spontaneous termination of the tachycardia by a second mechanism. In some patients, treatment with propranolol did not significantly reduce the initial rate of the tachycardia, but it slowed the rate of recovery of blood pressure so that insufficient activation of vagal tone occurred and hence spontaneous termination of the tachycardia did not transpire. This was undoubtedly due to a decrease in the heart's contractile response to augmented adrenergic tone.[25] In FIGURE 8 five consecutive episodes of tachycardia terminated within 32 seconds or less. Following 10 mg of propranolol, the induced initial tachycardia rate and hypotension are quite similar to control panels. However, the blood pressure recovery was slowed, resulting in an insufficient augmentation of vagal tone, and consequently the tachycardia did not terminate. A summary of the hemodynamic effects of beta-adrenergic blockade in patients with spontaneous termination is shown in FIGURE 9. Propranolol reduced the initial tachycardia rate, reduced the reflex increase in heart rate, reduced the initial fall in blood pressure, prolonged the time for the blood pressure to recover to a stable level, and reduced the blood pressure overshoot following the tachycardia's termination. Thus spontaneous termination of paroxysmal supraventricular tachycardia requires an adequate initial hypotensive stimulus and an intact cardiac adrenergic mechanism in order to generate a brisk rise in blood pressure.

One can draw an analogy between the mechanism of spontaneous termination of supraventricular tachycardia and the reflex changes that follow a Valsalva maneuver.[27] The period immediately following the onset of a tachycardia may provide a powerful enough afferent stimulus to elicit an appropriate rise in efferent sympathetic tone which in turn may promote a sufficient rise in blood pressure to reflexly terminate the tachycardia. However, if the events at the onset of the tachycardia fail to cause spontaneous terminate of tachycardia, the arrhythmia equilibrates and it may continue indefinitely until its equilibrium is disturbed. A Valsalva maneuver can cause such a disturbance. By inhibiting the return of blood to the heart, the Valsalva maneuver activates powerful sympathetic reflexes which in turn cause an overshoot in blood

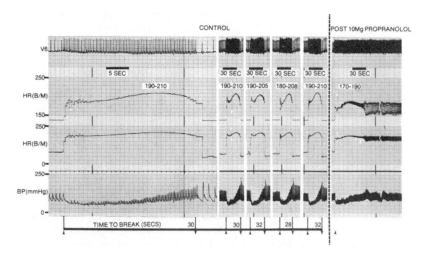

FIGURE 8. This is a simultaneous recording of ECG lead V6, beat-to-beat heart rate on two scales, and blood pressure from a patient with paroxysmal supraventricular tachycardia. The up-going arrows denote the administration of a premature atrial beat while the down-going arrow denotes spontaneous termination of the induced tachycardia. During control conditions, five consecutive episodes of paroxysmal supraventricular tachycardia were initiated, all of which terminated spontaneously within 32 seconds or less. Each episode of tachycardia was accompanied by considerable hypotension. As the blood pressure recovered, the rate initially accelerated and then slowed, leading to termination. Following propranolol, another episode of tachycardia was induced, and the tachycardia rate was mildly slowed compared to the control conditions. One sees the same degree of hypotension as was present during the control records. However, the rate of recovery of blood pressure in this case was considerably attenuated. As a consequence, the tachycardia did not exhibit spontaneous termination. Beat to beat heart rate alternans developed. (Reproduced with permission from Reference 8.)

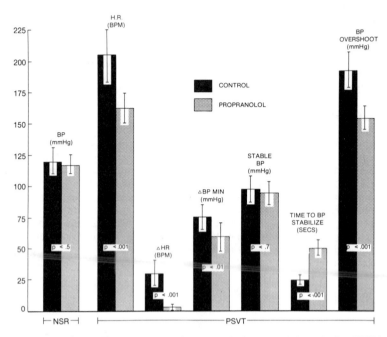

FIGURE 9. This is a plot of the resting blood pressure during normal sinus rhythm (NSR) and the hemodynamic parameters during paroxysmal supraventricular tachycardia (PSVT) in eight patients before and after propranolol. These patients showed spontaneous termination prior to the administration of propranolol. (Reproduced with permission from Reference 8.)

pressure following release of the strain phase, and this in turn can terminate the tachycardia.[27] The similarity between the Valsalva maneuver and spontaneous termination of tachycardia is illustrated in FIGURE 10. In panel A, supraventricular tachycardia was initiated, and within 22 seconds, it terminated spontaneously. One observes considerable hypotension at the onset of the tachycardia and the reflex mechanisms initiated by the hypotension raised the rate, increased the blood pressure, and in turn, this activated vagal tone which slowed and terminated the tachycardia. In panel B, another episode of tachycardia was initiated, but it did not terminate spontaneously and remained stable for 5 minutes. Following the release of a Valsalva strain of 40 mmHg held for 10 seconds, one sees a considerable overshoot in blood pressure, but this was insufficient to terminate the tachycardia. In panel C, the same tachycardia was still ongoing, and following release of another Valsalva maneuver one observes a brisk rise in blood pressure, which in turn caused reflex slowing and termination of the tachycardia. In panel D, during another stable episode of supraventricular tachycardia a Valsalva maneuver was performed, and the tachycardia terminated. It is useful to observe the remarkable similarity of the heart rate and blood pressure records on panels A, C, and D. In panel A, appropriate sympathetic and vagal reflexes were initiated spontaneously, whereas in C and D, the superimposition of an additional stimulus to activate sympathetic tone (i.e., the Valsalva maneuver) was necessary to raise the blood pressure and terminate the tachycardia.

TRANSFORMATION OF PAROXYSMAL SUPRAVENTRICULAR
TACHYCARDIA TO ATRIAL FIBRILLATION

Individuals suffering from paroxysmal supraventricular tachycardia may also experience episodes of atrial fibrillation. This is particularly well appreciated in patients with WPW syndrome, since the transformation of paroxysmal supraventricular tachycardia to atrial fibrillation may result in a rapid ventricular rate and ventricular fibrillation.[30] The mechanism of transformation of paroxysmal supraventricular tachycardia to atrial fibrillation, particularly in patients with WPW syndrome, is thus of more than academic interest. If the transformation from supraventricular tachycardia to atrial fibrillation is in some way connected mechanistically, then one expects that transection of the bypass tract will result not only in the cure of the supraventricular tachycardia, but also eliminate the transformation to atrial

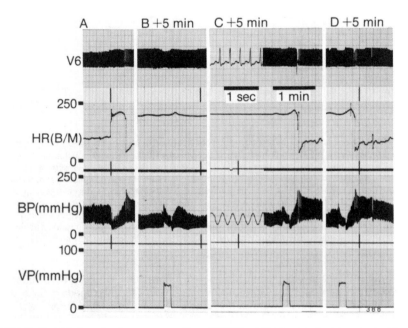

FIGURE 10. This is a simultaneous recording of ECG lead V6, beat-to-beat heart rate, blood pressure, and Valsalva pressure (VP) from a patient with paroxysmal supraventricular tachycardia. In panel A, an induced episode of supraventricular tachycardia resulted in considerable hypotension and the tachycardia broke spontaneously. There was a brisk overshoot in blood pressure following the termination of the tachycardia and this caused reflex bradycardia. During another episode of tachycardia (panel B), a Valsalva maneuver (held pressure of 40 mmHg) performed for 10 seconds caused a modest overshoot in blood pressure following release of the strain, but the tachycardia did not terminate. In panel C, another Valsalva maneuver was performed, and now release of the strain resulted in a dramatic rise in blood pressure, which reflexly terminated the tachycardia. In panel D, another Valsalva maneuver during an episode of tachycardia terminated the arrhythmia as a consequence of the reflex overshoot in blood pressure. It is important to note the similarity in heart rate and blood pressure records in panels A, C, and D. (Unpublished observations, M. B. Waxman.)

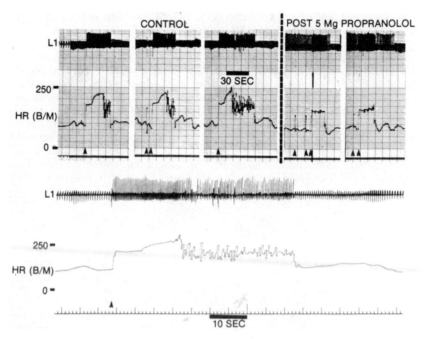

FIGURE 11. This is a simultaneous recording of surface ECG lead 1 and beat-to-beat heart rate from a patient with WPW syndrome. During control conditions, premature atrial beats (arrowheads) were administered, and three episodes of supraventricular tachycardia were initiated. In each case, the tachycardia rate accelerated from its initial value to over 225 beats per minute and it transformed into atrial fibrillation and then terminated spontaneously. The enlargement at the bottom is a blow-up of the third episode of tachycardia. Following pretreatment with propranolol, episodes of supraventricular tachycardia were initiated, but the rates were much slower and there was no acceleration and hence no transformation to atrial fibrillation. Both episodes of tachycardia terminated spontaneously within 25 seconds. (Reproduced with permission from Reference 16.)

fibrillation.[31] On the other hand, if the atrial fibrillation develops by a different mechanism, possibly as a consequence of atrial disease, then interruption of the bypass tract would not be expected to affect the recurrence rate of atrial fibrillation.

We have observed transformation of paroxysmal supraventricular tachycardia to atrial fibrillation in individuals whose reflex response to supraventricular tachycardia is brisk and who manifest a large acceleration in the supraventricular rate within the first 30 seconds of the onset of the tachycardia.[16] As has been stated, the period immediately following the onset of the tachycardia is accompanied by marked hypotension and intense sympathetic compensation to restore the blood pressure. The rise in sympathetic tone inevitably exerts a facilitatory effect on the AV node, and this accelerates the tachycardia rate at the same time as the blood pressure is being restored. It is during this phase of tachycardia acceleration that we have observed the transformation of supraventricular tachycardia to atrial fibrillation. Interventions that reduce the rate of supraventricular tachycardia or reduce the reflex response to the tachycardia inhibit the transformation to atrial fibrillation. Specifically, we have studied a group of individuals who have exhibited reflex transformation of supraventricular tachycardia to atrial fibrillation before and after the administration of propranolol. We found that propranolol blocks this transformation (FIGURE 11).

On the basis of these observations, we hypothesized that the transformation of supraventricular tachycardia to atrial fibrillation is secondary to the large rate rise during supraventricular tachycardia. In keeping with this concept we have observed that one can induce atrial fibrillation in the same individuals by other maneuvers that activate the adrenergic system and raise the rate of the supraventricular tachycardia. Thus, in cases where atrial fibrillation has not developed spontaneously, reflex increases in adrenergic tone may induce atrial fibrillation (FIGURE 12).

CONCLUSIONS AND FURTHER DIRECTIONS

The majority of experimental and clinical attention in the arrhythmic field has been directed toward an understanding of the electrophysiologic mechanisms underlying arrhythmias and the basis of drug action. Remarkably little attention has been paid to the reflex neural responses that develop consequent to a tachycardia, and how these are affected by the state of the heart and blood vessels and the concomitant use of drugs including antiarrhythmic agents. The ability of the circulation to weather the tachycar-

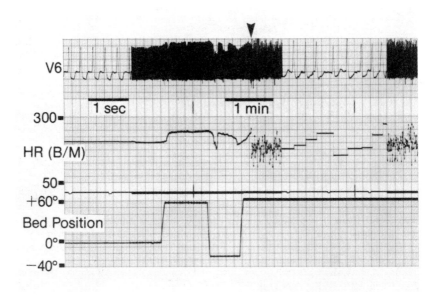

FIGURE 12. This is a simultaneous recording of surface ECG lead V6, beat-to-beat heart rate and bed position from a patient with paroxysmal supraventricular tachycardia. During an ongoing episode of tachycardia, the patient was passively tilted to +60° and the tachycardia rate accelerated from 215 beats per minute to 250 beats per minute. When the patient was turned to −20°, the tachycardia initially slowed dramatically and then stabilized at approximately 200 beats per minute. Following another passive tilt to +60°, the tachycardia rate accelerated to 250 beats per minute and it transformed (at the arrowhead) to atrial fibrillation (note the irregular heart rate intervals). (Unpublished observations, M. B. Waxman.)

dia is at least in part related to the intactness of the response of the autonomic nervous system. These reflex changes may also be responsible for terminating, sustaining, or transforming a tachycardia.

REFERENCES

1. FREEMAN, G. L., W. C. LITTLE & R. A. O'ROURKE. 1987. Influence of heart rate on left ventricular performance in conscious dogs. Circ. Res. 61: 455–464.
2. SCHLEPPER, M., H. G. WEPPNER & H. MERLE. 1978. Hemodynamic effects of supraventricular tachycardias and their alteration by electrically and verapamil induced termination. Cardiovasc. Res. 12: 28–33.
3. LIMA, J. A. C., J. L. WEISS, P. A. GUZMAN, M. L. WEISFELDT, P. R. REID & T. A. TRAILL. 1983. Incomplete filling and incoordinate contraction as mechanisms of hypotension during ventricular tachycardia in man. Circulation 68: 928–938.
4. LINDERER, T., K. CHATTERJEE, W. W. PARMLEY, R. E. SIEVERS, S. A. GLANTZ & J. V. TYBERG. 1983. Influence of atrial systole on the Frank-Starling relation and the end-diastolic pressure-diameter relation of the left ventricle. Circulation 67: 1045–1053.
5. MANCIA, G., A. FERRARI, L. GREGORINI, R. VALENTINI, J. LUDBROOK & A. ZANCHETTI. 1977. Circulatory reflexes from carotid and extracarotid baroreceptor areas in man. Circ. Res. 41: 309–315.
6. SCHER, A. M. 1977. Carotid and aortic regulation of arterial blood pressure. Circulation 56: 521–528.
7. NAKANO, J. 1964. Effects of atrial and ventricular tachycardia on the cardiovascular dynamics. Am. J. Physiol. 206: 547–552.
8. WAXMAN, M. B., A. D. SHARMA, D. A. CAMERON, F. HUERTA & R. W. WALD. 1982. Reflex mechanisms responsible for early spontaneous termination of paroxysmal supraventricular tachycardia. Am. J. Cardiol. 49: 259–272.
9. LEVY, M. N. & P. J. MARTIN. 1979. Neural control of the heart. In Handbook of Physiology, Cardiovascular System. R. B. Berne, N. Sperlakis & S. R. Geiger, Eds. 1: 581–620. William & Wilkins. Baltimore, Md.
10. WAXMAN, M. B., D. A. CAMERON, R. W. WALD & G. R. LASCAULT. 1983. The use of autonomic maneuvers for diagnosis and treatment of cardiac arrhythmias. In Cardiac Arrhythmias. G. S. Wagner, R. A. Waugh & B. W. Ramo, Eds. (Chapter 4): 57–108. Churchill Livingstone. New York, N.Y.
11. THOREN, P. 1979. Role of cardiac vagal C-fibers in cardiovascular control. Rev. Physiol. Biochem. Pharmacol. 86: 1–94.
12. BISHOP, V. S., A. MALLIANI & P. THOREN. 1983. Cardiac mechanoreceptors. In Handbook of Physiology: the Cardiovascular System. J. T. Shepherd, F. M. Abboud & S. R. Geiger, Eds.: 497–556. Williams and Wilkins. Baltimore, Md.
13. WAXMAN, M. B., J. F. BONET, J. P. FINLEY & R. W. WALD. 1980. Effects of respiration and posture on paroxysmal supraventricular tachycardia. Circulation 62: 1011–1020.
14. TIKKANEN, I., K. METSARINNE & F. FYHRQUIST. 1985. Atrial natriuretic peptide in paroxysmal supraventricular tachycardia. Lancet 2: 40–41.
15. MAACK, T. & H. D. KLEINERT. 1987. Renal and cardiovascular effects of atrial natriuretic factor. Biochem. Pharmacol. 35: 2057–2064.
16. WAXMAN, M. B., R. W. WALD & D. CAMERON. 1983. Interactions between the autonomic nervous system and tachycardias in man. Cardiol. Clin. 1: 143–185.
17. WAXMAN, M. B. & R. W. WALD. 1984. Effects of autonomic tone on tachycardias. In Tachycardias. B. Surawicz, C. P. Reddy & E. N. Prystowsky, Eds. (Chapter 4): 67–102. Martinus Nijhoff. Boston, Mass.
18. UDELSON, J. E., R. O. CANNON III, S. L. BACHARACH, T. F. RUMBLE & R. O. BONOW. 1989. β-Adrenergic stimulation with isoproterenol enhances left ventricular diastolic performance in hypertrophic cardiomyopathy despite potentiation of myocardial ischemia: comparison to rapid atrial pacing. Circulation 79(2): 371–382.

19. BOURDILLON, P. D., B. H. LORELL, I. MIRSKY, W. J. PAULUS, J. WYNNE & W. GROSSMAN. 1983. Increased regional myocardial stiffness of the left ventricle during pacing-induced angina in man. Circulation **67:** 316–323.
20. FIFER, M. A., P. D. BOURDILLON & B. H. LORELL. 1986. Altered left ventricular diastolic properties during pacing induced angina in patients with aortic stenosis. Circulation **74:** 675–683.
21. CHIDSEY, C. A. & E. BRAUNWALD. 1966. Sympathetic activity and neurotransmitter depletion in congestive heart failure. Pharmacol. Rev. **18:** 685–700.
22. ECKBERG, D. L., M. DRABINSKY & E. BRAUNWALD. 1971. Defective parasympathetic control in patients with heart disease. N. Engl. J. Med. **285:** 877–883.
23. GINSBURG, R., M. R. BRISTOW, M. E. BILLINGHAM, E. B. STINSON, J. S. SCHROEDER & D. C. HARRISON. 1983. Study of the normal and failing isolated human heart: depressed response of failing heart to isoproterenol. Am. Heart J. **106:** 535–540.
24. BILLMAN, G. E., P. J. SCHWARTZ & H. L. STONE. 1982. Baroreceptor reflex control of heart rate: a predictor of sudden cardiac death. Circulation **66:** 874–880.
25. FELDMAN, T., J. D. CARROLL, F. MUNKENBECK, P. ALIBALI, M. FELDMAN, D. L. COGGINS, K. R. GRAY & T. BUMP. 1988. Hemodynamic recovery during simulated ventricular tachycardia: role of adrenergic receptor activation. Am. Heart J. **115:** 576–587.
26. THE NORWEGIAN MULTICENTER STUDY GROUP. 1981. Timolol-induced reduction in mortality and reinfarction in patients surviving acute myocardial infarction. N. Engl. J. Med. **304:** 801–807.
27. WAXMAN, M. B., R. W. WALD, A. D. SHARMA, F. HUERTA & D. A. CAMERON. 1980. Vagal techniques for termination of paroxysmal supraventricular tachycardia. Am. J. Cardiol. **46:** 655–664.
28. IRISAWA, H., W. M. CALDWELL & M. F. WILSON. 1971. Neural regulation of atrioventricular conduction. Jpn. J. Physiol. **2:** 15–25.
29. WAXMAN, M. B., R. W. WALD, R. MCGILLIVRAY, D. A. CAMERON, A. D. SHARMA & F. HUERTA. 1981. Continuous on line beat-to-beat analysis of AV conduction time. PACE **4:** 262–273.
30. KLEIN, G. J., T. M. BASHORE, T. D. SELLERS, E. L. C. PRITCHETT, W. M. SMITH & J. J. GALLAGHER. 1979. Ventricular fibrillation in the Wolff-Parkinson-White syndrome. N. Engl. J. Med. **301:** 1080–1085.
31. SHARMA, A. D., G. J. KLEIN, G. M. GUIRAUDON & S. MILSTEIN. 1985. Atrial fibrillation in patients with Wolff-Parkinson-White syndrome: incidence after surgical ablation of the accessory pathway. Circulation **72:** 161–169.

Index of Contributors

Subject Index